Symposium on malignancies
of the head and neck

Contributors

Jerome E. Adamson, M.D.

Chief, Department of Plastic and Reconstructive Surgery, Norfolk Medical Center Hospital, Norfolk, Virginia

Robin Anderson, M.D.

Professor and Head, Department of Plastic Surgery, Cleveland Clinic Educational Foundation, Cleveland, Ohio

Donald W. Benson, M.D., Ph.D.

Professor of Anesthesiology, The Johns Hopkins University School of Medicine, Baltimore, Maryland

Edwin G. Beven, M.D.

Head, Department of Vascular Surgery, Cleveland Clinic Educational Foundation, Cleveland, Ohio

David E. Bytell, M.D.

Associate, Department of Otolaryngology and Maxillofacial Surgery, Northwestern University–McGaw Medical Center, Chicago, Illinois

James H. Carraway, M.D.

Associate, Eastern Virginia Medical School; Attending Surgeon, Department of Plastic Surgery, Norfolk Medical Center Hospitals; Norfolk, Virginia

William J. Catalona, M.D.

Clinical Associate, Surgery Branch, National Cancer Institute, National Institutes of Health, Bethesda, Maryland

Robert G. Chambers, M.D.

Assistant Professor of Surgery, Assistant Professor of Plastic Surgery, The Johns Hopkins University School of Medicine, Surgeon-in-charge, Tumor Clinic, The Johns Hopkins Hospital; Chief, Head and Neck Service, Greater Baltimore Medical Center; Baltimore, Maryland

Paul B. Chretien, M.D.

Head, Tumor Immunology Section, and Assistant Chief, Surgery Branch, National Cancer Institute, National Institutes of Health, Bethesda, Maryland

Lester M. Cramer, D.M.D., M.D.

Professor and Chairman of Plastic Surgery, Temple University Health Sciences Center, Philadelphia, Pennsylvania

George Crile, Jr., M.D.

Emeritus Consultant, Department of Surgery, Cleveland Clinic Educational Foundation, Cleveland, Ohio

Norris K. Culf, M.D.

Professor of Plastic Surgery, Temple University Health Sciences Center, Philadelphia, Pennsylvania

Milton T. Edgerton, M.D.

Professor and Chairman, Department of Plastic Surgery, University of Virginia Medical Center, Charlottesville, Virginia

Bruce D. Edison, M.D.

Department of Otolaryngology, United States Air Force Medical Center, Lackland Air Force Base, Texas

Ray A. Elliott, Jr., M.D.

Associate Clinical Professor of Plastic Surgery and Associate Clinical Professor of Orthopedics (Hand), Albany Medical College; Attending Plastic Surgeon, Albany Medical Center Hospital, Veterans Administration Hospital, St. Peter's Hospital, Memorial Hospital, and The Child's Hospital, Albany, New York; Attending Plastic Surgeon, Cohoes Memorial Hospital, Cohoes, New York; Consulting Plastic Surgeon, New York State Department of Health, Sunnyview Rehabilitation Center, Schenectady, New York, and Putnam Memorial Hospital, Bennington, Vermont

John C. Gaisford, M.D.

Chief, Division of Surgery, The Western Pennsylvania Hospital, Pittsburgh, Pennsylvania

Nicholas G. Georgiade, D.D.S., M.D.

Professor of Plastic, Maxillofacial, and Oral Surgery, Duke University Medical School, Durham, North Carolina

William P. Graham III, M.D.

Director, Division of Plastic and Reconstructive Surgery, The Milton S. Hershey Medical Center of the Pennsylvania State University, Hershey, Pennsylvania

K. Guler Gursu, M.D.

Associate Professor and Chief of Plastic Surgery, Hacettepe University Medical School, Ankara, Turkey

Dwight C. Hanna, M.D.

Director, Plastic Surgery Department, Western Pennsylvania Hospital, Pittsburgh, Pennsylvania

Ronald L. Hansing, B.S.

Medical Student, George Washington University, Washington, D. C.

Charles C. Harrold, Jr., M.D.

Assistant-Attending, Head and Neck Service, Memorial Cancer Center, New York, New York

Shattuck W. Hartwell, Jr., M.D.

Associate Professor, Department of Plastic Surgery, Cleveland Clinic Educational Foundation, Cleveland, Ohio

William A. Hawk, M.D.

Head, Department of Pathology, Cleveland Clinic, Cleveland, Ohio

John E. Hoopes, M.D.

Professor of Surgery, Division of Plastic Surgery, The Johns Hopkins University School of Medicine, Baltimore, Maryland

Charles E. Horton, M.D.

Professor of Surgery (Plastic), Eastern Virginia Medical School, Norfolk, Virginia

Stuart J. Hulnick, M.D.

Assistant Professor of Plastic Surgery, Temple University Health Sciences Center, Philadelphia, Pennsylvania

Alfred S. Ketcham, M.D.

Professor and Chief, Division of Oncology, Department of Surgery, University of Miami School of Medicine, Miami, Florida

Magdi S. Kodsi, M.D.

Assistant Professor of Plastic Surgery, Temple University Health Sciences Center, Philadelphia, Pennsylvania

Harvey J. Lerner, M.D.

Assistant Professor of Surgery, University of Pennsylvania; Head, Section of Chemotherapy, Division of Surgery, Pennsylvania Hospital; Philadelphia, Pennsylvania

Herbert Lipshutz, M.D.

Clinical Professor of Plastic Surgery, University of Pennsylvania Hospital; Head, Section of Plastic Surgery, Division of Surgery, Pennsylvania Hospital; Philadelphia, Pennsylvania

John M. Loré, Jr., M.D.

Professor and Chairman, Department of Otolaryngology, State University of New York at Buffalo, Buffalo, New York

William S. MacComb, M.D.

Surgeon and Emeritus Professor of Surgery, Department of Surgery, The University of Texas, M. D. Anderson Hospital and Tumor Institute, Houston, Texas

Frederick J. McCoy, M.D.

Clinical Professor of Surgery (Plastic), University of Missouri School of Medicine at Kansas City; Chief of Plastic Surgery, Kansas City General Hospital and Medical Center; Chief of Plastic Surgery, The Children's Mercy Hospital; Kansas City, Missouri

Richard A. Mladick, M.D.

Attending Plastic Surgeon and Director of Head and Neck Tumor Clinic, Norfolk General Hospital; Faculty, Eastern Virginia Medical School; Consultant, Hampton Veterans Administration Hospital, Portsmouth Naval Hospital, and Bethesda Naval Hospital; Norfolk, Virginia

Joseph H. Ogura, M.D.

Lindburg Professor and Head, Department of Otolaryngology, Washington University School of Medicine, St. Louis, Missouri

David S. Postlewaite, M.D.

Norfolk, Virginia

George J. Richards, Jr., M.D.

Chief of Radiology, Greater Baltimore Medical Center, Baltimore, Maryland

Ronald H. Rosillo, M.D.

The Piersol Rehabilitation Center, The Department of Physical Medicine and Rehabilitation and Psychiatry, The University of Pennsylvania, Philadelphia, Pennsylvania

Norman G. Schaaf, D.D.S.

Chief, Department of Dentistry and Maxillofacial Prosthetics, Roswell Park Memorial Institute, Buffalo, New York

Donald G. Sessions, M.D.

Associate Professor of Otolaryngology, Washington University Medical School; Assistant Otolaryngologist, Barnes Hospital Group; Section Head of Otolaryngology, St. Louis City Hospital; Consultant in Otolaryngology, Veterans Administration Hospital, Jewish Hospital, and St. Louis County Hospital; St. Louis, Missouri

Donald P. Shedd, M.D.

Chief, Head and Neck Surgery, Roswell Park Memorial Institute, Buffalo, New York

John N. Simons, M.D.

Formerly Head, Section of Plastic Surgery, Mayo Clinic, Rochester, Minnesota

George A. Sisson, M.D.

Professor and Chairman, Department of Otolaryngology and Maxillofacial Surgery, Northwestern University–McGaw Medical Center and Northwestern Memorial Hospital; Attending, Department of Otolaryngology, Cook County Hospital, Children's Memorial Hospital, and Veterans Administration Research Hospital; Chicago, Illinois

Elliot W. Strong, M.D.

Attending Surgeon and Chief, Head and Neck Service, Memorial Sloan-Kettering Cancer Center; Associate Professor of Surgery, Cornell University Medical College; New York, New York

Patrick L. Twomey, M.D.

Clinical Associate, Surgery Branch, National Cancer Institute, National Institutes of Health, Bethesda, Maryland

Tolbert S. Wilkinson, M.D.

Clinical Assistant Professor and Head, Division of Plastic and Reconstructive Surgery, University of Texas Health Science Center; Consultant, Audie Murphy Veterans Administration Hospital and Texas State Chest Hospital; San Antonio, Texas

Preface

The Symposium on Cancer of the Head and Neck, of which this volume is the collection of presented papers, was held in Baltimore in September, 1973. It was the fifteenth symposium conducted since 1967 under the auspices of the Educational Foundation of the American Society of Plastic and Reconstructive Surgeons, Inc. It was the third symposium on the general subject of head and neck cancer surgery; the first was held in Pittsburgh in 1969 and the second in Denver in 1972. Several papers presented in Denver have been included in this volume.

The purpose of these courses has been to educate at a sophisticated postgraduate level, but with a definite orientation toward the surgical resident and the young practicing surgeon. No attempt was made to limit participation to plastic surgeons; in fact, considerable effort was expended to achieve good representation of the three specialties on the participating faculties involved in surgery of the head and neck: plastic surgery, otolaryngology, and general surgery. In the symposiums, the speakers were selected on the basis of their preeminence in specific facets of head and neck cancer surgery, and the scope of their presentations has been wide enough to provide excellent reviews of the field as a whole.

As plastic surgeons, we wish to thank our colleagues from allied specialties who contributed time and effort to make the symposium a success. As members of the sponsoring Educational Foundation, our participation is expected and contributed without hesitation. That our otolaryngologic and general surgical associates have been equally willing to use jealously hoarded meeting time for this purpose is greatly appreciated. Our thanks also go to Miss Susan Clifton of The Johns Hopkins Medical Institutions for her superb handling of the technical aspects of the meeting.

Robin Anderson, M.D.
John E. Hoopes, M.D.

Contents

Symposium on malignancies
of the head and neck

Chapter 1

Radiation therapy in cancer of the head and neck

George J. Richards, Jr., M.D.

Four years after the discovery of the x-ray by William Roentgen, the first report of a successful radiation treatment came from the United States.[6] In 1899, interestingly enough and quite appropriate to this symposium, a malignant tumor of the nose was treated. Radiation therapy, perhaps more than any other field of medicine, has witnessed remarkable technological progress in the past two decades. The armamentarium of the radiation therapist has come to provide him with a wide choice of weapons. Although the weapons have changed, however, the fundamental tactics employed in cancer therapy have remained the same. Radiation therapy has become one of the primary modalities for the treatment of malignant disease.

CLINICAL AIMS OF RADIATION THERAPY
Curative

When a tumor is still confined to a small volume of tissue, the objective of treatment is to eradicate the entire neoplastic tissue. Most tumors exhibit a degree of radioresponsiveness, and a favorable result can be achieved with a dose ranging from 5,000 to 7,000 rads, administered over a period of 5 to 8 weeks. Radiocurability depends on the radioresponsiveness of the tumor, its actual physical volume, and the proximity of the tumor to other radiosensitive structures. Generally speaking, a tumor that is still confined to the organ of origin lends itself to radical radiotherapy.

Adjunctive to surgery

Preoperative. Radiation therapy is administered as a preliminary to a projected surgical procedure. Certain principles outlining our conception of preoperative irradiation have been developed. It is applied chiefly to apparently resectable cancers. The field of irradiation should encompass the primary tumor site, the area through which metastases might pass, and the lymph nodes to which the tumor might have spread. To reduce the total volume of tissue being irradiated, lymph nodes are either treated as a separate field of irradiation, or the fields are restricted to those lymph nodes grossly presenting tumor tissue. While other authors[2] may subscribe to the principle that the dose is rarely of a curative level, all of our patients receiving preoperative irradiation received a cancericidal dose in accordance with the appropriate time-dose relationships. Supervoltage irradiation was exclusively used except where supplemented by intraoral cone deep x-ray therapy. A recovery period of 6 to 8 weeks prior to definitive surgery is felt to be essential. This delay permits maximum tumor recession and adequate tissue recovery.

The aims of preoperative irradiation are to render locally nonresectable cancers resectable, to render nonviable any malignant cells that happen to be implanted in the wound or circulatory system during surgery, thereby reducing the index of metastatic take, and to decrease the incidence of recurrence. Once viable cells have been transected and dissemi-

1

nated in a wound, the task of irradiation becomes more difficult. As a cancer mass enlarges, its supporting tissues and vascular bed are incapable of maintaining adequate oxygenation and nutrition. Peripheral cells are well oxygenated, nourished, and mitotically active; thus a nonresectable periphery may be rendered resectable by preoperative irradiation. Many primary cancers of uncertain extent may have undetected or occult local extension beyond the limits of proposed surgery. We have found that preoperative irradiation frequently enables a modification of the original composite surgical plan by a complete eradication of the primary tumor. In these cases simple local excision of the primary site and removal of the lymph nodes by radical neck dissection have resulted in a cure without the need for the extensive destructive composite surgical procedure. It has been said that preoperative irradiation impairs wound healing and delays a curative surgical procedure, providing an added opportunity for metastases, and that the gross shrinkage of the cancer mass may tempt a surgeon to perform a less radical resection or a patient to refuse surgery.[3] We have found none of these factors to be a deterrent. The adherence to the prescribed recovery period, the careful surgical handling of tissues, and the use of delayed surgical flaps where indicated have resulted in an incidence of fistula, necrosis, and other complications no greater than in similar cases treated without preliminary irradiation.

Postoperative. In the treatment of certain cancers of the head and neck that are not particularly suited for preoperative irradiation, because of their cellular radiation response or the proximity of the tumor to vital structures or other tissues with relatively lower radiosensitivity, patients may receive postoperative irradiation. Since many of these tumors have a high rate of local recurrence, high doses of postoperative irradiation are usually necessary to accomplish a cure. In this category we generally include all tumors of the major and minor salivary glands, certain olfactory tumors such as esthesioneuroblastoma, and tumors of sarcomatous origin other than lymphomas. Another group of patients referred for postoperative irradiation are those in whom advanced cancer has been found or has extended beyond the limits of surgical excision. In these cases extension may be vague, and transection may have disseminated neoplastic cells. The results of postoperative irradiation in these patients is sometimes unsuccessful because the transected cancer cells may be protected by hypoxia created by changes in vascularity as the result of the surgical procedure. Irradiation administered immediately following surgery is more likely to succeed than when regrowth is clinically obvious.

Palliative

It is often apparent in the first assessment of a malignancy that a fatal issue is unavoidable. To attempt to cure such a case may not only shorten the life but may also impair the quality of life that remains. As therapists, our purpose is to prolong human life but not to prolong death or to make the remaining life of a patient more miserable. The desire to prolong human life should not be allowed to overrule the clinician's better judgment, and he should always satisfy himself that his intervention will make life more tolerable; the prospects of benefit should be weighed against the discomforts of local radiation reaction, radiation sickness, and possible radiation necrosis. Palliative doses should be kept below the full radical level and should be pursued only until the symptoms for which pallation is sought are relieved. To achieve amelioration of symptoms, it must be accepted that often only part of the disease may need to be eradicated.

RADIOTHERAPEUTIC AIMS

The radiotherapist must decide whether the treatment is to be by external irradiation, by x-rays or gamma rays, by surface or intracavitary radium, or by interstitial radium or radioisotope therapy. This decision will be determined by the type of tumor, its site, its extent, and its accessibility. Associated with this selection are problems concerning the duration of treatment and the fractionation of dosage. Having decided upon the treatment policy, the radiotherapist must plan the details of his application so that he may know precisely the dose sustained at every point of tissue in and near his target area.

Therapeutic irradiation

X-rays and gamma rays of radium, cobalt, and other radioactive substances are identical in nature, differing only in origin. While x-rays are produced by the collision of accelerated electrons striking a target, gamma rays result from nuclear emissions produced by the spontaneous radioactive decay of atoms. X-rays and gamma rays have a penetrating power that varies with the voltage at which they are produced. This voltage is expressed in terms of kilovolts or megavolts.

Low-voltage therapy. Rays with energies over a

range of 50 to 100 kv. will be used extensively for the treatment of malignant diseases of the skin and the conjunctiva.

Medium-voltage therapy (deep x-ray therapy). For several decades the workhorse of radiation therapy departments was the machine that generated radiations over a range of 200 to 400 kv. The penetrating qualities of this beam are sufficient to allow an attempt at the treatment of deep-seated tumors. The disadvantages of radiation therapy at these voltages are the severity of the skin and mucosal reactions, excessive dosages in bone (where bone is traversed), and bone absorption, resulting in partial shielding from radiation any disease that lies behind it. Intraoral cone therapy, as an adjunctive to external teletherapy, utilizes energies in this range.

Supervoltage therapy. This is a term generally reserved for radiations in excess of 1 mev. Supervoltage x-rays, generated by linear accelerators and electron beams of 8 to 100 mev., are available for use. A cobalt 60 teletherapy source falls under this classification, producing two gamma rays of 1.3 and 1.17 mev.

Radium and isotopes

Radium and other radioactive isotopes emit three kinds of irradiations: alpha, beta, and gamma. The alpha irradiations have so little penetrating power that they have little application in clinical therapy. The beta rays, derived from radium, phosphorus, strontium, and other isotopes, have a wide range of energies and are used as external applicators in the treatment of diseases of the eye, skin, mucosal surfaces of the mouth, and the nasopharynx.

Intracavitary therapy. Other beta particles, phosphorus and gold, can be placed directly into body cavities or can enter a malignant cell or a diseased organ with the parent radioactive isotope, as in the case of iodine 131 in the treatment of thyroid malignancies. The gamma rays, radium, and other radioactive isotopes, among which are cobalt 60 and cesium, lend themselves to introduction in suitable containers into the accessible body cavities. This intracavitary therapy is used in the treatment of malignancies of the accessory nasal sinuses, nasopharynx, ear, and esophagus.

Interstitial therapy. This is the introduction of radioactive needles or seeds directly into the tissues. This type of application is frequently utilized in treating tumors of the tongue, floor of the mouth, buccal mucosa, tonsil, and those metastatic to the lymph nodes in the neck. Interstitial radium is used in the treatment of cancer of the head and neck as a primary modality or as an adjunctive to external beam therapy. In some institutions, radium is used in a molded apparatus for surface therapy.[6]

BIOLOGICAL CONSIDERATIONS

The total dose and time over which the total course of treatment is extended are interdependent. In any treatment of cancer in which the objective is curative, it is imperative that the largest tolerated dose be given with regard for the site, the extent of the disease, and the age and condition of the patient. This is because the carcinomatous lethal dose is so close to the lethal dose of normal tissue. A carcinoma is a radioresponsive tumor.

Radiosensitivity

The sensitivity of the tumor cells to irradiation influences the radiation dose. A radiosensitive tumor such as a lymphosarcoma, certain embryonal tumors, and the majority of lymphomas will regress rapidly and may completely disappear with a dose of 3,000 rads in 4 weeks. A local recurrence is improbable, and it is doubtful that anything is to be gained by a higher dose with this type of tumor. An extreme degree of radiosensitivity usually carries with it an unfavorable prognosis since it implies early dissemination of the tumor cells of a multifocal nature. The moderately radiosensitive (or radioresponsive) tumors are all squamous cell carcinomas of the head and neck, mucodermoid tumors of the salivary glands, transitional cell tumors, esthesioneuroblastomas, and most other head and neck cancers. From this group are derived the best and the most curable results from radiotherapy. Radiocurability depends, in addition, on the reaction of the tumor bed and the host response. Radioresistant tumors are unlikely to be controlled or restrained by a dose of under 6,000 rads. The tolerance of these tumors may exceed the tolerance of the surrounding tumor bed.

For a number of years radiation therapists have sought a radiosensitizing substance that would enhance the effect of ionizing irradiation on malignant cells. Ideally these would render radioresistant tumors more responsive and radioresponsive tumors more curable. Many agents have been used with limited effectiveness. The enhancement of the irradiation effect by increased oxygen saturation of the malignant cell and its tumor bed led to the development of the hyperbaric chamber and the local infusion of peroxidase. The knowledge that actively dividing cells are more radiosensitive than resting cells led to attempts to stimulate mitotic activity by means of various hormones and known cell stimulants. Attempts have been made to alter cellular metabolism by either speeding up metabolic activity, as in treatment with thyroxin, or by producing injury or death to cells concomitantly with irradiation effect, as in treatment with antimetabolites and alkylating agents.[7]

We have attempted to improve the results of treatment of cancer of the head and neck by using chemotherapeutic agents either concomitantly with radiotherapy or prior to radiotherapy. In many cases we have continued the use of chemotherapeutic agents for many months and years after the completion of the combined radiotherapy and surgery. It has long been noted that the radiosensitivity of cells undergoing division is not uniformly increased over the entire mitotic cycle. The stage of the equatorial plate is generally considered to be the most sensitive phase. Thus an ideally radiosensitizing agent would be one that could destroy relatively radioresistant cells in the "S" stage and synchronize other cells in a relatively radiosensitive stage, permitting irradiation to be more effective. Experimentally, hydroxyurea appears to have such properties.[8,9] Since 1966 at the Greater Baltimore Medical Center, all patients with epidermoid carcinoma of the head and neck have received hydroxyurea concomitantly with irradiation either prior to surgery or during the postoperative period. The administration of hydroxyurea has been continued for several years in most patients in whom surgery was modified because of the excellent preoperative response or in whom extensive persistent disease was encountered at the time of surgery.

Complications of radiation therapy

Skin. There is little that can be done before treatment starts to improve the condition of the skin. With the utilization of high-energy sources, erythema and dry epidermitis do not usually progress to wet epidermitis. The daily use of Septisol lotion throughout the entire treatment course and in the postoperative period has minimized skin reactions. Skin reactions heal quickest if kept dry, exposed to air, and away from temperature changes and irritating preparations. Shaving is restricted to the use of an electric shaver to avoid skin trauma. In certain situations, where medium voltage irradiation is used and exposed areas have become moist, a 1% solution of aqueous gentian violet is useful because of its coagulant action and its formation of a crust, which protects the reacting area. Exposure to sunlight, even for many years after treatment, is not recommended, because the exposed areas are susceptible to damage from excessive exposure of sunlight. Delayed skin reactions occur from the effect on blood vessels. The nutrition of the treated skin is not as good as that of the normal surrounding areas. If the surface breaks down, an area of necrosis is likely to develop, resulting in a chronic indolent ulcer. This type of ulceration usually requires surgical excision with a full-thickness skin flap reconstruction.

Mucous membranes. It is imperative that patients undergoing irradiation to the head and neck refrain from smoking and drinking alcoholic beverages, because both contribute to the accentuation of the normally induced radiation edema. Initially, a dryness of the mouth and throat is produced. This condition is followed by a slight edema, and by the tenth day a patchy, yellowish radiation membrane appears. Dysphagia usually occurs during the third week of treatment and may become extremely painful. It is best ameliorated by having the patient gargle with strong, black tea or by using local anesthetics such as lidocaine hydrochloride (Xylocaine Viscous) and benzonatate (Tessalon). Poor nutrition accentuates the reaction, and patients are urged to utilize high-protein, high-caloric fluid feedings. Radiation necrosis of the soft tissues, with ulceration and tenacious slough, may occur. There is also a danger of hemorrhage from ulceration and sloughing at the tumor site. Hoarseness develops with lesions in the area of the larynx and may last for many months after completion of treatment. Indirect laryngoscopy shows residual edema of the mucous membrane. Instrumentation and biopsy should be avoided at this stage unless there is frank evidence of recurrence, because repeated biopsies tend to precipitate latent necrosis. Dryness of the mouth, loss of taste, and tenacious secretions may last for several months.

Teeth and bone. The decay of teeth, frequently seen after irradiation, may result directly from the action of irradiation on the tooth or its alveolar bed or indirectly from the alterations of the amount and chemical characteristics of the saliva. The most frequent type of dental caries seen after irradiation is the decay of the neck of the tooth. The caries spread superficially around the neck of the tooth, gradually extending deeper, and eventually causing complete amputation of the tooth. A milder change is the gradual wearing away of the cutting or masticating surface of the teeth. Extraction of teeth following irradiation requires protection against infection by the use of antibiotics before and after extraction and by careful reconstruction of the alveolar ridge to avoid sharp or irregular spicules. Suturing is recommended to avoid exposure of the bone. We do not recommend prophylactic removal of teeth within the field of irradiation, for we consider it a danger to the integrity of the overlying protective gum and synovial membrane. Patients who have had extensive irradiation have had little difficulty with subsequent dental extractions. We feel that this situation is because of the high quality of dental education in this community, which insists upon meticulous oral hygiene, skillful dental surgery, and the utilization of all modern medical adjunctives in combating infection. In the event that a radio-osteonecrosis occurs, the treatment is one of intensified oral hygiene and irrigation, combined with antibiotics administered locally and systemically. Dead bone should not be removed until it is loose enough to fall out by itself or to be lifted out. If healing does not occur within a few months, surgical resection of the devitalized bone is then indicated.

Eye. In head and neck irradiation, treatment fields should be meticulously planned in order to avoid, where possible, the eye and its adjacent structures. In the treatment of cancer of the accessory nasal sinuses, the eye frequently must be included in the treatment field. In these patients a small shield to minimize the extent of acute conjunctivitis, scleritis, and painful corneal ulceration should be utilized. Irradiation to the cornea will result in corneal keratinization and a punctate keratitis. Vitreous hemorrhages may occur from 5 to 21 months after completion of treatment to the region of the eye, a serious complication in the treatment of retinoblastoma. Vascular damage to the retina may cause a subsequent loss of vision, secondary glaucoma, and atrophy of the globe. Cataracts may occur from 2 to 4 years after exposure to irradiation.

Much has been written concerning the cataractogenic dosages of irradiation.[6] It is generally accepted that fractionation of irradiation delays the onset of cataracts and results in fewer opacities. The minimum cataractogenic exposure is 200 rads in a single dose, 400 rads fractionated over a period of 3 weeks to 4 months, and 1,000 rads in divided treatments of more than 4 months.[4]

Irradiation delivered to an enucleated socket usually leads to a progressive fibrosis and a socket contracture unless an implant is worn from the beginning of the irradiation.

Ear. The acute complications of irradiation to the ear are fullness, earache, tenderness, loss of hearing, hyperemia of the drum, slight retraction, bulging of the eardrum, and moderate conductive hearing loss, which results from a radiation otitis media and is usually treated in the same fashion as a bacterial otitis media. Ten percent of patients show a necrosis and breakdown of the external auditory canal. As a rule these complications usually clear up within a few weeks. The late changes of irradiation to the ear are the result of an obliterated endarteritis with impaired blood supply to the cochlea, labyrinth, and ossicles, which usually results in a nerve type of deafness.

Cartilage. Chondritis and perichondritis are painful, disabling complications that may occur as a result of infection associated with neoplastic invasion of the cartilage of the nose and ear. Irradiation in these areas may be contraindicated. If it is tried and fails, the appendage may have to be removed. Radiochondritis is rarely seen in the absence of a tumor. In the glottis, especially the epiglottis, most patients with neoplastic cartilage invasion develop chondritis, which subsequently leads to necrosis and slough with hemorrhage. A patient who initially has normal cartilage may develop chondritis during or following irradiation. The infection causes devitalized cartilage and may be the result of overtreatment or poor technique. In the case of the larynx and epiglottis, the treatment is total laryngectomy.

Laryngeal. Every patient who receives a cancericidal dose of irradiation to the glottic area will develop some degree of edema. This complication is worse when large fields are used and the fractionation is less than 4 weeks. Usually the edema is slight and diminishes within a few months. If it persists beyond that point, one should suspect residual carcinoma. Edema often necessitates a tracheostomy. Multiple biopsies should be avoided because these frequently lead to increased edema and necrosis.

Central nervous system. Radiation in the head and neck through anterior and posterior fields should be avoided to prevent the spinal cord's inclusion in the field of irradiation. Radiation myelitis is rare. It may not manifest itself for 1 to 3 years. It varies in its degree of clinical manifestations from simple paresthesia to complete loss of motor function. Intensified corticosteroid and vitamin B_{12} therapy may be of value in limiting the progressive loss of neurologic function.

CLINICAL EVALUATION
General principles

Certain generalities can be applied to all patients with cancer of the head and neck.

Clinical staging. Clinical staging was based on the classification recommended by the International Committee of Stage Grouping in Cancer and is described elsewhere.[7]

Radiation therapy. All patients receiving irradiation were treated with a cobalt 60 source utilizing fixed fields. The fields were designed to include the primary site of treatment and additional regional involvement. The entire lymph node areas were not prophylactically treated unless there were definite signs of clinical involvement. All patients received a time-dose–related cancericidal therapy.

Hydroxyurea therapy. All patients treated at the Greater Baltimore Medical Center with epidermoid carcinomas of the head and neck were treated concomitantly with hydroxyurea. All of these patients received a daily dose of 1,500 mg.

Surgery. Except in early cases of laryngeal carcinoma and cancers of the nasopharynx, where radiation therapy alone may have been the principle modality, all other tumor sites were treated by a combination of surgery and irradiation. The surgical procedures consisted of varieties of operation, each designed to fit the individual case, staging, and response.

Specific sites

While the general principles of radiation therapy discussed heretofore apply to all primary sites of cancers of the head and neck, there are certain local considerations that are applicable to specific tumor sites.

Tongue. Seventy-five patients were seen with lesions of the base of the tongue. Only six were seen with neoplasms of the anterior two thirds, a primary surgical lesion, and are not included in this discussion. Sixty-nine percent (52/75) had clinically positive lymph nodes. Carcinoma of the base of the tongue is usually an advanced lesion when detected. Approximately 82% of our patients had T3 and T4 lesions. The advanced staging of these lesions does not lend itself to a surgical approach. Only 19 of our patients were operated on after being treated with irradiation and hydroxyurea. This area is not readily accessible to interstitial implantation of radioisotopes, surface mold application, or intraoral cone therapy. External beam therapy via bilateral parallel opposing fields is the chief method of therapy and should include all of the involved lymph nodes. Survival rates of 36% of patients receiving radiation therapy, hydroxyurea, and surgery and 29% in patients receiving only radiation therapy and hydroxyurea com-

pare favorably with results of 6% to 50% reported by other authors.[1]

Floor of mouth. This area readily lends itself to treatment by one or more modalities. Superficial or locally advanced lesions can be treated either by external beam, interstitial implantation, or intraoral cone therapy. Because 50% of our patients had positive lymph nodes, we preferred to treat these lesions by a combination of external beam therapy, utilizing a full cancericidal dose of 6,000 rads in 6 to 7 weeks, augmented by intraoral cone therapy (2,000 rads in 2 weeks) to the primary site, thus delivering approximately 8,000 rads to the primary site in 8 to 9 weeks. The combination of radiation therapy, hydroxyurea, and surgery resulted in an 80% survival rate. Preliminary irradiation usually results in a less radical surgical procedure, eliminating the need for elaborate repairs of the floor of the mouth and resection of the mandible.

Buccal mucosa–lower gingiva. Thirty-nine percent (6/19) of our patients had clinically palpable lymph nodes when first seen. Accessible lesions in the anterior or central portion of the buccal mucosa may be treated by intraoral cone, a combination of intraoral cone and external beam therapy, or an interstitial radium needle implant. Posterior lesions adjacent to the tonsillar fossa are treated with unilateral or bilateral external beam therapy. These lesions have a higher incidence of nodal metastasis; therefore, the fields of irradiation must include the cervical lymph nodes. An overall survival rate of 37% was seen in 19 patients with primary epidermoid tumors arising in this site. Sixty percent (6/10) of those undergoing radiation, hydroxyurea, and surgery survived. Two cases of rhabdomyosarcoma in children under 5 years of age, arising in the buccal mucosa from the orbicularis oris muscle, were successfully treated by irradiation following two or more surgical recurrences.

Tonsil. The tonsillar fossa does not readily contain barriers to the spread of malignancy. Of 86 patients, only one had a T1 lesion. Sixty percent had clinically positive lymph nodes. The main objective of treatment should be to irradiate the primary site with an adequate margin of surrounding tissue and the immediate regional lymph nodes. At least one external skin field to cover the primary site and the involved lymph nodes is used. A tumor dose of 7,000 rads utilizing cobalt 60 teletherapy is given over a period of 6 to 8 weeks. Occasionally, opposing right and left lateral beams are used in extensive tumors. Other techniques include an oblique wedge pair,[4] a combination of an intraoral cone (2,500 rads) and an external supervoltage beam (6,000 rads) in 6 to 8 weeks. Our usual technique is to reduce the size of the primary tumor by external cobalt 60 therapy and then to cone in on the residual. The survival rate of patients with tumors in this site was 50% (42/86). Sixty-eight percent (29/46) of our patients who received radiation therapy, hydroxyurea, and surgery survived. Our survival statistics for carcinoma of the tonsil compare favorably with those reported by other authors (15% to 37½%).[2]

Soft palate. Lesions in this area are treated in a manner similar to that described for carcinomas of the tonsil. The soft palate is readily cross-fired through parallel opposing external beam portals, including both the primary site and lymph node drainage areas. Occasionally the external therapy is augmented by the use of an intraoral cone. Fifty-two percent (10/19) of our patients with tumors in this site survived. Of these, only three had surgery after irradiation.

Larynx. The anatomical limits of the larynx were defined as recommended by the American Joint Committee for Cancer Staging.[10]

Glottic. Although much controversy surrounds the selection of the modality of treatment for glottic carcinomas, we feel that the criteria for the use of radiation therapy as a primary modality for the treatment of glottic lesions are easily defined. Radiation therapy should be considered as the primary treatment of cancer of the true cords, where no fixation is present. All stage I lesions were treated with radiation therapy utilizing small-field cobalt 60 external beams to a total tumor dose of approximately 6,000 rads in 6 to 7 weeks. Eighty-seven percent of these patients survived. Stage II lesions were treated by radiation therapy and hydroxyurea as a primary modality; the survival rate was approximately 75%. Close observance of these patients after treatment, with rebiopsy where indicated, is essential in order that radiation failures may be salvaged by subsequent laryngectomy. The more advanced lesions of the glottis were treated with radiation therapy, hydroxyurea, and total laryngectomy with radical neck dissections. One hundred percent of these patients (9/9) survived.

Supraglottic. The presence of lymph node metastases in 41% (33/81) of patients with squamous carcinomas arising in the supraglottic area makes survival rates differ significantly from those of the glottic region. Sixty percent (18/30) of patients receiving radiation therapy, hydroxyurea, and sur-

gery survived. The overall survival rate was 43% (35/81). Thirty patients were operated on after having received radiation therapy and hydroxyurea; 27 had composite resections, and 3 had limited resections. Preoperative irradiation is most essential in this area because of a high rate of recurrence following attempts at primary curative surgery. Of 15 patients seen with recurrence following surgery, 3 were saved by subsequent treatment with radiation therapy and hydroxyurea.

Subglottic. Effective irradiation is justifiable in the treatment of small infiltrating lesions with no cartilage invasion or palpable adenopathy. Six of nine patients seen with lesions in this area have survived. Of these, four received irradiation, hydroxyurea, and surgery, and one received hydroxyurea and irradiation.

Hypopharynx. As in the case of lesions of the tonsil and base of the tongue, the lack of barriers to the spread of cancer of the hypopharynx results in more advanced staging. Eighty-four percent of our patients had T3 and T4 lesions, and 85% (61/72) had lymph node involvement. These patients were treated in a fashion similar to that for advanced carcinomas of the larynx; large fields were utilized to encompass all tissues from the inferior border of the mandible to the clavicle and from the anterior tip of the thyroid cartilage to the mastoid line. All received concomitant hydroxyurea therapy. Because surgery is usually difficult in this area, only 12 patients underwent a radical pharyngeal resection. Fourteen had local resections, with no tumor reported in the primary site. Fifty-three percent (14/26) of our patients who received radiation therapy, hydroxyurea, and surgery survived. Of all patients seen, 36% (26/72) have remained tumor free.

Nasopharynx. Historically, the primary modality of treatment of lesions of the nasopharynx has been radiation therapy. This method was based on the inaccessibility of the primary site and the principal regional lymph node drainage areas (sphenopalatine) to surgery. Survival rates reported by various authors, ranging from 25% to 33%, suggest that other methods of treatment should be explored.[1] Bilateral external beam therapy including the base of the skull, the sphenopalatine fossa, and the entire nasopharynx is combined with lateral or tangential fields encompassing the cervical lymph nodes. The survival rate for patients who received this type of radiation therapy and hydroxyurea was 64% (14/22). Recently we have explored the use of the radical neck dissection of all clinically involved nodal areas, followed by radiation therapy augmented by hydroxyurea. The survival rate for this group of patients was 80% (8/10).

Nasal fossa. Of nine patients with tumors arising in this site, four were seen with esthesioneuroblastomas. Two of these were treated by an intracranial nasal approach, one with preliminary irradiation and the other with postoperative irradiation; one was treated with radical antrectomy with orbital exenteration after preliminary irradiation and cyclophosphamide (Cytoxan) therapy; and one was treated by irradiation. All are alive.

Maxillary sinus. This area is usually characterized by rather extensive primary involvement of the maxillary and ethmoid sinuses as well as of the turbinates. Twenty-six of our 30 patients had T3 and T4 lesions, and only 13% (4/30) had lymph node metastases. Because of the extensive bony destruction, surgery after preliminary irradiation augmented by hydroxyurea therapy is our favorite mode of treatment. AP and lateral wedge fields are utilized. These include the involved maxillary antrum, the nasal fossa, and the ethmoid air cells bilaterally. Where there is involvement of the bony orbit, the entire contents of the orbit are included; only the cornea is shielded to prevent painful corneal ulceration. In those cases where the eye is to be surgically spared, the entire orbital contents are shielded. A 53% (16/30) survival rate is reported. Twelve patients had either radical antrectomies with orbital exenteration (seven patients) or local maxillary resections (five patients) after irradiation and hydroxyurea therapy. No viable tumor remained in four patients.

Parotid and minor salivary glands. Forty-nine malignant epithelial tumors of the parotid gland were treated. Pathologically, a wide distribution of mucoepidermoid, squamous, adenoid cystic, adenocarcinoma, and anaplastic carcinoma was diagnosed. Thirty percent of these patients had clinically involved lymph nodes and had a survival rate of 40% (6/15). Seventy-three percent of these patients were treated with radical surgery, simple or radical parotidectomy, with or without neck dissection as indicated and with facial nerve graft where necessary and feasible. All patients were irradiated postoperatively with concomitant hydroxyurea therapy. Eighty-six percent (31/36) survived. This unusually high survival rate in this usually unfavorable disease was due to the radical approach used. These patients had radical surgery, total or radical parotidectomy, followed by extensive radiochemotherapy for T1 or T2 lesions, rather than the simple proce-

dures so often done for parotid lesions. They received approximately 4,500 rads in 3 weeks, utilizing a combination of deep x-ray therapy (400 kv.) and cobalt 60.

CONCLUSION

Successful treatment of cancers of the head and neck requires close cooperation and teamwork. All patients are seen by the surgeon and radiation therapist together at the onset of treatment and weekly or biweekly during the course of radiation therapy and in the immediate postradiation recovery period. Together the surgeon and radiation therapist plan the entire course of treatment, deal with complications promptly as they arise, and modify treatment plans as the clinical response or lack of it unfolds. Postsurgical follow-ups and chemotherapy management are joint projects. It is through this method of two physicians acting in unison that these excellent results in carcinomas of the head and neck have been achieved.

REFERENCES

1. Ariel, I. M.: Treatment of tumors of the tongue, nasopharynx and the parotid salivary gland. In Pack, G. T., and Ariel, I. M., editors: The treatment of cancer and allied diseases, New York, 1959, Paul B. Hoeber, Inc.
2. Berven, E. G. E.: Radiation therapy of malignant tumors of the palatine tonsil. In Pack, G. T., and Ariel, I. M., editors: The treatment of cancer and allied diseases, New York, 1959, Paul B. Hoeber, Inc.
3. Moss, W. T., and Brand, W. N.: Therapeutic radiology, St. Louis, 1969, The C. V. Mosby Co.
4. Murphy, W. T.: Radiation therapy, ed. 2, Philadelphia, 1967, W. B. Saunders Co.
5. Philips, F. S., Sternberg, S. S., Schwartz, H. S., Cronin, A. P., Sodergran, J. E., and Vidal, P. N.: Hydroxyurea. I. Acute cell death in proliferating tissues in rats, Cancer Res. **27:**61-74, 1967.
6. Raven, R. W.: Cancer, vol. 5, London, 1959, Butterworth & Co. (Publishers) Ltd.
7. Richards, G. J., and Chambers, R. G.: Hydroxyurea; a radiosensitizer in the treatment of neoplasms of the head and neck, Am. J. Roentgenol. Radium Ther. Nucl. Med. **55:**555-656, 1969.
8. Sinclair, W. K.: Hydroxyurea; differential lethal effects on cultured mammalian cells during cell cycle, Science **150:**1729-1731, 1965.
9. Sinclair, W. K.: Hydroxyurea; effects on Chinese hamster cells grown in culture, Cancer Res. **27:**297-308, 1967.
10. Smith, R. R., Caulk, R., Frazell, E., Holinger, P. H., MacComb, W. S., Russell, W. O., Schulz, M. D., and Tucker, G. F.: Revision of the clinical staging system for cancer of the larynx, Cancer **31:**72-79, 1973.

Chapter 2

Chemotherapy of head and neck cancer

Herbert Lipshutz, M.D.
Harvey J. Lerner, M.D.

Except in cases of highly specific tumor growths, such as rhabdomyosarcoma, the use of chemotherapeutic agents in the treatment of head and neck malignancies has been reserved for far-advanced lesions. Therefore, careful examination of the patient to determine the size of the tumor, as well as the presence or absence of enlarged cervical lymph nodes, is of the utmost importance. Fortunately, a standard has been set for staging and classifying lesions[3] (Table 2-1). In general, tumors of the buccal mucosa, anterior tongue, and floor of the mouth tend to be less aggressive than those in the posterior oropharynx, nasopharynx, or hypopharynx. Thus in most instances the use of chemotherapeutic agents has been reserved for the treatment of T3 and T4 lesions with nodal involvement. Practically all of these patients are inoperable when originally seen.

Treatment by a single modality of x-ray or surgery is reserved for smaller lesions, either T1 or T2, where they would be most effective. It appears that combinations of treatments offer a higher percentage of survivors. It is obviously redundant to say that cure rates for far-advanced lesions are poor. The overall survival rates in T3 and T4 lesions range from 3% to 34%,[5] although there is some evidence that extenuating factors such as anatomic site, histologic grade, and the presence or absence of nodes may be influential.

To simplify the discussion of the use of chemotherapy in the treatment of head and neck cancer, it seems logical to categorize this use into treatment with drug alone, combination drug therapy, combination drug and radiation therapy, and combination drug and radiation therapy with surgery.

DRUG THERAPY ALONE

The category of drug therapy alone can be further divided into systemic and local treatments. Most of the agents that are now in use both clinically and experimentally are noted in the following outline:

DRUGS USED IN THERAPY OF HEAD AND NECK CANCER

I. Antimetabolites
  A. Methotrexate (MTX)
  B. 5-Fluorouracil (5-FU)
  C. 6-Mercaptopurine (6-MP)
  D. 6-Thioguanine (6-TG)
  E. 1-B-D-Arabinosyl cytosine (ARA-C)
II. Alkylating agents
  A. Nitrogen mustard (HN$_2$)
  B. Chlorambucil
  C. Melphalan

Table 2-1. Staging table for malignancies of the head and neck

	Tumor size and involvement		Regional lymph node involvement
T1	2 cm. or less	N0	No clinically palpable cervical nodes
T2	2 to 4 cm.	N1	Palpable homolateral nodes (not fixed)
T3	Greater than 4 cm.	N2	Palpable bilateral nodes (not fixed)
T4	Huge	N3	Palpable bilateral nodes (fixed)

D. Thio-TEPA
E. Cyclophosphamide
F. Busulfan

III. Antibiotics
   A. Adriamycin
   B. Daunorubicin
   C. Dactinomycin
   D. Mithramycin
   E. Bleomycin

IV. Miscellaneous drugs
   A. 1,3-Bis(2-chloroethyl)-1-nitrosourea (BCNU)
   B. L-Asparaginase
   C. 1,1-Dichloro-2(*o*-chlorophenyl)-2(*p*-chloro-phenyl)ethane (*op'*-DDD)
   D. Vinca alkaloids
      1. Vincristine sulfate
      2. Vinblastine sulfate
   E. Hydroxyurea
   F. Procarbazine hydrochloride

Methotrexate (MTX), cyclophosphamide (Cytoxan), bleomycin sulfate, and hydroxyurea are the single agents reported to produce an objective response in 30% to 40% of patients with advanced squamous cell carcinoma of the head and neck.[2] MTX is the agent that has been most studied to date and apparently is most effective in systemic, intermittent (q. 4 to 7 days), or high dosage therapy with citrovorum factor (Leucovorin). Although regional infusions (intra-arterial) give a large amount of drug to a local area, the value is diminished by a high frequency of lesions beyond the arterial supply, and there is also a high complication rate.[11] However, agents used in this manner have achieved better response rates. The complications include faulty placement of catheters, bleeding and embolization, and a high toxicity rate. The use of dichloromethotrexate (DCM) has been recommended to reduce the toxicity, and the dosage is 10 mg. per day. This is metabolized in the liver, but in so doing, it has a slightly lower blood level. The limiting toxicity of DCM is stomatitis similar to other intra-arterial drug infusion reactions.

One note on the placement of the intra-arterial catheter: it is best placed in a superficial temporal artery. The placement of the catheter can be checked by the injection of fluorescein and by using a Wood's light to determine the actual extent of the blood supply.

Livingstone and Carter,[7] in reviewing single-agent chemotherapy, stated that there is considerable difficulty in compiling statistics because of the small number of patients. In their study of a series of single drugs, using MTX, 5-fluorouracil (5-FU), 6-mercaptopurine (6-MP), vinblastine sulfate, procarbazine hydrochloride, chlorambucil, and mechlorethamine hydrochloride, they showed a response varying from 7½% to 39%. Complete remissions were usual; partial responses were short. The mean response time was 1 to 5 months. The information available on the newer drugs is extremely meagre and at this time meaningless, although some antineoplastic responses have been achieved with the following drugs: the nitrosoureas, Adriamycin, and cytosine arabinoside.

Bleomycin sulfate, however, is being studied much more extensively.[10] So far, there is an overall response rate of approximately 36%. Interest in the drug is great because it has a low toxicity to the bone marrow and thus may be extremely useful in a drug combination, reducing overall reactions. However, total drug dosage is limited because of severe pulmonary toxicity.

At the present time there is no data comparing primary site and response with a particular agent.

As stated previously, the largest amount of collected data is with MTX, and the best results are with the drug being given intermittently, either orally or intravenously, every week or twice a week. Bertino[2] stated that 50% of patients had a greater than 50% reduction in a tumor mass, with 15% showing complete disappearance of a tumor. In monthly 5- to 10-day courses 44% responded; of these, 29% had greater than 50% reductions, and there were no complete disappearances.

In addition to the previously stated complications, one may include white blood cell count (WBC) depression, bleeding, and infection, with low serum folate levels.[4] MTX, when given orally, releases slowly and erratically from the intestines and results in longer elevated serum concentrations. Excretion may be delayed by kidney disease. Because MTX alone can produce renal damage as well as hepatic damage, the protection of citrovorum factor is needed. This is given at the end of the MTX therapy q. 6h. for 4 doses.

DRUG COMBINATIONS ALONE

Here also, published series and studies are few in number. The responses, when present, are of short duration, and complete remissions are extremely rare. The combinations can be endless and variable, as are the results, and are highly toxic. Almost all of these combinations are given intravenously and intermittently, with the patients hospitalized and closely observed.

Bertino reported on the various combinations and results that he used. The combination of bleomycin and MTX[8] showed a greater than 50% regression in only 2 of 4 patients. The same response rate was noted in the combination of MTX and vincristine sulfate in 15 of 28 patients. A greater than 50% regression was noted with bleomycin and adriamycin in 4 of 8 patients. Similar responses with the combination of cyclophosphamide, MTX, vincristine, and 5-FU in 10 patients resulted in 1 complete and 7 partial regressions. The following combination used with a total of 82 patients showed 45 patients with a greater than 50% regression: vinblastine sulfate, streptonigrin, thiophosphoramide, chlorambucil, 6-MP, MTX, and procarbazine.[2]

Oberfield, Cady, and Booth[9] reported on the drug combination of floxuridine (FUDR), 5-FU, MTX, and folinic acid given as an intra-arterial infusion to 94 patients. Seventy-one percent had catheters in the common carotid and 13.8% had catheters in the external carotid. The results were as follows: 48% exhibited a 50% tumor regression, and 26% achieved a 100% regression objectively. They also showed that patients with increased toxicity had increased responses but decreased survival rates. Mild to moderate toxicity produced optimal responses to the survival ratio. They showed no correlation among the total cumulative drug dosage, response, and survival toxicity. They stated that 31% of the patients survived 1 year from the onset of chemotherapy. The complications recorded were that 8.9% had cerebrovascular accidents (CVA's) (some transient), 45% had severe systemic drug toxicity, 30% had severe local toxicity, and 2% died from drug or catheter toxicity, or both. Their assumption was that the toxicity was related to the condition of the patient, not to the drug dosage.

On our chemotherapy service the drug combination that seems to be showing some promise is that of hydroxyurea and 5-FU. This combination has been used in approximately 10 patients. Actual statistics are unavailable because of too short a time period, but an early response rate has been noticed in all 10 patients.

Those patients with far-advanced cancers that did not initially respond to drugs, radiation, or surgery, or a combination of these have been given the following group of drugs: vincristine sulfate, hydroxyurea, cyclophosphamide, MTX, and 5-FU. To date, these patients have shown early response, but there have been no long-term survivors. This multidrug combination is extremely toxic and has been used in approximately 25 patients. In some instances prednisone has been given also, somewhat empirically, to prevent bone marrow depression.

DRUG TREATMENTS IN COMBINATION WITH RADIATION THERAPY OR SURGERY, OR BOTH

MTX and radiation, which has been the combination drug and radiation therapy under study for the longest period of time, has seemingly prolonged remissions, but cures over long periods of time are questionable.

Ansfield[1] reported that 5-FU caused an increase in median survival figures; he also noted that results were better in anterior intraoral lesions that in posterior ones. This is the only study that clearly defines or suggests that the biology of the disease in specific sites may be a primary determinant of the response to the drug alone or to the drug in combination with radiation therapy.

Our intermittent drug and radiation therapy program, which has recently completed a 6-year follow-up,[6] is the only long-term intermittent drug treatment that has been reported to date. It consists of the following data:

A total of 82 patients with proved advanced epidermoid carcinomas of the head and neck were treated with intermittent hydroxyurea and radiation and, when the patients would submit, surgery. The administration of hydroxyurea is continued indefinitely after the completion of the radiation and surgery. The drug is discontinued temporarily only if the WBC falls below 2,000 per cu. mm.[2]

In all 82 patients there was a regression of the primary tumor. Maximum regression was demonstrated 6 to 8 weeks after completion of the radiotherapy. Fifty-three of the 82 patients have been clinically free of the disease for periods ranging from 3 to 72 months. Sixty-five of the 82 patients showed a 100% regression in tumor size, 9 patients had an 80% or more regression, and 8 patients had a 50% or more regression. If one eliminates deaths from intercurrent causes, the survival rate increases for those patients undergoing combined therapy plus surgery.

The drug combination with radiation does cause stomatitis and intraoral mucositis. However, it has the following advantage: since the drug is given orally and intermittently, the therapy does not require hospitalization, and blood counts taken weekly will determine if the patients are taking the drug. If the WBC is normal, the patient is not taking the drug. If the WBC is too low, the drug is temporarily discontinued, and the leukocyte count rapidly rebounds.

So far, the concomitant use of drug, radiation, and surgery has worked best and given the highest survival rate.

One can therefore conclude that the drug combinations are probably more effective than single-unit treatments and that new drug combinations and more combined therapies are needed if we are to significantly increase the survival rate.

REFERENCES

1. Ansfield, F. J., Ramirez, G., Davis, H. L, Korbitz, B. C., Vermund, H., and Gollin, F. F.: Treatment of advanced cancer of the head and neck, Cancer **25**:78-82, 1970.
2. Bertino, J. R., Mosher, M. B., and DeConti, R. C.: Chemotherapy of cancer of the head and neck, Cancer **31**:1141-1149, 1973.
3. Clinical staging system for carcinoma of the oral cavity, Chicago, American Joint Committee for Cancer Staging and End Results Reporting, 1967, pp. 1-12.
4. Hellman, S., Dannotti, A. T., Bertino, J. R.: Determination of the levels of serum folate in patients with carcinoma of the head and neck treated with methotrexate, Cancer Res. **24**:105-113, 1964.
5. James, A. G.: Cancer prognosis manual, New York, American Cancer Society.
6. Lipshutz, H., and Lerner, H. J.: Six year observation of the combined treatment for far-advanced cancer of the head and neck, Am. J. Surg. **126**:519-522, 1973.
7. Livingston, R. B., and Carter, S. K.: Single agents in cancer chemotherapy, New York, IFI/Plenum Publishing Corp., 1970.
8. Mosher, M. B., DeConti, R. C., and Bertino, J. R.: Bleomycin Therapy and advanced Hodgkin's disease and epidermoid tumors, Cancer **30**:56-60, 1972.
9. Oberfield, R. A., Cady, B., and Booth, J. C.: Regional arterial chemotherapy for advanced carcinoma of the head and neck (a ten year review), Cancer **32**:82-88, 1973.
10. Ohnuma, T., Selawry, O. S., Holland, J. F., DeVita, V. T., Shedd, D. P., Hansen, H. H., and Muggia, F. M.: Clinical study with bleomycin; tolerance to twice weekly dosage, Cancer **30**:914-922, 1972.
11. Watkins, E., Jr., and Sullivan, R. D.: Cancer chemotherapy by prolonged arterial infusion, Surg., Gynecol., Obstet. **118**:1-19, 1964.

Chapter 3

Immunologic defects associated with squamous carcinoma

Paul B. Chretien, M.D.
Patrick L. Twomey, M.D.
William J. Catalona, M.D.
Ronald L. Hansing, B.S.

One of the most important recent contributions in clinical oncology has been the demonstration that cancer patients have immune defects early in the clinical evolution of their tumors and that this impairment correlates with prognosis after clinically definitive tumor therapy.[4,6] These data suggest that measurement of immune reactivity in cancer patients may be useful in determining mechanisms of tumor development and progression, detecting early primary or recurrent malignancy, understanding and augmenting immune defense mechanisms, and guiding both conventional and immunotherapy.

With the development of relatively precise methods of quantitating in vitro lymphocyte reactivity to phytohemagglutinin (PHA)[2] and in vivo contact sensitivity to dinitrochlorobenzene (DNCB)[1], such studies now appear feasible. As an initial step in discerning the usefulness of these assays in determining the tumor status of treated cancer patients, immune reactivity was assessed in over 100 postoperative cancer patients with sufficiently long intervals after treatment of their tumors without recurrence to be considered cured. The immune reactivity was then compared with that of over 200 preoperative patients who had tumors of the same histologic type and with that of a large population of healthy volunteers in the same age range.

This report focuses on a major finding in this study: that patients with squamous carcinoma of the head and neck region and female pelvic organs are unique, compared with patients with sarcomas, melanomas, and adenocarcinomas, in that immune defects present in tumor-bearing patients occur in similar incidence among clinically cured patients.

MATERIALS AND METHODS
Cured patients

Over 100 patients who had been treated for histologically proved malignancies at the Surgery Branch, National Cancer Institute, were studied. All were in good general health at the time of the study; each had undergone a physical examination within 3 months of the study and were considered clinically cured of tumor at that time. Only patients with a normal hematocrit, white blood cell count (WBC), sedimentation rate, and other appropriate laboratory studies were included. Patients who had undergone postoperative chemotherapy or radiation therapy were excluded. No patients taking medications known to alter immune reactivity were included, and all abstained from medications for 24 hours before blood sampling.

The patients were divided into five groups according to the histologic type of tumor excised.

1. Head and neck squamous carcinoma. These patients had been treated by wide excision of the

primary site and in almost every instance, radical neck dissection. Although most had been heavy smokers preoperatively, only 7 of the 21 patients in this group admitted to tobacco use in any form when studied. Patients with a history or other evidence of alcohol abuse postoperatively were excluded. Their disease-free interval ranged from 4 to 17 years (median 10 years).

2. Pelvic squamous carcinoma. Twenty-five patients had primary cervical carcinoma, and 2 had carcinoma of the vulva. Nineteen cervical cancer patients had been treated by radical hysterectomy, and the remainder by total pelvic exenteration. Patients with chronic urinary tract infections were excluded. Their disease-free interval was 6 to 17 years (median 10 years).

3. Sarcomas. In this group there were 3 patients with osteosarcomas, 4 with chondrosarcomas, 2 with liposarcomas, 5 with fibrosarcomas, and 2 with myosarcomas. All had been treated by radical excision of the primary tumor. The disease-free interval for the group ranged from 4 to 12 years (median 6 years).

4. Melanomas. The 16 patients in this group had been treated by wide excision of the primary site and regional node dissection. Their disease-free interval was 5 to 14 years (median 7 years).

5. Adenocarcinomas. Among the 21 patients in this group, 10 had adenocarcinoma of the breast, 9 of the large intestine, and 1 each of the salivary gland and paranasal sinus. All had been treated by standard surgical resection. Their disease-free interval was 5 to 14 years (median 8 years).

Preoperative patients

Over 200 patients were studied who had the same histologic types of tumors as the cured group and who were admitted to the Surgery Branch, National Cancer Institute, for definitive surgical resection. Only patients with clinically operable tumors were included. In some, metastases were found in the course of preoperative evaluation or during surgical exploration. Patients who had undergone surgery, chemotherapy, or radiation therapy within the previous 3 months or those with chronic diseases, drug ingestion, or active infections were excluded.

Control subjects

Over 400 healthy volunteers were solicited from the employees of the National Institutes of Health and from residents of a retirement community. Their ages ranged from 20 to 80 years and were almost equally distributed in each decade represented. They were screened to exclude those who had chronic disease, those who were taking any medications, and those who had a recent illness or history of malignant disease. All had a normal hematocrit, total WBC and differential count, and erythrocyte sedimentation rate.

Lymphocyte reactivity to PHA

White cell suspensions were obtained by sedimenting whole blood specimens with methylcellulose, and lymphocytes were isolated by exposure to carbonyl iron. Individual cultures contained 5×10^6 lymphocytes per ml. in 90% RPMI-1640 and 10% AB serum. All studies were conducted with a single pool of AB serum obtained from healthy volunteers. Phytohemagglutinin-P (Difco Laboratories, Detroit, Michigan) was added in four concentrations ranging from 3.1 to 50 μg. of protein per ml. of culture. The cultures were incubated for 54 hours; then tritiated thymidine (300 mCi./mM., 30 μCi./ml. of culture) was added; and after a 3-hour labeling period, the cultures were frozen in liquid nitrogen. The nuclear protein was precipitated with trichloroacetic acid, washed with saline, and solubilized in Soluene (Packard Instrument Companies, Inc.). The preparation was neutralized with acetic acid and transferred to scintillation-counting vials with washes of toluene-Liquifluor (New England Nuclear), Boston, Mass.). Incorporation of tritiated thymidine by the lymphocytes was quantitated in a Packard Tri-Carb scintillation counter, and the absolute activity was expressed in disintegrations per minute (DPM). Cultures with each dose of PHA and controls without PHA were prepared in triplicate.

Assay of serum effect on lymphocyte reactivity

The effect of serum from normal volunteers and cancer patients on the reactivity of normal lymphocytes to PHA was compared with the reactivity of the same lymphocytes in the pooled AB serum. The quotient of the former determination divided by the latter was termed the lymphocyte reactivity index (LRI).

Determination of normal lymphocyte reactivity

The lymphocyte reactivity of 284 normal volunteers in the same age range of the cancer patients (20 to 80 years) was derived by determining the mean distribution of lymphocyte reactivity $\pm$ 1 standard deviation (SD) for each decade.[2] Lymphocyte reactivity was then arbitrarily defined as *normal* if it did not differ from the mean for the age group by more than 1 SD, *high* if it exceeded the mean for the age group by more than 1 SD, and *low* if it was below the mean for the age group by more than 1 SD.

DNCB contact sensitivity

The method employed for quantitating DNCB reactivity incorporates the spontaneous flare reaction that occurs at the site that DNCB is applied 7 to 14 days beforehand.[3] Doses of 2,000 μg. and 50 μg. of DNCB are applied to the upper arm and forearm, respectively. A spontaneous flare at both the 2,000-μg. and 50-μg. sites by 14 days is scored 4+. A spontaneous flare at the 2,000-μg. site only is scored 3+. If neither site develops a spontaneous flare by 14 days after application of DNCB, a challenge of 50 μg. is applied to the opposite forearm. If a delayed cutaneous hypersensitivity reaction (DCH) occurs at this site within 48 hours, it is scored 2+. An equivocal reaction that requires biopsy for confirmation is scored 1+ if the histologic features of DCH are present. If these changes are not seen or if no grossly visible reaction occurs, the subject is considered anergic to DNCB.

Statistical methods

The lymphocyte reactivity and lymphocyte reactivity index for each cancer patient were determined and compared with those of the appropriate age group of the normal population. Comparisons of lymphocyte reactivity and serum effect on lymphocyte reactivity were done by chi-square analysis and standard error of the difference between means, respectively. Comparisons of DNCB reactivity of the patient groups and the normal population were done by chi square analysis.

RESULTS
Lymphocyte reactivity to PHA

As in a previous study,[2] the lymphocyte reactivity of preoperative patients correlated with tumor histology. In the present study, among patients with squamous carcinomas of the head and neck region and female pelvic organs, with sarcomas, and with melanomas, there was a greater incidence of low reactivity than among the control group (Table 3-1).

The lymphocyte reactivity of patients cured of cancer also correlated with tumor histology. Among patients previously treated for squamous carcinoma of the head and neck region and female pelvic organs, there was an increased incidence of patients with low reactivity similar to that found in preoperative patients. Among patients previously treated for sarcomas, melanomas, and adenocarcinomas, however, the incidence of high reactivity exceeded that of the normal population.

The effect of the serum of the cancer patients on the reactivity of normal lymphocytes also correlated with tumor histology. Serum from both

Table 3-1. Comparison of in vitro lymphocyte reactivity of preoperative and cured cancer patients with normal controls

Patient group	Number of patients	Percent low*	Percent normal†	Percent high‡	Distribution differs from normal group§
Normal	284	16	68	16	
Head and neck squamous carcinoma					
Preoperative	47	38	57	4	Increased low, p < .01
Cured	21	38	57	5	Increased low, p < .025
Pelvic squamous carcinoma					
Preoperative	30	36	57	7	Increased low, p < .02
Cured	24	38	46	16	Increased low, p < .025
Sarcoma					
Preoperative	46	33	54	13	Increased low, p < .025
Cured	15	0	47	53	Increased high, p < .01
Melanoma					
Preoperative	36	28	69	3	Increased low, p < .05
Cured	16	0	62	38	Increased high, p < .05
Adenocarcinoma					
Preoperative	33	15	70	15	Not significant
Cured	18	11	50	39	Increased high, p < .05

*Low: < 1 standard deviation below mean of controls.
†Normal: ± 1 standard deviation from mean of controls.
‡High: > 1 standard deviation above mean of controls.
§Statistical differences by chi-square analysis.

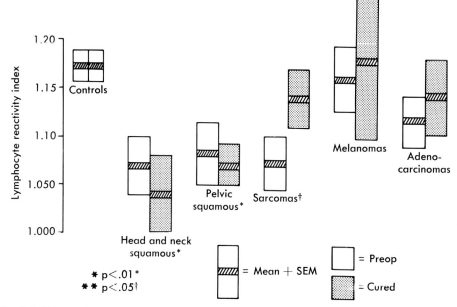

Fig. 3-1. Effect of serum from patients with preoperative and cured cancer and a normal control group on reactivity of normal lymphocytes.

preoperative and cured patients with squamous carcinomas significantly inhibited normal lymphocyte reactivity. Serum suppressants were demonstrated in preoperative sarcoma patients, but not among cured patients. Serum from patients with melanomas and adenocarcinomas, both preoperative and cured, did not have an inhibitory effect on lymphocyte reactivity (Fig. 3-1).

DNCB contact sensitivity

Among 143 control subjects ranging in age from 20 to 80 years, 138 or 96.5% developed a spontaneous flare reaction within 14 days of DNCB sensitization. One additional subject reacted to DNCB challenge, and four were anergic.[1] These data indicate that the normal reaction to DNCB contact sensitization is a spontaneous flare (3 and 4+) and reactions that require a challenge to elicit (1 and 2+) are abnormal.

As demonstrated in a previous study,[1] preoperative patients have a significantly impaired DNCB reactivity. The incidence of abnormal DNCB contact sensitivity was highest among patients with squamous carcinomas. The combined incidence of anergy and impaired positive reactivity (1 and 2+) among preoperative patients with squamous carcinomas of the head and neck region and female pelvic organs was greater than any other preopera-

tive group. Patients cured of tumors of this histologic type displayed similar incidences of abnormal DNCB reactivity. The incidence of anergy and impaired positive reactivity among preoperative patients with sarcomas, melanomas, and adenocarcinomas, although less than among patients with squamous carcinomas, was still significantly higher than among normal subjects. The distribution of DNCB reactivities among patients cured of tumors of these histologic types, however, did not differ significantly from those of the normal group (Table 3-2).

DISCUSSION

The most significant finding in this study is the relationship of the immune reactivity of cured cancer patients to the histologic type of tumor previously excised. Cured squamous carcinoma patients had a high incidence of cellular defects similar to that found in preoperative patients, while patients successfully treated for sarcomas, melanomas, and adenocarcinomas, unlike their preoperative counterparts, had normal or heightened cellular immunity.

The persistence of immune defects in cured squamous carcinoma patients provokes questions concerning the role of genetic and environmental factors in the genesis of these tumors. For instance, are these patients from a cohort of the population with preexisting and perhaps genetically determined

Table 3-2. Comparison of DNCB reactivity of preoperative and cured cancer patients with normal controls

Patient group	Number of patients	Percent anergic	Percent impaired positive (1-2+)	Percent normal (3-4+)	Distribution differs from normal group*
Normal	143	3	1	96	—
Head and neck squamous carcinoma					
Preoperative	44	27	14	59	p < .01
Cured	21	10	19	71	p < .01
Pelvic squamous carcinoma					
Preoperative	41	44	23	32	p < .01
Cured	22	27	5	68	p < .01
Sarcoma					
Preoperative	44	18	18	64	p < .01
Cured	12	0	0	100	Not significant
Melanoma					
Preoperative	41	12	29	59	p < .01
Cured	12	8	8	84	Not significant
Adenocarcinoma					
Preoperative	31	29	23	48	p < .01
Cured	18	6	6	88	Not significant

*Statistical differences by chi-square analysis.

abnormalities of thymus-dependent lymphocyte function? Do the preexisting immune defects then predispose the patients to cancer by increasing susceptibility to environmental carcinogens? Is a preexisting immune impairment a prerequisite for induction of cancer by agents that have been linked to squamous carcinogenesis, such as tobacco[12] and herpesvirus infection?[8]

An alternative possibility to account for the persisting defects in these patients is that putative carcinogens associated with squamous carcinoma exert their effect indirectly by suppressing host immunity. Support for this speculation is the recent finding that the most common nonlymphoid malignancy in immune-suppressed transplant patients is squamous carcinoma.[13] If such carcinogens are directly immune suppressant, however, our findings would imply a permanent alteration of immune reactivity by these agents, either by their direct action, or by predisposing the patients to the action of agents (for example, viruses), which then have immunosuppressant effects that are permanent.

The serum suppressants of lymphocyte reactivity found in preoperative and cured squamous carcinoma patients have not yet been further identified. Antigen-antibody complexes isolated from the sera of tumor-bearing hosts inhibited both immune lymphocyte destruction of target cells[14] and tumor-antigen stimulation of lymphocytes,[15] and therefore may also inhibit PHA-stimulated lymphocyte transformation; but it seems unlikely that these complexes would persist in the sera of cured patients.

Serum alpha globulins suppress in vivo immune reactivity[10] and in vitro lymphocyte reactivity to PHA.[5] Since increased serum alpha globulin levels occur in both experimental and human cancer hosts, they are reasonable candidates for the serum factors demonstrated in this study.[9] The present concept that alpha globulins have an "immunoregulatory effect," combined with our findings of serum suppressant factors in cured squamous carcinoma patients, provokes the speculation that inappropriately high serum levels of these factors preceded the malignancies and were an important factor in tumor induction.

The high incidence of impaired cellular immunity in squamous carcinoma patients may serve as a rational basis for selection of radiotherapy or surgery for lesions that are appropriately treated by either modality. In view of the evidence for an immunosuppressive effect of radiotherapy,[11] patients with impaired immunity might be selected for surgical treatment, while those with normal reactivity may be more favorable candidates for radiotherapy. The determination of immunologic reactivity may be particularly important in the selection of chemotherapeutic agents and the regulation of drug dosage[7] for these patients.

In an effort to determine the role of genetic and environmental factors in the induction of squamous carcinoma, studies are being conducted to assess the immune reactivity of relatives of these patients, persons with chronic cigarette consumption, and women with premalignant gynecologic disease. The present findings alone, however, appear to justify the caution that persons with impaired immune reactivity, particularly, should avoid agents that have been implicated in the induction of squamous carcinoma.

SUMMARY

Cellular immune competence was quantitated in 200 preoperative cancer patients, 100 postoperative cancer patients considered clinically free of tumor, and over 400 normal persons. Immunity was assessed by in vitro PHA-induced lymphocyte reactivity and in vivo DNCB contact sensitivity. Patients cured of sarcomas, melanomas, and adenocarcinomas had lymphocyte reactivity higher than both their preoperative counterparts and normal subjects and did not display the abnormalities of DNCB contact sensitivity present in the comparable preoperative groups. Patients cured of squamous carcinomas, however, had high incidences of impairment of lymphocyte reactivity and DNCB contact sensitivity similar to that found in preoperative patients. Furthermore, a suppressant effect on lymphocyte reactivity of sera from preoperative patients with squamous carcinomas also occurred with sera from cured squamous carcinoma patients. The persisting high incidence of impaired cellular immunity in patients cured of squamous carinomas indicates the need for investigation of genetic and environmental factors that may be responsible for the defects and determination of their relationship to tumor induction. Treatment of these tumors may be improved by monitoring immune reactivity during therapy and by regimens that correct these defects.

REFERENCES

1. Catalona, W. J., and Chretien, P. B.: Abnormalities of quantitative dinitrochlorobenzene sensitization in cancer patients; correlation with tumor stage and histology, Cancer **31:**353-356, 1973.
2. Catalona, W. J., Sample, W. F., and Chretien, P. B.: Lymphocyte reactivity in cancer patients; correlation with tumor histology and clinical stage, Cancer **31:** 65-71, 1973.
3. Catalona, W. J., Taylor, P. T., Rabson, A. S., and Chretien, P. B.: A method for dinitrochlorobenzene contact sensitization; a clinicopathological study, N. Engl. J. Med. **286:**399-402, 1972.
4. Chretien, P. B., Crowder, W. L., Gertner, H. R., Sample, W. F., and Catalona, W. J.: Correlation of preoperative lymphocyte reactivity with the clinical course of cancer patients, Surg. Gynecol. Obstet. **136:** 380-384, 1973.
5. Cooperband, S. R., Davis, R. C., Schmid, K., and Mannick, J. A.: Competitive blockade of lymphocyte stimulation by a serum immunoregulatory alpha globulin (IRA), Transplant. Proc. **1:**516-523, 1969.
6. Eilber, F. R., and Morton, D. L.: Impaired immunologic reactivity and recurrence following cancer surgery, Cancer **25:**362-367, 1970.
7. Hersh, E. M., Whitecar, J. P., Jr., McCredie, K. B., Body, G. P., Sr., and Freireich, E. J.: Chemotherapy, immunocompetence, immunosuppression and prognosis in acute leukemia, N. Engl. J. Med. **285:**1211-1216, 1971.
8. Hollinshead, A. C., Lee, O., Chretien, P. B., Tarpley, J. L., Rawls, W. E., and Adam, E.: Antibodies to herpesvirus nonvirion antigens in squamous carcinomas, Science **182:**713-715, 1973.
9. Hsu, C. C. S., and LoGerfo, P.: Correlation between serum alpha globulin and plasma inhibitory effect on PHA-stimulated lymphocytes in colon cancer patients, Proc. Soc. Exp. Biol. Med. **139:**575-578, 1972.
10. Kamrin, B. B.: Successful skin homografts in mature non-littermate rats treated with fractions containing alpha globulins, Proc. Soc. Exp. Biol. Med. **100:** 58-61, 1959.
11. McCredie, J. A., Inch, W. R., and Sutherland, R. M.: Effect of postoperative radiotherapy on peripheral blood lymphocytes in patients with carcinoma of the breast, Cancer **29:**349-356, 1972.
12. Moore, C.: Cigarette smoking and cancer of the mouth, pharynx, and larynx; a continuing study, J.A.M.A. **218:**553-558, 1971.
13. Penn, I., and Starzl, T. E.: Malignant tumors arising de novo in immunosuppressed organ transplant recipients, Transplantation **14:**407-417, 1972.
14. Sjogren, H. O., Hellstrom, I., Bansal, S. C., and Hellstrom, K. E.: Suggestive evidence that the "blocking antibodies" of tumor-bearing individuals may be antigen-antibody complexes, Proc. Natl. Acad. Sci. USA **68:**1372-1375, 1971.
15. Vanky, F., Stjernsward, J., Klein, G., and Nilsonne, U.: Serum-mediated inhibition of lymphocyte stimulation by autochthonous human tumors, J. Natl. Cancer Inst. **47:**95-103, 1971.

Chapter 4

A brief review of anesthesia for head and neck surgery

Donald W. Benson, M.D., Ph.D.

In the discussion of anesthesia for cancer surgery of the head and neck, it is interesting to recall that the first appropriately reported clinical use of ether anesthesia was for the removal of a tumor of the neck.[1] This operation, performed at the Massachusetts General Hospital in 1846, was very likely for the removal of a scrofulous lymph node, but it was the beginning of a long series of surgical events that have developed into the very complex and arduous procedures of cancer control by surgery in the region of the head and neck.

It is also appropriate to recall that yet another claimant to the first use of clinical anesthesia, Dr. Crawford Long of Georgia, used ether anesthesia for the removal of a tumor of the neck.[1] This surgery was performed on one James Venable in March of 1842. These two events have been the source of much controversy ever since as to who had the prior right for claiming the first use of ether anesthesia. Interestingly enough, neither source made any claim to the initiation of head and neck surgery.

Undoubtedly there are many historical vignettes that recount the history of head and neck surgery and the anesthesia attendant thereto. None is more exciting than the account of the two surgical procedures performed on President Grover Cleveland in the summer of 1893.[5] The country at that time was in the throes of a monetary crisis, and President Cleveland felt it very necessary, as did his cabinet, that there be no indication made of any illness that he might have. A diagnosis had been made of probable cancer in an ulcer on the hard and soft palate of his mouth. Under great secrecy President Cleveland submitted to surgery by a team of surgeons under Dr. Joseph D. Bryant on July 1, 1893, on a yacht proceeding at half speed on the East River near New York City. The entire proceedings and the attendant problems were described in a 1917 issue of the Saturday Evening Post. The article was written by William W. Keen, M.D., an emeritus professor of surgery at the Jefferson Medical College in Philadelphia, who had been present at the surgery. Dr. Keen was also one of the physicians who had worked with Dr. Weir Mitchell in the writing of the report on nerve injuries during the Civil War, which culminated in the classic description of causalgia.

The following is Dr. Keen's report of the surgery and anesthesia:

The anesthetic troubled us. Our anxiety related not so much to the operation itself as to the anesthetic and its possible dangers. These might easily arise in connection with the respiration, the heart, or the function of the kidneys, etc., dangers which are met with not infrequently as a result of administering an anesthetic, especially in a man of Mr. Cleveland's age and physical condition. The patient was 56 years of age, very corpulent, with a short thick neck, just the build and age for possible apoplexy—an incident which had actually occurred to one of my own patients. He was also worn out mentally and physically by four months of exacting labor and the office seekers' importunities. Twenty-four years ago we had not the refined methods of diagnosis, nor had we the greatly improved methods of anesthesia which we have today. After canvassing the whole matter we decided to perform at least the early steps of the operation under nitrous oxide and then later if necessary under ether. Doctor Hasbrouck was of the opinion that we could not keep the patient well anesthetized with nitrous oxide long enough to complete the operation satisfactorily. . . .

Doctor Hasbrouck first extracted the two left upper bicuspid teeth under nitrous oxide. Doctor Bryant then made the necessary incisions in the roof of the mouth, also under nitrous oxide.

At 1:14 P.M. ether was given by Doctor O'Reilly. During the entire operation Doctor Janeway kept close watch upon the patient's pulse and general condition. Doctor Bryant performed the operation assisted by myself and Doctor Erdman.[5]

No other mention was made of the conduct of the anesthesia, but undoubtedly it was complicated by the fact that because no endotracheal tube was in place, an airway had to be maintained by the surgeon. In all likelihood it was an exciting procedure.

As anesthetic procedures for surgery of the head and neck have developed, it has become more and more apparent that the anesthetic agents used are of less importance than the maintenance of homeostasis of the cardiovascular system and especially the respiratory system because more often than not, the airway is compromised preoperatively by disease, during the operation by the surgeon, incidental to the surgical procedure, or by dressings in the postoperative period.

PREOPERATIVE EVALUATION AND PREPARATION

Patients with cancer of the head and neck can have a variety of difficulties or none at all. However, it is prudent to consider in each patient a few points that consistently cause difficulty during anesthesia and surgery. The first of these is the adequacy of circulating blood volume.[6] An impaired ability to eat and drink in a normal fashion can be a severe problem, leading to a pronounced weight loss, which results in an intravascular capacity that is potentially considerably greater than the blood volume present. It must be borne in mind that one of the major effects of almost any anesthetic agent is a production of some vasodilation, which may result in a rapid drop in blood pressure in the event that not enough fluid is available to fill the intravascular space. Although blood volume measurement tends to go in and out of fashion, any patient who has a long history of inadequate food intake with weight loss deserves a measurement of blood volume and the correction of any deficit. With a well-hydrated patient whose hematocrit may be a little low, in the region of 30% to 35%, I usually recommend packed red cells because they tend to expand the intravas-

cular volume in a physiologic fashion without loading, which can occur when whole blood is used to build up intravascular volume.

The second area of import, especially when restoring blood volume, is the heart itself. Most patients will in all likelihood have no difficulty. It must be kept in mind, however, that a prolonged surgical procedure is in store for these individuals, and a history of cardiac disease warrants a special consultation. Appropriate digitalization where it is indicated should be undertaken well in advance. Cardiac medications of any type, such as antihypertensive drugs and antiarrhythmic drugs, should be withdrawn if indicated, or appropriate notice should be given of their presence when the patient comes for surgery, and if necessary, adjustment of anesthetic techniques should be made for these. This adjustment is rarely necessary, but it must be borne in mind. A baseline electrocardiogram should be available, not so much for the discovery of disease, but for comparison with intraoperative or postoperative electrocardiograms in case of hypotension, arrhythmias, or other cardiac function impairment.

The lungs should be assessed for both their mechanical function and their possible state of disease.[4] Many head and neck cancer patients have histories of an inability to cough, an upper airway obstruction, aspirations of secretions, and the like. In patients with known pulmonary disease some measurement of their pulmonary function, such as vital capacity, maximum breathing capacity, FEV_1, and blood gases should be obtained. In the event that there is chronic lung disease, which can be helped by a few days of pulmonary preparation, it is wise to proceed with such preparation aggressively because there is good evidence that it does improve the postoperative course if these patients do not start out with incipient pneumonia.

Inasmuch as pulmonary complications are relatively common in these patients, it is also wise to have good baseline x-ray films of the chest for comparison when necessary.

ANESTHETIC PROCEDURE

For the anesthetist these surgical procedures can usually be considered as one entire procedure or as being divided into two sections. In the first instance there is usually an insertion of an endotracheal tube at the beginning of the procedure, and this is maintained as the airway throughout. In the second case, however, the larynx may be isolated, separated, or even removed, at which time the airway will be compromised and have to be changed to another position. Thus the establishment of the airway is of prime importance in the anesthetic procedure.

Before the case begins, the surgeon and the anesthesiologist must discuss whether or not an endotracheal tube shall be placed either through the nose or the mouth and possibly thus through or past a lesion, either as the airway for the entire procedure or as the initial airway. Still another choice is beginning the procedure with a tracheotomy. This technique, once very popular, seems to be used less often now. Tracheotomy under local anesthesia, however, is a very favorable method of handling situations that may present undue difficulties, either for intubation or because of unknown surgical situations that may arise. Thus there are two initial choices for the anesthetist: (1) general anesthesia with intubation, followed by a tracheotomy, which may or may not be done sometime during the procedure, and (2) a tracheotomy performed with the patient under local or general anesthesia with a face mask and the operation continuing with the tracheotomy as the major airway. Whichever of these routes are taken, there must be a clear understanding between the surgeon and the anesthesiologist as to which method will be used during the procedure. The techniques are usually unique to an institution or to a surgical team, and aside from pointing them out, they need not be discussed here except as general principles. The airway must be very positive at all times. The separation of the endotracheal tube from its various connectors when unrecognized can be disastrous. It must be kept under constant surveillance by both the surgeon and the anesthetist, for it is the patient's life line, from the standpoint of both anesthesia and respiratory homeostasis.

Oral or nasal endotracheal intubation is relatively routine. The matter of intubating through the open tracheotomy site and then leading the airway to an outside position is less well understood. The tracheotomy site is usually somewhere in the middle third of the trachea, which places the tracheotomy relatively low in the trachea and allows for a very short distance between the tracheotomy site and the carina. Tubes that are available are frequently too long and inadvertently slide into the right main stem bronchus. The patient must be constantly observed for this undesirable action.

The types of tubes also depend tremendously on the team itself. Interestingly enough, in our own institution there has been a gradual evolution to the use of very simple cuffed anode tubes for oral or nasal intubation or for direct tracheotomy intubation. These tubes have very short cuffs and therefore do not extend far down into the trachea and thence into a bronchus. They are also very flexible so that they can be moved readily from one position to another in the surgical field. In each operative procedure an appropriate full-length, relatively new anode tube and a short extension tube with a male and female endotracheal slip joint connector on the ends are gas sterilized to be placed with the equipment on the table for the surgical procedure. At the time of the tracheotomy the surgeon merely places the fresh endotracheal tube into the distal portion of the trachea, attaches it to the extension, and passes it out under the drapes, where the anesthetist then hooks it up to his regular anesthetic equipment and carries on without interruption. At this time the anesthetist must be certain that both lungs are ventilating.

There are a tremendous variety of tubes available for the tracheotomized patient. Again, the type used will depend greatly on the desires of the team and what they get used to. It is far more important that they settle on one device rather than continuously try out new things and have frequent inadvertent accidents.

ANESTHETIC DRUGS AND TECHNIQUES

General anesthesia is the rule. Only rarely does a surgeon perform radical head and neck surgery with the patient under local anesthesia. The drugs available are many and varied. The halogenated hydrocarbons are excellent choices in most instances, but where any evidence of sensitivity exists, they should not be utilized. They have the distinct advantage of allowing the patient to breathe nearly continuously on his own, with or without some assistance. Probably in more common use are the narcotic, relaxant, and nitrous oxide techniques. Here, a wide variety of narcotics and occasionally small amounts of barbiturates are utilized for the maintenance of anesthesia. This again is often a choice based on personal experience of the anesthetists, and a precise technique does not warrant discussion.

One simple principle, however, should be borne in mind. In procedures around the neck, where tracheotomy is utilized, skin flaps are frequently raised that come right up to and are sutured onto the trachea itself. In the event that a patient happens to be placed on a respirator postoperatively, great care must be taken to prevent subcutaneous emphysema. I have recently seen a patient who needed postoperative respiratory support wherein the tracheotomy tube was raised by subcutaneous emphysema to such a position that it became obstructed, and the patient asphyxiated, had a cardiac arrest, and died. It is far better that the patient be left with some capability for managing respirations on his own.

Inasmuch as these procedures tend to be protracted, artificial ventilation or assisted ventilation is in order. There is a strong tendency toward lung collapse, and atelectasis is frequently found at the end of the procedure. It is our habit to utilize a respirator with a humidifier and maintain relatively large tidal volume ventilation with a humidified atmosphere of nearly 100% saturation and a temperature slightly below body temperature throughout the procedure. This practice tends to minimize the postoperative pulmonary complications.

MONITORING AND SUPPORT

The anesthetist must be on guard against a variety of complications. A primary one may occur when the surgical procedure itself (not uncommonly) extends into the fossae on either side of the neck or inadvertently into intercostal spaces. It is possible to provoke a pneumothorax, which if of the tension type and if unrecognized, can be fatal. This situation must be monitored at all times.

Controlled hypotension may be valuable in selected patients. Certainly this is the case in the resection of certain vascular tumors. Patients without cardiac disease or indication of peripheral vessel arteriosclerosis should be selected; otherwise, the complications make the technique unacceptable. Careful measurement of arterial pressure with either an indwelling arterial catheter or an oscillometer-type sphygmomanometer is essential. Pressure should be lowered no more than necessary to sharply decrease the oozing type of bleeding. Full advantage should be taken of the patient's position by elevating the head 5 to 10 degrees to allow for peripheral pooling.

A variety of techniques and drugs are available for producing hypotension.[2] Trimethaphan camphorsulfonate is probably the most common. Sodium nitroprusside has recently been reintroduced. Before it is used, the technique should be investigated in more detail than can be given here. The anesthetist who does handle head and neck cases, however, should be well versed in the different methods because they can sometimes mean the difference between a success and a failure.

Bradycardia is an arrhythmia frequently seen in radical neck surgery. Usually this is associated with manipulation of the carotid sinus and is prevented by simple infiltration with 0.5% lidocaine hydrochloride. However, it is best to be certain that manipulation of the carotid sinus is the cause before administering 0.2 to 0.5 mg. of atropine sulfate intravenously. Bradycardia is also a symptom of hypoxia, which must be ruled out.

All monitoring techniques that are available should be utilized. The electrocardiogram is of great value throughout the case, as is an occasional monitoring of venous pressure, and for some people, an occasional hematocrit. In especially long cases, those taking 6 or more hours, a simple expedient that indicates adequate tissue perfusion is the measurement of urine output. An effort should be made to maintain an output of about 50 ml. per hour.

Fluid support is dependent on the fluids that are lost and on fluid shifts.[6] Blood should be replaced with blood or with packed cells when whole blood is not available. The use of volume expanders such as plasma derivatives or albumin can be very helpful, but it should be kept in mind that neither of these are substitutes for whole blood when there is a need for oxygen-carrying capacity. Depending on the patient's general condition, fluids should be utilized to such a degree as to maintain an adequate central venous pressure and urine output. I give approximately 5 ml./kg./hr. during the first 3 to 4 hours of the procedure and then drop down to 2 or 3 ml. per hour. These fluids are generally salt-containing solutions, commonly ringers lactate or 5% dextrose with 0.2% sodium chloride.

The monitoring of body temperature is also necessary. With protracted procedures in rather cold operating rooms, patients tend to lose body heat. They become unstable and at the end of the procedure often do not awaken properly. Cooling much below 36 C. should be avoided. If a lower temperature is indicated, there must be some technique available for warming if indicated. By far a greater danger, however, is that of malignant hyperthermia, and the only way that this can be detected is by monitoring the temperature. This simple technique of temperature monitoring is warranted in every case.

Anesthesia, then, consists mainly of the establishment of an airway, the maintenance of ventilation, and the maintenance of circulatory hemeostasis, plus continuous monitoring and maintenance of the various physiologic parameters.

POSTOPERATIVE CARE

In the immediate postoperative period, not uncommonly the head and neck cancer patient must breathe through a tracheotomy. This abrupt change in the aerodynamics of his airway can result in a strong tendency for alveolar collapse and atelectasis. It has been our habit recently to place all of these individuals on a regimen of low constant end expiratory pressure.[3] This is done by connecting the patient's cuffed tracheotomy tube to a source of compressed air or compressed air and oxygen with adequate humidity that is in series with a bag and has a flow that exceeds the minute volume respiration of the patient. The patient then inhales from the bag and exhales through an underwater seal with usually somewhere between 2 and 5 cm. of water. This provides an end expiratory pressure, or PEEP, as it is commonly known, which helps greatly to maintain a normal alveolar stability and is a normal ventilation perfusion ratio.

CONCLUSION

Although anesthesia for head and neck surgery does not usually take any great skill, it does require constant attention to small detail. The proper selection of an anesthetic agent to fit the patient's general condition, an airway system that is commensurate with the surgical procedure, and a technique that allows for maintenance of good pulmonary dynamics are mandatory. A clear understanding and a good relationship between the surgeon and the anesthetist is vital for the patient. Knowing what each other is doing rules out the occasional mix-ups that can result in inadequate ventilation, airway obstruction, or some other disaster that might bring death to the patient. Constant vigilance and attention to the details of physiologic and pharmacologic homeostasis usually make for a good anesthesia result, which is important to the long-term result of the surgical procedure.

REFERENCES

1. Boland, F. K.: The first anesthetic; the story of Crawford Long, Athens, Ga., 1950, University of Georgia Press.
2. Eckenhoff, J. E.: A technique of deliberate hypotension, Anesth. Analg. **44**:779, 1965.
3. Galvis, A. G., and Benson, D. W.: Spontaneous continuous positive airway pressure (CPAP) breathing in the management of acute pulmonary edema in infants, Clin. Pediatr., **12**:265, 1973.
4. Hodgkin, J. E., Dines, D. E., and Didier, E. P.: Preoperative evaluation of the patient with pulmonary disease, Mayo Clin. Proc. **48**:114, 1973.
5. Keen, W. W.: The surgical operations on President Cleveland in 1893, Philadelphia, 1917, G. W. Jacob and Co.
6. Underwood, P. S.: Body fluid shifts associated with radical cancer surgery. In Howland, W. S., and Schweiger, O., editors: Clinical anesthesia, vol. 9(1), Philadelphia, 1972, F. A. Davis Co., pp. 9-31.

Chapter 5

Classification of head and neck tumors

William S. MacComb, M.D.

The need for an acceptable form of classification of cancer of the head and neck has long been necessary. Many authors have reported end results for specific anatomical sites, but have neglected to give adequate details for comparison with reports by other authors from other institutions. Members of the (UICC) International Union Against Cancer have recently made an effort to attain some uniformity on this subject. An international committee has formed task forces for each individual anatomical site.

Classification is of vital concern to all those who participate in the treatment of patients with these tumors. Classification involves the clinician, the pathologist, the radiologist, the surgeon (general or plastic) or otolaryngologist, and the radiotherapist. On the contribution of each depends the final decision about therapy for the patient, his prognosis, and the end result, at which point the epidemiologist also enters the scene.

The need for a uniform method of classification of tumors of the head and neck areas was recognized for many years by otolaryngologists and surgeons before radiotherapists became interested. The need for a more uniform classification seemed even more urgent when the latter group of physicians entered the sphere of cancer therapy.

From the literature on end results of treatment of patients with cancer of the head and neck area by surgical therapy or radiotherapy preceding, during, and following World War II, one is left in considerable doubt about the superiority of one discipline over the other. The results of treatment for laryngeal cancer demonstrate this fact most clearly. Reports by both European and American radiation therapists of those early years after the publication of Coutard's[2] results of treatment for cancer of the larynx with x-ray therapy were most encouraging, even enthusiastic. Pursuing Coutard's example, many physicians treated patients with cancers of the larynx by radiotherapy consisting of a daily dose of 300 R to each side of the neck on alternate days over a 3-week period. Because some of these patients did not have early lesions, they should perhaps have had surgical therapy or, in cases of advanced disease, should not have been treated at all. In reviewing these reports, one is unable to determine the stage of the disease, since no attempts were made to define the extent of the border of the tumor. In some instances, results would be reported in which surgical therapy alone was used with astonishingly good results. No mention was made of the selection of patients or whether any were denied treatment because of the extent of disease. Similarly, radiation therapists were reporting their good results and failing to give the complete picture of the size of the tumor. Certainly, the results could not be compared because of this lack of uniformity.

The otolaryngologists were also reporting excellent results in the management of glottic lesions by surgical therapy. Obviously, however, only patients with early lesions were being treated. When one attempts to compare the statistical results of surgical therapy and radiotherapy, one soon reaches the conclusion that any definitive comparisons are impossible because of various factors, chiefly the lack of definition of the position, size, and extent of the lesions.

The reports on treatment for laryngeal cancer are only an example of similar accounts for other

24

cancers of the head and neck area, but they clearly demonstrate the need for uniformity in classifying all tumors in order that some conformation might be obtained to compare the end results achieved by similar disciplines, various writers, or different institutions.

The need for a uniform classification of cancer had been recognized for many years before any definitive action was taken. Reports on end results from various specialists, institutions, and countries emphasized this necessity, which was more pronounced during the years after World War II. The need for uniformity of some type became more and more apparent. Certainly a contributing factor was the increasing interest in the disease itself. With better demographic findings being published every year, the need for obtaining more consistent and reliable statistical information on end results became apparent.

The UICC had been interested for many years in the problem of clinical classification. The basic requirements of any system, were it to be adopted on a worldwide scale, were simplicity, adaptability, and practicality. The idea of a TNM system was born to P. F. Denoix[5] in 1943. By 1953 a UICC committee on tumor nomenclature and statistics, under the chairmanship of Isabella Perry[5] of the United States, had been appointed. In that year this committee met with the International Congress of Radiology. Agreement was reached on a general technique for classification, staging, and presentation of results of treatment.

Later, the UICC appointed a permanent committee for classification and staging of all tumors. Denoix[5] acted as the first chairman; later, M. H. Harmer of the United Kingdom filled this office.

For some time, the crude survival rate had been determined from the results obtained by dividing groups of patients into those treated for early and late cancer. This division implied a correlation of progression of the disease with time, ignoring other factors included in the TNM manual, published by the UICC in 1968.[5] These factors were (1) the rate of growth, (2) the extension of the neoplasm, (3) the type of tumor, (4) the tumor-host relationship, and (5) the interval of time between the first symptom or sign recognized by the patient and the time of diagnosis or treatment.

The members of the committee recognized that including all these variables presented an insurmountable obstacle to a perfect classification, an entirely different conception to staging but also a challenge

to the recording of precise information on the extent of the disease as to make possible a clinical description which may serve a number of related objectives. These are, briefly, to aid the clinician in the planning of treatment, in making a prognosis, in assisting in the evaluation of the resuls of treatment, and perhaps most important of all, facilitating the exchange of information between centers and individual specialists.[5]

The general policy of the UICC was to propose a classification for a trial period of 5 years, after which revisions might be considered. This policy has been followed with beneficial results as shown in the second, revised staging of laryngeal cancer, published in July 1972.[1]

One may possess divergent opinions on some feature of staging on any designated anatomical site. Many believe that the staging as published by task forces of the UICC might be improved, and perhaps it should. Those who have not participated on one of these task forces can have no idea of the difficulties facing a group of so-called specialists attempting to assemble a program for staging cancer of any designated site, to be applied to all countries. Surgeons, radiotherapists, and pathologists are usually involved in these programs. Surgeons may be general surgeons, cancer surgeons, plastic surgeons, or otolaryngologists. The task of obtaining uniform agreement has appeared formidable and, at times, impossible to attain.

Many have their own individual ideas about what criteria are deemed important and essential, even to such minor items as how the exact measurements of a tumor could be accurately determined. Only a seasoned diplomat could steer a group of individuals of diverse opinions to final agreement and the ultimate goal. Certainly, adequate recognition and acknowledgment have never been granted to Robert R. Smith, formerly of the National Cancer Institute, who acted as chairman for the task force committee on staging of the anatomical sites of cancer of the head and neck areas.

The staging of cancer of the head and neck areas should be done by the clinician who first examines the patient. Usually this is the surgeon or the otolaryngologist.

An essential rule of the system is that the TNM description of a tumor is applied to cases not previously treated and that the extent of the disease must be determined and recorded on clinical examination only. Clinical examination includes diagnostic radiology of any sort and endoscopy of any type.[5]

Experience has shown that if the examiner is requested to put his clinical impression on first examination in writing and to classify and stage the tumor, his views after radiologic examinations will tend to be more specific in clearly defining the picture as he sees it, either in writing or by diagrams, or both.

Once the clinician has staged a tumor, that stage must not be changed later, except, as previously stated, after radiologic studies, such as tomograms or laryngograms, are completed. Achieving uniformity of staging between the clinician (usually the surgeon) and the radiotherapist, should the patient be referred for radiotherapy, is often difficult.

The ultimate aims of accurate staging of cancer on first examination are (1) to determine by staging the best approach to treatment (surgical therapy, radiotherapy, or a combined approach using both disciplines), (2) to give a more definitive prognosis to the patient or his family, as well as to the referring or family physician and to the staff of the hospital service who will be directly responsible for his treatment, and (3) when records are assembled for statistical analysis, to make the end results more meaningful, since all cases have been staged on initial examination.

No uniform end result reporting system was suggested until 1935, when Martin and Pflueger[4] published a proposed method that they called "determinate reporting." One objection to this method,

the inclusion of those patients lost to follow-up but free of disease, was covered by Eleanor Macdonald in 1948.[3] She proposed classifying these patients as an indeterminate group and subtracting the number from the total. This system gave a more definitive picture of the survival group and the percentage thereof, but it did not give a fair percentage for the entire series or the so-called total experience.

Classification or staging should be as simple as possible. Therefore, restaging for all anatomical sites should be considered at least at 5-year intervals, when entirely new members should be appointed to the task forces.

REFERENCES

1. Clinical staging system for carcinoma of the larynx, Chicago, July 1972, American Joint Committee for Cancer Staging and End Results Reporting.
2. Coutard, H., and Baclesse, F.: Roentgen diagnosis during the epitheliomas of the larynx and hypopharynx, Am. J. Roentgenol. Radium Ther. Nucl. Med. 28:293, 1932.
3. Macdonald, E. J.: The present incidence and survival picture in cancer and the promise of improved prognosis, Bull. Am. Coll. Surg. 33:75, 1948.
4. Martin, H. E., and Pflueger, O. H.: Cancer of the cheek (buccal mucosa), Arch. Surg. 30:731, 1935.
5. TNM classification of malignant tumors, Geneva, 1968, Imprimerie C. de Buren S. A.

Chapter 6

Transsternal radical neck dissection (mediastinal approach)

George A. Sisson, M.D.
David E. Bytell, M.D.
Bruce D. Edison, M.D.

The disease had obviously made progress, the local malady having increased and adjacent parts having become more infiltrated. The advisability of an operation was again discussed and rejected. The wisdom of such a decision was manifested in sparing him unnecessary mutilation and allowing him to pass the remainder of his days in comparative comfort. Relatively, however, it meant suffering for him until the end.[4]

These were the words of George F. Shrady, eminent physician and editor of the New York Medical Record who, in 1885, attended General Ulysses S. Grant. His patient had carcinoma of the tongue with metastasis to the neck. The barriers to successful surgery in the head and neck were awesome. These barriers have been in large part overcome in the past century by men like Crile, McGill, and Flemming. The overwhelming morbidity and mortality associated with extirpation of tumors in the laryngopharynx could not be decreased until the advent of blood replacement, rational treatment of shock, antibiotics, and endotracheal anesthesia. Surgical approaches and management have improved, as have methods for immediate reconstruction.

The rationale for radical surgical technique is that en bloc resection of the site of the primary tumor and contents of the neck with wide borders will control or cure cancer. Presently, there remain only a few adjacent anatomical barriers that prevent en bloc removal of head and neck malignancies. Head and neck neoplasms are controllable provided that vital vessels, the base of the skull, the cervical vertebrae, or the mediastinum are not involved. In addition, there should be no evidence of distant metastasis. One of these barriers, the mediastinum, has been a target for clinical investigation by one of us (G.A.S.) for many years. The clavicle and the manubrium frequently prevent the surgeon from obtaining good margins of safety in patients who have advanced lesions of the larynx or cervical esophague. These same barriers are also present and limiting in cases of stomal laryngeal cancer, advanced cancer of the thyroid, and recurrent nodal cancer resulting from primary intraoral disease. Animal experiments by Johner[3] support previous clinical reports by Bailey and Pressman,[1] Fisch and Sigel,[2] and Rouviere[5] that nodes at the jugulosubclavian venous angles in the neck, as well as in the paratracheal chain, are critical stations linking the spread of disease to the mediastinum and lung.

These studies suggest that it would be reasonable to include this area in the treatment of any low-lying cancer in the neck. Usually, removal of the jugulosubclavian venous nodal stations is not included in a classical neck dissection, because it lies below the manubrium and clavicular heads. If the manubrium is split and tumor or soft tissue removed, a large dead space is created. Since most of these patients have received large amounts of irradiation, this space more often than not becomes infected. Abscesses form, and major arterial hemmorhage can take place during the immediate postoperative period.

Removal of the clavicle and the manubrium may produce insurmountable problems. The chest can become flailed. Healing of the opened upper mediastinum is slow, increasing the patient's susceptibility to infection and hemorrhage. While rotated muscle flaps help obliterate the dead space, they, too, can fail when blood supply is poor. Patients with advanced cancers in the lower neck usually have been treated prior to referral by surgery or radiation, or both. Tissues of the neck and mediastinum may already be fibrosed again, decreasing vascularity and impairing healing.

HISTORICAL BACKGROUND

In 1962 Sisson and Straehley reported six cases in which one-stage mediastinal dissections and relocations of the trachea were performed for stomal recurrences after laryngectomy. While five of these patients survived the immediate postoperative period, serious problems were encountered with the next six patients. In each instance innominate blowout occurred because the blood supply to the flaps was poor as a result of previous surgery and irradiation. Mediastinitis was always associated with cases of large vessel blowout.

In 1968 the technique was revised by performing the operation in two stages. The skin and muscle flaps were delayed 3 weeks before the definitive surgery. At this same time the clavicular heads and upper third of the sternum were resected, with care taken to preserve the periosteum of the internal manubrium. Pectoralis muscle flaps were also prepared and rotated medially 180 degrees. The definitive resection, including repositioning of the trachea, was performed 3 weeks later. Even since the development of the two-stage operation, in selected cases we still perform a modification of the early one-stage procedure. The reason for this will be clarified as we discuss selection of flaps and present indications for staging.

GENERAL INDICATIONS

The mediastinal or extended radical neck dissection has proved to be useful in the following cases:

1. Stomal recurrences after laryngectomy
2. Carcinoma of the cervical esophagus when the inferior border is 2 cm. or less above the sternal notch
3. T4, N1, or N2 lesions of the larynx

4. Primary carcinoma of the subglottic region or trachea
5. Carcinoma of the larynx with subglottic extension
6. Low nodal metastasis from intraoral pharyngeal carcinoma
7. Substernal infiltrating papillary adenocarcinoma, follicular, alveolar or medullary carcinoma of the thyroid gland

SELECTION OF SKIN FLAPS AND INDICATIONS FOR STAGING

When the neck tissues are healthy and there is little evidence of radiation effects, a one-stage procedure may be considered. The flap of choice for a one-stage procedure is the bipedicle swing chest flap, used in early stomal recurrences when the esophagus is not involved, in lower nodal recurrent cancer from primary intraoral disease, in primary T4, N1, or N2 lesions of the larynx, and in substernal thyroid cancer.

If it is suspected that a segment of the cervical esophagus must be resected, or if the esophagus is to be entered, experience has shown that the flaps should be delayed. A deltopectoral flap and a large laterally based chest flap (nipple flap) are the flaps of choice when esophageal reconstruction is contemplated. At the same time these chest flaps are delayed, the mediastinum is marsupialized by removing the upper segment of the sterum and the clavicular head on the same side from which the nipple flap was raised. The clavicular head on the side of the deltopectoral flap is removed during the second stage because removal earlier might jeopardize integrity of the deltopectoral flap. The bony segments of the manubrium and clavicle are carefully dissected and rongeured to make certain that the deep periosteum is left intact.

Muscle flaps

When bipedicle chest flaps are selected, the pectoralis muscles, based medially and rotated 180 degrees on themselves, are sutured together in the midline, obliterating the defect caused by the bony removal. When a combination deltopectoral and lateral thoracic flap (nipple) is utilized, a broadly based single pedicle pectoralis flap is raised from the side from which the laterally based chest flap was taken. It would not be prudent to raise a pectoralis muscle flap on the same side from which the deltopectoral flap is formed, because this would impede the blood supply to the latter.

Completion of the operation

If the operation is unstaged, the inner periosteum is opened after removal of the bony fragments. If the operation is staged, the muscle flaps, when two are raised (as in the case of the bipedicle swing chest flap), are sutured together in the midline and positioned into the defect caused by the bony removal. These are dissected free at the time of the second operation, and the deep periosteum is carefully incised along its inferior border, which allows entry into the superior mediastinum. The arch of the aorta, the innominate artery, and left carotid artery serve as landmarks once the mediastinal space is entered, and these must be identified before the dissection is carried superiorly. If the thoracic duct is encountered, it must be carefully ligated. Occasionally it is necessary to do this by utilizing the operating microscope, which assures identification of the small ramifications and tributaries.

The recurrent tumor around the stoma, esophagus, or in the neck is widely resected. By initiating the dissection inferiorly, the surgeon avoids previously irradiated and fibrotic tissue and can identify the proper dissection plane. Also, the en bloc concept is maintained by dissecting inferiorly toward the tumor. When this dissection is complete, one can establish a safe margin from the tumor before transecting the trachea. After the trachea is mobilized, it is then pulled up from the mediastinum and sutured to the edges of the muscle flaps and the deltopectoral and lateral thoracic skin flaps. With the use of a bipedicle chest flap, the repositioned superior flap resurfaces the lower neck and sternal clavicular area. In this situation the trachea, once transected, is repositioned and sutured into the center of the flap. The donor area created by elevation of the bipedicle swing chest flap is covered by elevating a 12 cm. wide inferior bipedicle chest flap and transposing it superiorly. When considerable skin has been removed from the neck, the final defect along the inferior border of the lower bipedicle chest flap is covered by a split-thickness skin graft from the leg. The donor areas created when combination flaps are used are covered for 48 hours by Telfa and a light dressing. Split-thickness skin grafts delayed at the time of surgery are transferred to the chest flaps in a minor procedure performed in the patient's room. This method saves time in the operating room and is 95% to 100% successful. The 48-hour delay for both the donor and the recipient sites apparently is of great benefit to prompt wound healing.

The correct positioning of the Hemo-vac drainage tubes is important. Two complete sets of medium-sized tubes are necessary. Seldom during the first 4 or 5 days is either a tracheostomy or laryngectomy tube needed. These tubes are not efficient, because the new position of the trachea creates an acute angle that makes it difficult to insinuate a conventional tube. For patients in whom the esophagus or portions of it must be removed and immediate reconstruction is not attempted, care is taken to bring an esophagostoma through the skin at a distance as far as practical from the new tracheostoma. The pharyngostoma is completely closed in layers, forcing the patient to suction his saliva from the mouth. Salivary output is reduced after the pharyngostoma is closed for several days. Patients are given broad-spectrum antibiotics to prevent infection, and nutritional requirements are maintained by a nasogastric or gastrostomy tube for 10 to 12 days. In cases of severe nutritional deficiences, the feeding gastrostomy is performed prior to surgery.

CONCLUSIONS

After reviewing 50 cases performed during the past 10 years, we have reduced the problem of great vessel hemorrhage during the immediate postoperative period by staging and selecting the appropriate skin flaps for reconstruction of the upper mediastinum. In addition, the use of dermal grafts to cover all the great vessels has proved beneficial. Most important is the hour-to-hour care provided by the house staff and nursing personnel. These patients require meticulous attention to dressing changes and wound care. The problem inherent in operating on patients who have been heavily irradiated are difficult and perhaps unavoidable. Wound infection, secondary to fistulization, has been our primary problem during the past 5 years. Our good results achieved by employing controlled fistulas in the management of advanced recurrent cancer of the oral cavity and hypopharynx have led us to apply the benefits of the controlled fistula to cases of mediastinal dissection. While this does not apply to all cases, when it is practical we fashion a controlled fistula in conjunction with the mediastinal dissection. Review of our operative morbidities and mortalities has made us aware that had we applied this principle, perhaps our survival statistics would have been better. In heavily irradiated patients, the controlled fistula not only reduces the intraluminal esophageal pressure, which we believe to be one of the prime causes of fistula, but when planned and constructed properly, it will divert 95% of the salivary content away from the great vessels and mediastinum. We have successfully been able to close all of the gross pharyngeal defects created by the controlled fistula once the primary cancer has been controlled. Admittedly, in some cases it took as long as 24 months. These patients are most likely cured.

SUMMARY

Our experience during the past 7 years since implementation of the staged mediastinal resection has yielded a 5-year survival rate of approximately 20%. In addition, we have had 2- to 3-year survival rates of approximately 30%. Patients with advanced cancer of the cervical esophagus, thyroid, or larynx with both primary and recurrent disease have been successfully operated on in selected cases by the use of radical surgical techniques, including a dissection of the mediastinum with subsequent removal of the clavicular head and a portion of the manubrium. Survival rates, while low, are significant since all of these cases were one- or two-time losers with lethal disease. Postoperative complications, particularly the instance of immediate great vessel rupture, has been reduced by properly selecting flaps and staging the resection when possible. The use of the pectoralis muscle flaps to seal, obliterate, and promptly heal the mediastinum, while useful in most cases, may create other problems if primary healing is not evident. More work on the proper introduction of these muscle flaps is needed before perfection is achieved. Our major cause of morbidity during the past 5 years has been wound dehiscence and fistulization. Currently we are applying the principle of the controlled fistula, which we believe may be significant in decreasing this attendant morbidity.

REFERENCES

1. Bailey, B. J., and Pressman, J. J.: Dissection of the neck and mediastinum in continuity for carcinoma of head and neck, Trans. Am. Rhinol. Otolaryngol. Soc. 236-252, 1964.
2. Fisch, V. P., and Sigel, M. E.: Cervical lymphatic system as visualized by lymphography, Ann. Otol. Rhinol. Laryngol. **73:**869-882, 1964.
3. Johner, C., and Ranniger, K.: Mediastinal lymphography, Surg. Gynecol. Obstet. **127:**1313-1316, 1968.
4. Pitkin, T. M.: The captain departs, Carbondale, Ill., 1973, Southern Illinois University Press, 188.
5. Rouviere, H.: Anatomy of the human lymphatic system, Ann Arbor, 1938, Edwards Brothers.
6. Sisson, G. A., and Straehley, C. J., Jr.; Mediastinal dissection for recurrent cancer after laryngectomy, Laryngoscope **73:**1069-1077, 1962.

Chapter 7

Shoulder disability and neck dissection

Robin Anderson, M.D.

In 1906 George Crile[4] published his classic paper on radical neck dissection, describing the procedure that we carry out today, with literally no change, for removal of the regional node drainage area of the head and neck. An essential part of his plan of dissection was to extend the operative field to the trapezius muscle posteriorly, sacrificing the spinal accessory nerve. The inevitable sequela has been and remains paralysis of the trapezius muscle followed by pain in the shoulder.[6] It has been traditional to dismiss the complaint of shoulder pain in the patient who has had neck dissection as a minor annoyance far overshadowed by the curative value of the surgical procedure. In fact, this pain, while only rarely unbearable, is often described as unpleasant and occasionally severely disabling. If these symptoms can be relieved or prevented without decreasing the patient's chance of cure, it behooves us as surgeons to make the effort.

There is no way to know which patients will be distressed or disabled by loss of trapezius function after eleventh nerve removal. However, 75% or more complain of the problem to some degree, and at least 10% describe the disability as serious and one that interferes with the carrying out of important functions. There are some patients in whom the loss of trapezius function results in no symptoms whatsoever, presumably because the levator scapulae muscle, if its insertion on the scapula is sufficiently lateral, provides adequate shoulder support. In most instances trapezius function loss results in shoulder drop and inability to elevate the shoulder girdle, which provides abduction of the arm in its last 75-degree angle to the vertical position.

The spinal accessory nerve leaves the skull via the jugular foramen, in the sheath with the vagus nerve. It runs behind the digastric and stylohyoid muscles, through the sternomastoid muscle, and through the posterior triangle of the neck to the trapezius muscle. In the posterior triangle and within the substance of the trapezius, it is joined by sensory fibers of the second, third, and fourth cervical nerves, which make no contribution to motor function.

Three approaches are available to the surgeon for avoiding or modifying shoulder disability secondary to eleventh nerve palsy. The first and most obvious approach is to preserve the nerve and its function at the time of the neck dissection; the second is to sacrifice the nerve but restore its continuity by means of a free nerve graft; and the third is to surgically support the shoulder by means of muscle transfers and fascial slings.

PRESERVATION OF THE SPINAL ACCESSORY NERVE

The concept of carrying out a radical neck dissection without removing the spinal accessory nerve is not new. As early as 1944, Brown and McDowell[3] recommended saving the nerve in specific instances when there was no obvious node involvement in the posterior triangle. There has always been some question, however, as to whether leaving intact a structure running through the drainage area of the neck might not result in leaving cancer in the surgical field.

With this question in mind, Roy and Beahrs[9] employed this nerve-sparing procedure in 89 of 250 patients who underwent radical neck dissection during a 5-year period from 1960 through 1964 at the

Mayo Clinic. They selected their patients for the modified procedure, employing it only in those patients who had no disease along the course of the nerve or who did not require en bloc resections of tumor-bearing tissue in the jugulodigastric area. They found no difference between the two groups in either the incidence of tumor recurrence of the neck in the absence of primary tumor recurrence or in the overall survival rate.

There is no question that the use of this nerve-sparing operation requires the exercise of a high degree of surgical judgment. It is certainly not an operation to be considered for every patient. On the other hand, in the hands of the experienced head and neck surgeon, it is probably safe and justifiable for carefully selected patients.

REPLACEMENT OF THE SPINAL ACCESSORY NERVE

The use of a free nerve graft to bridge the defect created by removal of the spinal accessory nerve during neck disection is also not new. It was first proposed by Harris and Dickey in 1965.[7] In 1966 Ballantyne and Guinn[2] reported a high level of return of function following its use, and in 1969 we reported similar success in 19 instances.[1]

The technique is straightforward, the only potential difficulty being the identification of the proximal stump of the spinal accessory nerve at the upper limit of the dissection. This is not difficult if the area is not so involved by tumor as to force the surgeon to divide the nerve at such a high level as to preclude the possibility of technically carrying out a nerve anastomosis. It can be very frustrating to look for the proximal stump after the operation is completed; there is little problem if the surgeon keeps in mind that he may wish to use it subsequently and isolates the nerve as he carries his resection from the lateral aspect of the upper neck toward the midline. He is thus in a position not only to have it in view but to be certain that he has sufficient stump to permit suturing of the graft to it.

The graft of choice is the greater auricular nerve of the same side. If this is not available for whatever reason, any of the other cervical nerve branches at the base of the neck may be used, or the greater auricular nerve may be taken from the opposite side. The defect produced by nerve sacrifice is almost always less than 6 cm., and sufficient graft is always readily available. The graft is cut to fit the defect loosely and is sutured in place with three or four 7-0 silk sutures. The neck dissection wound is closed,

drained, and dressed in the usual manner. Replacement of the nerve by a free graft adds no more than 30 to 40 minutes to the operative time.

As is the case with repair or grafting of other pure nerves, grafts of the spinal accessory nerve do remarkably well. Return of trapezius function usually requires from 4 to 12 months, and we have had no instance in which shoulder disability was more than minimal. In all patients, trapezius function could be demonstrated by functional testing. In selected patients, electromyographic studies confirmed the clinical observations.

The question arises as to when free nerve grafting should be employed. It is obvious that the procedure is technically not possible in those patients whose tumors have invaded the upper neck. There are some patients for whom an additional 40 minutes

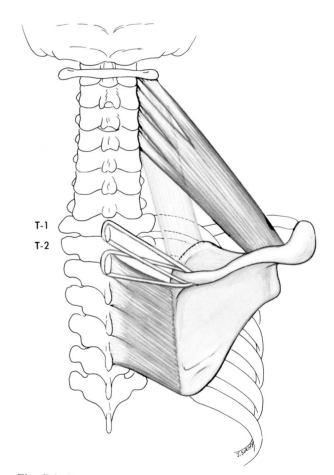

Fig. 7-1. Levator scapulae muscle transferred from normal medial position (stippled) to the lateral aspect of the scapula.[8] The medial border of the scapula is stabilized by loops of fascia lata.

of operating time is contraindicated. Furthermore, it is often possible to predict in advance from simple observation of the emotional behavior of the patient whether he is likely to be unhappy about a modest amount of aching and disability. On the other hand, there are three groups of patients for whom we should seriously consider doing the procedure in every instance: (1) the manual laborer whose job requires vigorous and powerful shoulder activity, (2) the anxious, hypersensitive patient who has already shown his preoccupation with multiple aches and pains before surgery, and (3) the young patient, particularly female, for whom the cosmetic deformity of a drooping shoulder would almost certainly be a severe blow.

ORTHOPAEDIC RECONSTRUCTION

Stabilization of the dropped shoulder girdle following trapezius denervation was first suggested by Dewar and Harris in 1950.[5] Another report of its successful use was presented by Hoaglund and Duthie in 1966.[8] The procedure consists of detachment of the levator scapulae muscle from its normal position at the medial aspect of the upper border of the scapula. It is then transferred to a more lateral position and fixed to the scapula with fascial strip sutures. The mechanical advantage of the muscle gained by this transfer permits it to function in the same manner as the upper portion of the trapezius and thus maintain reasonable elevation and stabilization of the shoulder girdle (**Fig. 7-1**).

The results have generally been reported as most satisfactory. Our own experience in only two cases is slightly less optimistic, since both patients had complete relief of disability for 1 to 2 years after the procedure but gradually developed increasing pain and disability thereafter. However, in neither instance was the developing problem as severe as it had been prior to surgery, and both patients expressed satisfaction with their results.

While complete and permanent relief of symptoms cannot be guaranteed, the procedure should be employed when either pain or disability is severe.

REFERENCES

1. Anderson, R., and Flowers, R. S.: Free grafts of the spinal accessory nerve during radial neck dissection, Am. J. Surg. **118:**796, 1969.
2. Ballantyne, A. J., and Guinn, G. A.: Reduction of shoulder disability after neck dissection, Am. J. Surg. **112:**662, 1966.
3. Brown, J. B., and McDowell, F.: Neck dissections for metastatic carcinoma, Surg. Gynecol. and Obstet. **79:** 115, 1944.
4. Crile, G.: Excision of cancer of the head and neck; with special reference to the plan of dissection based on one hundred and thirty-two operations, J.A.M.A. **47:**1780, 1906.
5. Dewar, F. P., and Harris, R. I.: Restoration of function of the shoulder following paralysis of the trapezius by fascial sling fixation and transplantation of the levator scapulae, Ann. Surg. **132:**1111, 1950.
6. Ewing, M. R., and Martin, H.: Disability following radical neck dissection; an assessment based on postoperative elevation in 100 patients, Cancer **5:**873, 1952.
7. Harris, H. H., and Dickey, J. R.: Nerve grafting to restore function of the trapezius muscle after radical neck dissection, Ann. Otol. Rhinol. Laryngol. **74:**880, 1965.
8. Hoaglund, F. T., and Duthie, R. B.: Surgical reconstruction for shoulder pain after radical neck dissection, Am. J. Surg. **112:**522, 1966.
9. Roy, P. H., and Beahrs, O. H.: Spinal accessory nerve in radical neck dissections, Am. J. Surg. **118:**800, 1969.

Chapter 8

The unknown primary

William S. MacComb, M.D.

The treatment of metastasis to cervical nodes from an unknown primary cancer of the head and neck region is one that has been under intensive discussion for many years. There is still no proved correct approach. Each writer appears to have had his own ideas and has tended to ignore previous publications on the subject.

In the early 1930's Hayes Martin was appointed Chief of the Head and Neck Service at Memorial Hospital. All those who trained under his guardianship or closely followed his writings soon became interested in his intense work in the treatment of head and neck cancer. Martin was an enthusiastic and dynamic leader in this area. Before he entered the field, a great deal of variation, if not indifference, had been evident. Great credit is due to him for his solutions of many individual problems concerning the treatment of malignant tumors of the head and neck.

The subject of metastasis to cervical nodes from unknown squamous cancer was of great interest to Martin. His first paper in 1944 was followed by others of the same character, and in each paper he was more definitive and emphatic in expressing his ideas on the subject. His first article in 1944, co-authored by Mason Morfit,[2] contains statements that are still pertinent. In this paper they reported on a series of 218 patients; the time of discovery of the primary site of cancer was as follows: before admission to Memorial Hospital, 35%; at the time of admission to Memorial Hospital, 34%; 1 to 2 weeks after the first examination in the Head and Neck Clinic, 22%; and within 1 to 54 months after repeated examinations in this clinic, 9%. However, in 55 patients no primary lesion was ever found.

No longer is the presence of metastasis to a cervical node or nodes from an unknown source considered unique. Since the paper by Martin and Morfit[2] was published, many articles have appeared on this subject.

In 1952 and again in 1961, Martin[1,4] emphasized one extremely important point that is often disregarded by the medical profession: a cervical node should not be immediately excised for the purpose of diagnosis.

In the 1961 article he stated, "An enlarged lymph node should never be excised as the first or even an early step in diagnosis." Later he added, "If, as a last resort, a cervical node must eventually be removed for diagnosis, the operation should be performed by a surgeon who is willing to treat the primary cancer if it is later found somewhere in the head and neck."[1]

In spite of Martin's plea, his clear-cut and concise recommendations are still almost universally ignored. Of 198 patients admitted to M. D. Anderson Hospital from January 1952 through September 1971 with the diagnosis of metastasis to cervical nodes (excluding the supraclavicular group), 77.5% had already had one or more cervical nodes removed elsewhere for microscopic examination. In other instances not only had nodes been removed for diagnosis, but biopsy specimens had been taken from an obvious primary site within the oral cavity or pharynx.

When should a cervical cancerous node be classified as being metastatic from an unknown primary site? The differing opinions in many publications regarding this essential fact make an honest comparison of statistics from such sources impossible. In fact, such end results may well be irrelevant.

DIAGNOSIS

Martin suggested in 1952[4] that the diagnosis of metastatic cervical cancer from an unknown primary site should be made only if the primary lesion has not been found after a thorough search extending over a period of at least 2 weeks. Now, 20 years later, it seems arbitrary to set a definitive or even approximate time during which the search for a primary source of the metastatic tumor should be made. The search for the primary tumor could be intensive or dilatory and might consist of one or more diagnostic approaches consuming various periods of time. The diagnosis of metastatic cervical cancer from an unknown primary source should be made only after all diagnostic measures to determine the site of the primary tumor have failed, regardless of the time consumed in the search.

The diagnosis of branchiogenic cancer formerly was frequently made for nodes in the neck in which no primary cancer had been located. Martin often stated that the degree of accuracy was evident by the number of diagnoses of branchiogenic carcinomas reported. The diagnosis of branchiogenic cancer has been discarded for the past 10 to 15 years.

Procedures of diagnosis

A patient with a mass or tumefaction in the cervical region may be presumed to have metastatic cancer until proved otherwise. A careful history should be obtained from the patient. Particular attention should be given to data on any previous treatment to skin lesions, especially moles, since the possibility of metastatic melanoma must always be considered. Questions pertaining to recurrent hoarseness, dysphagia, or any other abnormality may bring a response pertinent to the problem.

Examinations should be repeated if necessary, and often more than one examiner should be employed. Examination of the intraoral cavity, pharynx, and larynx is not satisfactory unless the patient is completely relaxed and cooperative. If necessary, examination should be done with the patient under light anesthesia.

No biopsy specimens should be taken, however, until all radiographic studies have been completed, since excision of tissue may result in distortion of the film. Radiographs should consist of the following:

1. Lateral soft tissue film of the neck. A film from this position may demonstrate abnormalities of the nasopharynx, base of the tongue, epiglottis, and preepiglottic regions.
2. Tomograms of the nasopharynx, larynx, or paranasal sinuses, as indicated.
3. Laryngograms. These films are of great value in glottic lesions and are of particular importance in demonstrating subglottic extensions of a true vocal cord tumor.
4. Esophograms. Such studies are of value in demonstrating early lesions of the pyriform sinus and postcricoid region.

A clinical diagnosis of metastatic carcinoma is best obtained by aspiration biopsy. A pathologist may be able to report definitely whether a tumor is squamous or glandular from the material obtained by aspiration biopsy. Supraclavicular nodes are not included in this discussion, since the primary lesion for such nodes invariably lies below the clavicle.

The possibility of a node being a lymphoma must always be kept in mind, although a single node is rarely lymphomatous. Pathologists can seldom make a diagnosis of a lymphoma of any specific nature unless an entire node is removed for this purpose. Often the pathologist requests removal of more than one node, and experience has shown that the chance of obtaining a specific diagnosis is better if a node of long duration is removed rather than a smaller node of more recent origin.

SITES OF UNKNOWN PRIMARY CANCERS

Originally, Martin and Morfit[2] reported the tongue, nasopharynx, and intrinsic larynx as the most frequent site of an unknown primary lesion. Their conclusion that the nasopharynx is the most likely site for the unknown primary metastatic cervical cancerous node seems to have been generally accepted, but this view was not confirmed in later reports.

The tendency within the past 10 years has been to take "blind" biopsies from the nasopharynx, base of the tongue, and tonsil in those patients in whom the neck node is proved metastatic squamous cancer but the primary site is unknown. Not infrequently, the primary site, which may or may not have been suspected but not proved, has thus been located. Because of this procedure, tumors of the nasopharynx, formerly listed as the most frequent site for an unknown primary metastatic cancerous node, may now be discovered earlier.

The records of 94 patients with cervical cancerous nodes other than the supraclavicular ones have been collected from the main part of the study, but these patients have not been followed for a sufficient period of time to yield any significant information. However, some facts are of interest.

In the 94 patients, only 8 primary sites of disease have been located to date. Two lesions were found to have started in the pancreas; both were found at autopsy. The base of the tongue, retromolar trigone, tonsil, pyriform sinus, and esophagus accounted for 1 primary site each. Another was presumably a small lip lesion that had previously been treated, but the conclusion was presumptive only because no microscopic examination had been made of the original lip lesion.

A further analysis of a group of 20 patients admitted from 1952 to 1963 revealed that a primary lesion had been subsequently found in 8 patients. Of these 8, 3 had primary lesions in the pyriform sinus, 2 in the base of the tongue, 1 in the retromolar trigone, and 1 in the esophagus. The eighth patient had lymphosarcoma.

TREATMENT

Of the group of 20 patients, 9 died of disease, 5 died of other causes, 3 are free of disease, and 3 were lost to follow-up at 13, 10, and 8 years after treatment. Surgical treatment predominated in the group of 20 patients.

Of the 17 patients followed, 14 were treated by surgical procedure and 2 were treated by radiation therapy (both having been treated as presumably having the primary site in the nasopharynx). One patient received surgical treatment followed by radiotherapy for lymphosarcoma.

The time of survival for these 17 patients ranges from 7 to 17½ years, with a mean of 11 years.

Contraindications for treatment of patients with metastatic cervical nodes as hidden primary lesions in the nasopharynx

In Martin and Morfit's report in 1944[2] and in a later one that they wrote with Ehrlich in 1950,[3] they showed the nasopharynx as the most likely site of an unknown primary cancerous lesion of the head and neck region.

Since that time many radiotherapists have come to believe that cervical nodes proved to contain metastatic squamous cancer from an unknown primary site represent metastasis from the nasopharynx and should be so treated. It has been my experience that these patients should not be treated with radiation therapy for a nasopharyngeal primary lesion.

Proposed definitive treatment for metastatic cervical nodes with unknown primary lesions

With no primary site proved, definite treatment should be instituted for the metastatic cancerous node. If a definitive microscopic report has not been obtained by aspiration biopsy, then, and then only, should the removal of the node for microscopic examination be considered. This procedure should be carried out in the operating room with the understanding and consent of the patient that if the diagnosis of metastatic cancer is confirmed, a surgical operation will be performed immediately.

Each patient represents an individual problem and should be so treated, but all require close and regular follow-up study, since hidden or occult primary lesions may not be found for months or years. If and when a primary lesion is ultimately discovered, the treatment should be devised with careful consideration if radiotherapy was originally employed and is being considered for the new primary lesion.

In some patients treated by radical neck dissection, the primary lesion is never found, not even at autopsy, a fact to which other writers have attested. These cases remain mysteries. In my own experience, one patient with metastatic squamous cancer of bilateral nodes treated by bilateral radical neck dissection developed pleural effusion from pulmonary and pleural metastases after 14 years and died with the primary cancer still undiscovered. Another patient, after undergoing bilateral radical neck dissection for metastatic squamous cancer in several nodes on each side of the neck, has survived more than 18 years after the operation. He remains free of disease, and no primary tumor has ever been found.

SUMMARY

A cervical node suspected of containing metastatic carcinoma should be aspirated by needle to prove that a tumor is present and, if possible, to find out what kind of tumor is present. Radiodiagnostic studies should be completed before any biopsy specimen is taken, since the removal of any tissue would cause distortion and might suggest misinformation to the radiologist.

Blind biopsies from the nasopharynx and base of the tongue are suggested. If the findings are negative, the cervical node may be removed for purposes of pathologic information. If squamous cancer is proved, a radical neck dissection is indicated at once. Radiotherapy is contraindicated without definite proof of the primary cancer. The complications of radiotherapy are too great to permit the use of the full dose required unless the patient can be assured that this administration and the aftereffects are necessary.

Close observation of the patient is essential, since primary cancers have been found 3 to 4 years after the neck dissection has been done. In one patient, 19 years have passed since a bilateral neck dissection was done with an unknown primary cancer. He has been examined at regular intervals, and a primary cancer has never been found. In another patient, death resulted from pulmonary metastases after a bilateral neck dissection for an unknown primary cancer; still, the primary site was never found.

Renewed activity in the neck of the patient with a previously excised node invariably appears in that region from which the node was excised for diagnostic purposes. This fact has been found too frequently to be ignored, and it occurs whether the patient has been treated by radiotherapy or by operation.

In conclusion, three points must be reemphasized.
1. To reiterate Martin's advice, repeated in several published articles, a cervical node should not be excised for diagnostic purposes until all other measures fail.
2. Every patient with a cervical node showing metastatic cancer should not be treated as having the nasopharynx as the primary site.
3. The possibility of subsequent discovery of a hidden primary tumor decreases with the passing of time.

REFERENCES

1. Martin, H.: Untimely lymph node biopsy, Am. J. Surg. **102:**17, July 1961.
2. Martin, H., and Morfit, H. M.: Cervical lymph node metastasis as the first symptom of cancer, Surg. Gynecol. Obstet. **78:**133, 1944.
3. Martin, H., Morfit, H. M., and Ehrlich, H.: The case for branchiogenic cancer (malignant branchioma), Ann. Surg. **132:**867, 1950.
4. Martin, H., and Romieu, C.: The diagnostic significance of a "lump in the neck," Postgrad. Med. **11:**491, 1952.

Chapter 9

Preoperative irradiation for head and neck cancer

Elliot W. Strong, M.D.

In the continuing search for more effective treatment of cancer, new modalities of therapy as well as combinations of well-established methods are being employed. Chemotherapy and immunotherapy have been more recently utilized, but their effects are diffuse and often nonspecific, and the results, particularly with head and neck cancer, are disappointing. Radiation and surgery represent the more conventional, well-established treatment methods. Their effects are specific and direct, and their results are predictable. However, with the leveling off of treatment results during the past 2 decades, plus the limitations of surgical and radiation therapy, it has been only logical to combine these two modalities, hoping thereby to enhance the subsequent results.

HISTORY

As early as 1914 Symonds[27] described how a large rectal cancer was shrunk so much by preoperative irradiation that its excision by a posterior approach was possible. Reporting from the Mayo Clinic in 1924, May[20] presented a detailed analysis of experience with combined radiation and surgery for the treatment of rectal cancer. He reported no undesirable side effects and described increased 2½-year survival rates. In 1930 Forssell[13] suggested that a

vast field for the further development of radiotherapy, is to reduce the size of the tumor and better limit the same from its surroundings by irradiation prior to operation and also to weaken the vitality of the tumor, thus diminishing the risk of local reimplantation or spreading the tumor throughout the operative interference.

He had treated patients with head and neck cancer with metastases with preoperative irradiation, surgery, and postoperative irradiation and had increased the survival rate of symptom-free patients from 0% after irradiation alone to 37%, 35%, and 40% at 1, 3, and 5 years, respectively, after combined therapy. In 1962 White and colleagues[30] reported their experience with irradiation and surgery for breast cancer. A comparable incidence of local recurrence in a group with more advanced disease was obtained, but survival rates were similar among patients subjected to preoperative irradiation and radical mastectomy, radical mastectomy alone, or radical mastectomy and postoperative irradiation.

Many other authors have described their clinical experience with combined therapy. In the older reports orthovoltage equipment and antiquated techniques were the rule. However, only one author has reported statistical documentation of a lower survival rate with preoperative irradiation, while some have described increased survival rates.[8] With modern high-energy equipment and current treatment methods, higher preoperative doses through larger treatment portals have been possible with less morbidity and shortened treatment intervals.

LABORATORY INVESTIGATION

Numerous experimental animal studies demonstrating the effectiveness of combined preoperative irradiation and surgery have been reported. It should be emphasized that these studies have generally involved artificially induced tumors in laboratory animals and that the extrapolation of such results to human experience may be erroneous.

Reinhart, Goltz, and Warner[23] reported that low dose irradiation of tumor cell suspensions prior to animal inoculation significantly increased the number of cells necessary to produce a given percentage of tumor "takes" and that the resultant tumors grew more slowly, taking longer to produce tumors of equal size, than did the nonirradiated control cells. In 1960 Agostino and Nickson[1] reported their studies on the effect of preoperative irradiation of simulated colon carcinoma in the rat. Animals were divided into control and irradiated groups. After the colon tumors were established, the irradiated group of animals received 200 R on 4 successive days. All animals then underwent colon resection if the tumor was resectable. The preoperatively irradiated group had a significantly higher percentage of operable tumors, an increased proportion free of disease at 9 weeks postoperatively, and a significantly lower local recurrence rate.

Inch and McCredie,[17] working with Walker carcinosarcoma 256, injected it into the subcutaneous tissues of rats irradiated 24 hours before or after wide local excision. A significant reduction in local recurrence at 50 and 100 days was obtained in both groups of animals, but to a greater degree in the group irradiated preoperatively. Similar results were obtained by using the same technique in another animal tumor system, but at 100 days only the preoperatively irradiated animals showed any benefit. One disconcerting fact of this second study was the higher incidence of pulmonary metastases in the animals irradiated preoperatively. However, these animals survived longer and thus possibly had a greater risk of developing such metastases.

Hoye and Smith,[16] working with several tumor systems in mice, artificially disseminated the tumor by surgical implant or intramuscular or intravenous injection 24 hours after irradiation of the tumor. Using amounts of irradiation insufficient to stop tumor growth or to produce tumor regression, they were able to decrease the growth of disseminated tumor cells by more than 90% with no increase in the incidence of pulmonary metastases.

Powers and Palmer,[22] in an excellent review of preoperative irradiation, cited a study where one third to one sixth of the 50% curative dose of radiation increased the survival rate when it was given as preoperative therapy in seven of ten mouse tumor systems. While the other three tumor model systems were not benefited by the preoperative irradiation,

apparently they were also not adversely affected.

The studies mentioned above are only a few of the many reported animal studies on the use of combined therapy. Generally, preoperative irradiation has been beneficial in the reduction of local recurrence or takes after artificial dissemination. Only scattered reports of increased bone, lymph node, and pulmonary metastases have been published, but these metastases have often occurred in those animals surviving longer. This may be related to alterations of tumorhost immunologic relationships, as well as to the factor of longer host survival.

GENERAL PRINCIPLES

To justify preoperative irradiation, certain principles must be satisfied.

1. There must be a significant tendency toward local recurrence, presumably because of viable tumor cells remaining in the treated area.
2. The preoperative radiation must be delivered to the entire area in which these local recurrences may occur.
3. The dose of radiation administered must be of such magnitude as to ensure that it will either destroy tumor cells or render them incapable of reproduction.

Preoperative irradiation is unlikely to be of value in certain situations. Generally, there is little to be gained by more adequate local tumor control in the presence of uncontrolled progressive distant metastases. While such local control may be desirable for palliation of pain, bleeding, or obstruction, it will probably not significantly prolong survival. Little benefit is likely to follow adjunctive irradiation in those tumors where conventional therapy already produces a very high (or a very low) cure rate. Such combined therapy is unlikely to alter the prognosis sufficiently to warrant its use. Examples of such tumors from the head and neck area include basal cell skin cancer, where conventional treatment methods produce cures in excess of 90% of patients, and in contrast, the highly lethal spindle and giant cell thyroid cancer, where in spite of any and all therapy, only a rare patient survives more than 6 months after diagnosis.

Adjunctive irradiation carries some disadvantages. The larger the radiation dose, the greater the time required for its delivery, the greater the expense, and the longer the rest interval needed before the definitive surgery. While some authors have concluded that preoperative irradiation does not increase postoperative complications, it is the experience of most surgeons that such adjunctive therapy does add to morbidity and does prolong time required for full recovery. Powers,[22] in an experimental animal model, documented the delay in healing of standard wounds in mice with increasing preoperative irradiation. Low doses of 1,000 to 2,000 rads produced little difference in the control animals, but doses of 4,000 rads produced profound delay in wound healing. With proper fractionation of dosage delivered by high-intensity radiotherapy equipment, with an appropriate recovery interval from irradiation prior to surgery, and with meticulous technique and attention to detail during surgery and the postoperative period, complications should not be excessive, provided that the radiation dose is not excessive.

IRRADIATION TECHNIQUES

Much debate and controversy surrounds what constitutes adequate preoperative irradiation. What constitutes optimum dosage, proper fractionation, and the ideal delay interval between completion of irradiation and surgery remain obscure. No well-controlled prospective clinical studies have yet been reported to conclusively answer these questions. Two general programs have evolved. The first one is the low dose, intensive, short course of irradiation, followed almost immediately by the appropriate surgery. Its advantages include lessened patient morbidity, shortened total treatment time with less expense, and possibly fewer postoperative complications. The major disadvantage may be that the full biologic potential of the radiation therapy is not realized at that low dose level. The second regimen is the high dose, necessarily protracted course of irradiation with its accompanying 4 to 6 weeks' delay prior to definitive surgery. The advantage may be the greater lethal effect of the larger dose of radiation on cancer. Possible disadvantages include increased and prolonged morbidity, greater expense, a much longer time interval required for completion of the full treatment plan, and a possible increase in postoperative complications. Hendrickson and Liebner,[15] in their study of the effects of 2,000 rads versus 5,000 rads given preoperatively for supraglottic larynx cancer, were unable to document the superiority of the low over the high dose.

CLINICAL EXPERIENCE

Many clinical studies of preoperative irradiation and surgery have been reported with varied and, at times, contradictory results. Unfortunately, almost no studies are randomized, almost none have concur-

rent untreated controls, and almost all are retrospective. With these limitations, it is still worthwhile to review the experience site by site.

Lip

Cancer of the lip mucosa is unique among head and neck cancers in that its natural history and response to treatment much more closely resemble that of skin cancer than mucosal cancer. Since conventional therapy is so highly successful in local control, there has been little interest in adjunctive therapy for lip cancer and no reports of its use. However, when the disease spreads to regional lymph nodes, it becomes as aggressive as any other head and neck mucosal cancer, with marked worsening of the prognosis. Under these circumstances preoperative irradiation to the neck prior to radical neck dissection may be beneficial.

To study the effect of preoperative irradiation on the incidence of local recurrence after radical neck dissection, a controlled prospective randomized study was instituted in 1960 at the Memorial Sloan-Kettering Cancer Center. All ward or service patients subjected to radical neck dissection for epidermoid carcinoma were randomized according to their birth dates. The treated group received 400 rads of supervoltage therapy to the neck on each of 5 successive treatment days. Radical neck dissection was carried out as soon as feasible after the completion of treatment. Some patients who should have received preoperative irradiation did not. These were included as "others," and as can be seen, behaved much like those in the control group. Table 9-1 documents the TNM staging of these three groups and illustrates their similarity.

No apparent differences in morbidity or complications could be identified among the three groups of patients (Table 9-2). A statistically significant reduction in local recurrence of cervical cancer was obtained in the preoperatively irradiated group (Table 9-3), and a highly significant decrease was noted in the patients with the greatest amount of metastatic disease, those with histologically positive nodes at multiple levels in the neck. Although this study does confirm a reduction in the incidence of local recurrence after combined therapy, it unfortunately has not been accompanied by a corresponding increase in survival rates.

Barkley and his group[3] at the M. D. Anderson Hospital, using a higher dose preoperative therapy, obtained similar beneficial reduction in recurrence of cervical cancer, in contrast with a study by Biller

Table 9-1. TNM staging of three groups of patients at the Memorial Sloan-Kettering Cancer Center

Stage	Control Number of patients	Control Percent	Treated Number of patients	Treated Percent	Other Number of patients	Other Percent
I	7	3.5	3	2.1	4	5.5
II	57	27.9	23	16.0	17	23.6
III	85	41.7	85	59.0	32	44.5
IV	27	13.2	19	13.2	3	4.2
Not staged	28	13.7	14	9.7	16	22.2
Totals	204	100.0	144	100.0	72	100.0

Table 9-2. Complications and morbidity of three groups of patients at the Memorial Sloan-Kettering Cancer Center

	Control		Treated		Other	
Number of patients with complications	70	34.3%	65	45.2%	24	33.4%
Carotid rupture	1		3		0	
Fistula closed spontaneously	13	} 13.7%	4	} 13.2%	7	} 16.7%
Fistula open on discharge or required secondary closure	15		15		5	
Chyle fistula	4		3		1	
Wound slough requiring secondary closure	3		3		0	
Average blood required during surgery	3.20 units		2.84 units		2.72 units	
Average duration of postoperative hospitalization	24.8 days		26.2 days		21.2 days	

Table 9-3. Recurrence rates of cancer in three groups of patients at the Memorial Sloan-Kettering Cancer Center

	Percent control	Percent treated	Percent other
Recurrence of primary cancer	31.8%	18.7%	23.6%
Recurrence of neck cancer	37.2%	23.6%	34.7%
Recurrence of neck cancer with positive nodes	54.2%	32.6%	49.1%

and colleagues[4] in St. Louis, who, utilizing either 1,500 or 3,000 R preoperatively, noted no difference in the incidence of recurrence of cervical cancer.

Oral cavity

The clinical behavior of cancer of mucous sites of the oral cavity are similar, and in most reports these have been grouped together. Relatively less emphasis on adjunctive therapy for oral cavity cancer is apparent. In our own experience, with a highly selected group of T1, T2, and a few T3 epidermoid cancers of the mobile tongue, without clinical evidence of metastases, local control of the primary T1 and T2 cancers by surgery alone was achieved in 80% of patients. There appears to be little indication for adjunctive therapy to the primary cancer in this

selected group of relatively early tongue cancers. However, in the same group of patients, failure to control later-appearing cervical metastases was significant, suggesting the need for more aggressive therapy to the neck. Biller and colleagues,[4] in a study of a very small selected group of patients with cancer of the floor of the mouth including the anterior two thirds and posterior one third of the tongue and tonsil, could not demonstrate any improvement in either local control or survival rates with preoperative irradiation of 3,000 rads in 3 weeks.

Krause, Lee, and McCabe,[19] however, in a study of a heterogeneous uncontrolled retrospective series of 472 patients with oral cancer including the tonsil and base of the tongue, reported increased survival rates among those patients having combined therapy (4,500 rads supervoltage) than among those treated by either irradiation or surgery alone, except for patients with buccal mucosal lesions. However, because of the relatively small numbers of patients in each individual category, the differences in survival rates were not felt to be statistically significant.

Roswit and colleagues,[25] reporting on a selected series of patients with advanced cancer of the oral cavity, pharynx, and larynx who were subjected to preoperative irradiation and surgery, were unable to document any significant increase in survival rates (in part because of the small numbers of cases) but did not note any increase in morbidity or mortality with combined therapy. There was no apparent difference in cure rates between those who received 4,000 rads or less and those who received more than 4,000 rads in this small series.

Tonsil

Roland and colleagues[24] have reported on a very small series of patients with moderately advanced cancers of the tonsil treated preoperatively with 4,000 to 4,500 rads and then subjected to combined resection. An excellent absolute survival rate of 56% was obtained. Other authors[11,21,28] have alluded to the desirability of combined therapy for certain selected patients with tonsil cancer, usually with the more advanced infiltrative lesions, but have not provided conclusive evidence for the benefit thereof. Biller and colleagues,[4] in their small series, noted no decrease in local recurrence rates or increase in survival rates after low dose preoperative irradiation.

Paranasal sinuses

Many authors have reported their experience with preoperative irradiation for cancer of the paranasal sinuses, but none have documented improved survival statistics. In 1965 Jesse[18] reported on a small series of patients with epidermoid carcinoma of the paranasal sinuses. He was unable to document any significant differences in local tumor control or in survival rates after surgery alone, preoperative irradiation and surgery, or surgery followed by postoperative irradiation. Much more information relative to this group of patients is needed before definitive conclusions can be reached.

Larynx and pharynx

The most solid evidence currently available supporting preoperative irradiation is that evidence relative to the treatment of cancer of the larynx and laryngopharynx. Several authors have reported their experiences. Goldman and his group in New York were among the first to publish their results. With a selected group of patients with advanced cancers of the larynx and laryngopharynx treated with 5,500 rads of cobalt teletherapy over a 5- to 6-week period followed in 3 to 6 weeks by radical surgery, their latest report documents a direct absolute 5-year survival rate of 66% and a determinate direct 5-year survival rate of 89%. Only 9 of the 64 patients in the series to date are known to have died of cancer, 4 died from local recurrence, and 5 died

from distant metastases. While the study is not controlled, the authors concluded that the regimen "has improved survival rates of patients with advanced cancer of the larynx and laryngopharynx."

Wang and colleagues,[29] in a study of combined therapy for supraglottic larynx and pyriform fossa carcinoma, concluded that treatment should be highly individualized, based on the extent of the disease. They noted little improvement in cure rates from combined therapy for those small exophytic tumors with clinically uninvolved cervical lymph nodes over radical curative radiotherapy alone. In the larger, more infiltrative T3 and T4 cancers, usually accompanied by cervical nodal metastases, combined therapy appeared to improve cure rates. Constable and colleagues[9] compared combined therapy to surgery alone for larynx cancer and from experience with 2 admittedly dissimilar groups, concluded that those patients subjected to combined therapy, using 5,000 rads in 5 weeks, had better local disease control and better survival rates with no significant increase in complications over those treated surgically only.

Biller and colleagues[5] reported their experience with low dose preoperative irradiation (1,500 or 3,000 rads in 2 to 3 weeks) to larynx and laryngopharynx cancers, followed by partial or total laryngectomy and radical neck dissection. The study was retrospective, and the criteria for selection of the patients for irradiation or no irradiation and the dose were not specified; but the treated and untreated groups were considered homogeneous and comparable. In this study preoperative irradiation had no influence on local or cervical recurrence rates of the glottic, transglottic, or supraglottic cancers, but a trend toward improvement in survival rates of those patients with pyriform sinus cancers without a corresponding decrease in local recurrence rates was noted. Combining the patients with cancer of the base of the tongue with those having pyriform sinus cancer resulted in a trend toward both decreased local recurrence rates and increased survival rates. In a different analysis of the series, combining all patients with stage III and IV cancers produced a statistically significant decrease in the incidence of local recurrence in the preoperatively irradiated patients.

Flynn, Jesse, and Lindberg,[12] describing their experience with supraglottic larynx cancer, reported that control of stage IV cancer was much improved by combined therapy, but they could not document a statistically significant difference in either survival or regional recurrence rates between irradiation alone, surgery alone, and combined therapy. A strong trend toward improvement in these two parameters in the combined therapy group was present, and it was postulated that as the series increases in numbers, the significance will increase also.

In their study of preoperative irradiation for larynx cancer, Bryce and Rider[7] were not able to document any significant increase in survival rates by utilizing combined therapy over surgery or irradiation alone. They suggested that irradiation be the primary treatment, with surgery reserved for the failures, thus preserving some larynxes rather than routinely subjecting all patients to total laryngectomy as part of a combined program. In another preliminary report Bryce[6] suggested that combined therapy might improve survival rates for hypopharyngeal cancer over those obtained from either surgery or irradiation alone.

Salivary gland

Little experience with combined therapy for salivary gland cancer has been reported. In Sweden Ahlbom[2] and Edvall[10] both stated that combined therapy was the treatment of choice and described a decreased incidence of local recurrence and increased survival rates in patients with both benign and malignant lesions. There appears to be little indication for adjunctive therapy of benign salivary gland tumors, and it is difficult or impossible to establish a specific histologic diagnosis prior to excisional surgery.

Thyroid gland

Almost no clinical experience with combined irradiation and surgery for thyroid gland cancer and head and neck sarcomas has been reported. Most of these tumors have been traditionally characterized as radio-resistant. The common well-differentiated thyroid gland cancers carry such an excellent prognosis after adequate surgical excision that adjunctive radiotherapy appears unjustified.

SUMMARY

A brief summary of some of the historical and laboratory experience with combined preoperative irradiation and surgery has been presented. General principles of combined therapy have been enumerated, and a discussion of the techniques of such therapy has been presented. Selected current clinical reports of combined therapy for head and neck cancer have been summarized. While statistically valid studies confirming the advantages of combined irradiation and surgery over either modality alone are lacking, there is increasing evidence to suggest that combined treatment is more effective in the eradication of advanced cancer of the laryngopharynx and in the control of cervical metastases. Such therapy may also be of value in the treatment of advanced oral and paranasal sinus cancer, but conclusive evidence is not yet available. Little justification exists for combined therapy in those patients whose cancers are satisfactorily controlled by conventional single modality treatment. There is an urgent need for well-controlled prospective studies to conclusively confirm the validity of combined therapy and the techniques to be employed. Advanced head and neck cancers offer a fertile field for such investigation, and while combined therapy may not dramatically improve survival rates, any benefit that may possibly be derived in the form of lessened morbidity and prolonged life is most desirable.

REFERENCES

1. Agostino, D., and Nickson, J. J.: Preoperative x-ray therapy in a simulated colon carcinoma in the rat, Radiology **74:**816-819, 1960.
2. Ahlbom, H. E.: Mucous and salivary gland tumors; a clinical study with special reference to radiotherapy, based on 254 cases treated at Radiumhemmet, Stockholm, Acta Radiol. Suppl. **23:**18, 1935.
3. Barkley, H. T., Jr., Fletcher, G. H., Jesse, R. H., and Lindberg, R. D.: Management of cervical lymph node metastases in squamous cell carcinoma of the tonsillar fossa, base of tongue, supraglottic larynx and hypopharynx, Am. J. Surg. **124:**462-467, 1972.
4. Biller, H. F., Harris, B. L., Cassisi, N. J., and Ogura, J. H.: Low dose preoperative irradiation for oral and oral pharyngeal cancers, Arch. Otolaryngol. **95:**464-466, 1972.
5. Biller, H. F., Ogura, J. H., Davis, W. H., and Powers, W. E.: Planned preoperative irradiation for carcinoma of the larynx and laryngopharynx treated by total and partial laryngectomy, Laryngoscope **79:**1387-1395, 1969.
6. Bryce, D. P.: Preoperative irradiation in the treatment of carcinoma of the hypopharynx, Can. Med. Assoc. J. **93:**1147-1151, 1965.
7. Bryce, D. P., and Rider, W. D.: Preoperative irradiation in the treatment of advanced laryngeal cancer, Laryngoscope **81:**1481-1490, 1971.
8. Cady, B.: Preoperative irradiation, Surg. Gynecol. Obstet. **126:**851-865 and 1091-1105, 1968.
9. Constable, W. C., Marks, R. D., Robbins, J. P., and Fitz-Hugh, G. S.: High dose preoperative radiotherapy and surgery for cancer of the larynx, Laryngoscope **82:**1861-1868, 1972.
10. Edvall, C. A.: Mucous and salivary gland tumors; a

presentation of 330 cases treated radiosurgically, Acta. Chir. Scand. **107:**313-320, 1954.

11. Fletcher, G. H., and Lindberg, R. D.: Squamous cell carcinomas of the tonsillar area and palatine arch, Am. J. Roentgenol. Radium Ther. Nucl. Med. **96:** 574-587, 1966.

12. Flynn, M. B., Jesse, R. H., and Lindberg, R. D.: Surgery and irradiation in the treatment of squamous cell cancer of the supraglottic larynx, Am. J. Surg. **124:**477-481, 1972.

13. Forssell, G.: Radiotherapy of malignant tumors in Sweden, Br. J. Radiol. **3:**198-234, 1930.

14. Goldman, J. L., Silverstone, S. M., Roffman, J. D., and Birken, E. A.: High dose preoperative radiation and surgery for carcinoma of the larynx and laryngopharynx—a 14 year program, Laryngoscope **82:** 1869-1882, 1972.

15. Hendrickson, F. R., and Liebner, E.: The results of preoperative radiotherapy for supraglottic larynx cancer, Ann. Otol. Rhinol. Laryngol. **77:**222-229, 1968.

16. Hoye, R. C., and Smith, R. R.: The effectiveness of small amounts of preoperative irradiation in preventing the growth of tumor cells disseminated at surgery, Cancer **14:**284-295, 1961.

17. Inch, W. R., and McCredie, J. A.: Effect of a small dose of x-radiation on local recurrence of tumors in rats and mice, Cancer **16:**595-598, 1963.

18. Jesse, R. H.: Preoperative versus postoperative radiation in the treatment of squamous carcinoma of the paranasal sinuses, Am. J. Surg. **110:**552-556, 1965.

19. Krause, C. J., Lee, J. G., and McCabe B. F.: Carcinoma of the oral cavity—a comparison of therapeutic modalities, Arch. Otolaryngol. **97:**354-358, 1973.

20. May, E. A.: Surgical and roentgen treatment of carcinoma of the rectum, Am. J. Roentgenol. Radium Ther. Nucl. Med. **11:**246-251, 1924.

21. Perez, C. A., Mill, W. B., Ogura, J. H., and Powers, W. E.: Carcinoma of the tonsil; sequential comparison of four treatment modalities, Radiology **94:**649-659, 1970.

22. Powers, W. E., and Palmer, L. A.: Biologic basis of preoperative radiation treatment, Am. J. Roentgenol. Radium Ther. Nucl. Med. **102:**176-192, 1968.

23. Reinhard, M. C., Galtz, H. L., and Warner, S. G.: The effect of radiation on transplantable mouse tumor cells, Cancer Res. **12:**433-437, 1952.

24. Rolander, T. L., Everts, E. C., and Shumrick, D. A.: Carcinoma of the tonsil; a planned combined therapy approach, Laryngoscope **81:**1199-1207, 1971.

25. Roswit, B., Spiro, R. H., Kolson, H., and Po, Y. L.: Planned preoperative irradiation and surgery for advanced cases of the oral cavity, pharynx and larynx, Am. J. Roentgenol. Radium Ther. Nucl. Med. **114:** 59-62, 1972.

26. Spiro, R. H., and Strong, E. W.: Epidermoid carcinoma of the mobile tongue; treatment by partial glossectomy alone, Am. J. Surg. **122:**707-710, 1971.

27. Symonds, C. J.: Cancer of the rectum; excision after application of radium, Proc. R. Soc. Med. **7:**152, 1914.

28. Terz, J. J., and Farr, H. W.: Carcinoma of the tonsillar fossa, Surg. Gynecol. Obstet. **125:**581-590, 1967.

29. Wang, C. C., Schultz, M. D., and Miller D.: Combined radiation therapy and surgery for carcinoma of the supraglottis and pyriform sinus, Laryngoscope **82:**1883-1890, 1972.

30. White, E. C., Fletcher, G. H., and Clark, R. L.: Surgical experience with preoperative irradiation for carcinoma of the breast, Ann. Surg. **155:**948-956, 1962.

Chapter 10

Complications and sequelae of surgery for cancer of the head and neck

Alfred S. Ketcham, M.D.

Surgery performed in the head and neck area is seemingly prone to result in complications, some of which are unique to this area and others that occur at an increased incidence over that noted with surgery performed in other anatomical areas. Familiarity with the literature indicates that too little is written on how to avoid such surgical morbidity,[1] yet there is abundant information to guide attempts at reconstruction and rehabilitation in the treatment of neoplasms of the head and neck.[3-5] Fortunately, major surgical alterations in this area cause few immediate physiologic disturbances other than those related to vascular, neurogenic, or respiratory influences. Therefore the usual postoperative problems noted after surgery in many other anatomical locations are often secondary in the head and neck area. Little attention need ordinarily be paid during the operation or in the convalescent period to electrolyte imbalance, shock, sepsis, major nutritional deficits, or urinary and bowel complications. However, some of the complicating situations that are more commonly encountered can be precipitously catastrophic if they are not recognized early and treated with the greatest of urgency. Among these are airway obstruction, carotid or major vessel hemorrhage, central nervous system and vascular collapse, and surprisingly enough, the acute problem of delirium tremors.

The head and neck surgeon deals with patients who are complication prone. The reasons for this are multiple, but two of the more commonly acceptable causes are a long history of alcohol and tobacco consumption and a history of treatment failure. These patients have cancer in a readily visible area, and the cosmetic and physiologic disturbances associated with treatment may well be significant considerations in the long-term rehabilitation. It is mandatory that the surgeon involved in the care of these patients have expertise similar to that of the artist who pays particular attention to details, the detective who never takes anything for granted, or the clergyman who takes pride in his accomplishments and is challenged by his failures. The surgeon who actually does aggressive head and neck surgery must be an experienced oncologist who has seen and treated enough cancer to allow him to be accurate in his diagnosis, comprehensive in his preoperative evaluation, and meticulous in his surgical judgment and management of both his extirpative and reconstructive endeavors. These considerations alone dictate who or what specialty groups should be treating patients with neoplasms of the head and neck. Treatment is not necessarily dictated by who first sees the patient or to which hospital service he is first admitted.

TREATMENT FAILURE

In spite of the justified alarm that accompanies the diagnosis of cancer and the sense of urgency that is usually associated with instituting treatment, the experience of most oncologists strongly suggest that "haste may make waste." The emergency is in making the diagnosis of cancer, but once it is made, then well-planned pretreatment evaluation with particular attention to the full extent of disease will pay multifold dividends. Only with this approach, with our present modalities of treatment being selectively offered, will one obtain the much sought-after increase in survival rates. Without careful evaluation to determine the true extent of tumor invasion and the anatomical areas involved, the most distressing, and in the large majority of instances, the most important complication and sequelae to head and neck cancer surgery will be failure to cure. This can be failure resulting from local recurrence, metastases, or a combination of both.

Local recurrence

Once the diagnosis of cancer is made, a meticulous evaluation of the organ site can do as much as any other one factor, including proper treatment, to ensure the success of cancer eradication. The experience at the National Cancer Institute is that 90% of the head and neck cancer patients are, or were at one time, excessive consumers of alcohol. Seldom, if ever, is such an individual without a similar history of tobacco exposure. These individuals have mucous membranes that are grossly abnormal in appearance and prone to developing multifocal cancer. Therefore, it is essential to carefully visualize and take a biopsy, sometimes even in multiple minimally suspicious areas, of the oral-pharyngeal mucosa. The instance of insidiously developing recurrent disease, whether it is actually recurrent or new or multiple primary cancer, may otherwise be discouraging and even disastrous. Similarly, it is advantageous to take small biopsies peripheral to the primary tumor itself to better delineate the local extent of the primary cancer and the evidence of unrecognized mucosal, submucosal, perineural, or vascular invasion. Although head and neck surgery is often referred to as heroic surgery, it would not be so critically viewed by many if primary treatment was more often successful without the high incidence of local recurrence. This success can best be achieved by accurately measuring the extent of local disease and then determining the feasibility of cure by en bloc resection with or without adjuvant treatment. Whether one should refer to cancer occurring in the area close to or adjacent to where the primary cancer was originally excised as local recurrence is controversial. It is cancer, and whether it is local recurrence or a new primary cancer, it will demand treatment just as the primary tumor did.

Multiple primary cancer

The identification of incidental large bowel clinically asymptomatic cancer in patients with cancer of the oral-laryngeal-pharyngeal cavity is indicative of what appears to be a greater trend toward multiple primary tumors in the gastrointestinal tract of patients with cancer of an embryonically similar developmental area. Wyse[22] reported a 17% multiple primary incidence with thyroid carcinoma, and Yashar[23] indicated an 8.4% incidence of multiple neoplasms in patients with malignant tumors of the oral cavity. The alarming increase in carcinoma of the lung and its association with smoking is similarly seen in patients with head and neck cancer and may justify a closer look at the pulmonary system before definitive treatment is offered to these patients. On an investigational basis, routine tomograms of the lung are being performed on many head and neck services before definitive cancer treatment is undertaken, to accurately identify the incidence of pulmonary lesions not seen on routine chest films. The present experience suggests that the time and expense of tomography as a preoperative evaluation of these patients is well justified.

Distant metastases

Nothing can be more disturbing to the oncologist than the identification, soon after treatment, of regional or distant metastases. Hoye[11] found a 55% incidence of distant metastases in patients who were dying of epidermoid carcinoma of the head and neck area; O'Brien[16] reported a below-the-clavical rate of metastases of 47%; and Gowen[8] indicated a distant metastases rate of 57%. (Most of these metastases were noted in the lung.) Again, the trend toward more accurate preoperative pulmonary screening of cancer patients may not lead to any increased survival rate, but it will identify more accurately those patients who can or cannot be offered a cure by conventional therapy.

REHABILITATIVE COMPLICATIONS
Oral hygiene

The patient with oral cancer commonly has distinctive evidence of poor oral hygiene, and such patients have an increased rate of wound breakdown, infection, and prolonged convalescent morbidity. Dental caries and gingivitis can definitely promote poor wound healing. The dentist[19] must function as part of the head and neck team because he also commonly serves as the prosthodontist who will structure such prosthesis as will be used to fill the palatal, orbital, and facial defect. The dentist sees the patient preoperatively and outlines a short but aggressive therapy program to bring the oral cavity to its maximum degree of dental health. Tooth extraction and control of dental plaque and caries can justify delaying surgery for as long as 1 to 2 weeks, depending on the location and magnitude of the anticipated surgery.

Nutrition

Although head and neck cancer patients are not commonly nutritional cripples unless the cancer is a locally advanced one that interferes with swallowing, there are a significant number of individuals whose alcoholic intake has interfered with good nutritional balance. In such instances a period of forced feeding or of hyperalimentation through the usual intravenous routes is indicated. Gastric intubation with hourly feedings restores nutritional disturbances quite effectively but less efficiently.

Cervical esophagostomy. The use of cervical pharyngoscopy[17] or the cervical esophagostomy[13] for tube feeding is usually reserved for postoperative nutritional maintenance. Occasionally, depending on the location, size, and site of the tumor, it is advisable to insert in the esophagus through a small stab wound in the lower contralateral neck a No. 18 plastic or rubber feeding tube through which nutritional balance can be rapidly obtained. At the time of definitive surgery, when the neck may be exposed, it is highly advisable to insert a lower esophageal feeding tube and bring it out the contralateral neck through a small stab wound alongside a small rubber drain. This procedure can be used for immediate postoperative gastric aspiration, although such aspiration is rarely indicated but is more commonly used for nutritional guidance. It can be left in place for an indefinite period of time if by chance multiple plastic reconstructive procedures might be planned and minimal care is required. It is a general policy to routinely use the cervical esophagostomy tube rather than nasal intubation if it is anticipated that oral feedings should be restricted for a period beyond 5 to 7 days. Removal of this tube is a simple matter, with the tract closing spontaneously, even when the tube has been left in place for several months.

Swallowing. One of the most difficult-to-handle postoperative complications of pharyngeal surgery is associated with swallowing.[15] Occasionally, bougie dilatations are necessary when the closure has been snug or when a contracture has developed because of delayed fistulization complicating the healing process. With the cooperative and understanding patient, almost all swallowing difficulties can eventually be corrected if intense repetitive guidance is offered to the patient by the dietician as well as by the responsible physician and nursing staff. Particularly after

glossectomy, positional instruction is most helpful, and some patients find that they require tilting the head posteriorly to assist the swallowing mechanism to function adequately. Almost all patients learn to swallow again, but those patients who continue to aspirate food become a real problem and sometimes require attempts at surgical correction,[15] occasionally leading to laryngectomy.

Taste and smell

Surgical resection of the oral-laryngeal-pharyngeal cavity more often than not will interfere significantly with the patient's ability to taste and smell.[9] It is common for the nutritionist and the responsible physician to be baffled by the patient's lack of desire to eat properly in the long-term postoperative convalescence.[10] Laryngeal surgery interferes with smell in spite of its remoteness from the olfactory fibers, and oral-pharyngeal surgery significantly interferes with both smell and taste. If these complications of head and neck surgery are kept in mind by both the patient and those who are preparing his food, either at the hospital or at home, as well as by those who are guiding this postoperative convalescence, many nutritional, swallowing, and other rehabilitative complications can be minimized.

OPERATIVE MANAGEMENT

Because of the embryonic stage of development of combined or adjuvant cancer treatment modalities, it is unwise to expect that the complication of local recurrence of cancer can be avoided without total gross tumor and even microscopic tumor resection. Total resection is best facilitated by accurate recognition of the extent of the tumor, but being able to conveniently excise the tumor mass is equally important. This can be done only if the surgeon uses his experience, clinical judgment, and expertise and has adequate operative exposure. The anesthetic techniques and surgical draping procedures are of utmost importance if complications of surgery are to be minimized.

Anesthetic cooperation

By tradition the anesthetist is usually situated directly at the head of the table, where he can closely monitor the patient's vital signs by touch and sight. Although this may be of importance, it has long been apparent to head and neck surgeons that the proximity of the anesthesiologist to the head and neck area during surgery makes exposure difficult and maneuverability impossible. It is strongly recommended that the cooperation of the anesthesiologist be obtained in the use of extension tubes on the endotracheal tube, which allows the anesthetist to move back from the patient. This system allows the surgeon to work in an unrestricted manner and for his assistants to be directly adjacent to the wound area. If a preliminary tracheostomy is used, the tubing is brought down over the chest wall and abdomen and is then brought out laterally to the opposite side of the patient's primary surgical exposure. This allows the surgeon and his assistants unrestricted mobility around the head and neck area. This apparent remoteness of the anesthesiologist from the patient is feasibly safe. At the least provocation the surgeon steps aside and allows the anesthesiologist direct access to the patient, a situation that seldom if ever occurs if preoperative planning is carried out, with adequate draping of the wound and the patient previously agreed on. Allowing relatively unrestricted closeness to the operative area is one of the better prophylactic measures available for ensuring adequate surgery and thus preventing local recurrence, as well as for controlling bleeding and other intraoperative complications that might develop.

Pulmonary ventilation

The minimization of surgical complications is measured directly by the surgeon's ability to develop a cooperative team effort among those who are working with him in the management of cancer patients. In no area is this more important than in head and neck surgery, where the surgeon and members of the anesthesiology and inhalation therapy team must have a mutual understanding of the principles of adequate pulmonary ventilation and carry them out preoperatively, intraoperatively, and postoperatively. While the anesthesiologist may not agree that anesthesia should be given by using long extension tubes and with him being relatively remote from the patient to allow adequate operative exposure and maneuverability, it has been repetitively shown that this is a safe approach to head and neck anesthesia. If the surgeon and the anesthesiologist are both alert to the potential development of tube kinking and compression or cardiac-pulmonary problems, the surgeon can respond rapidly, as unusual as the occasion might be, to such problems and move aside and allow the anesthesiologist to inspect and correct problems in the airway system.

The use of the many time-proved ventilatory assistants, such as the Bird respirator, can be regulated and monitored by the team effort of the inhalation therapist and the nurses. The toileting of the pulmonary tree, while the responsibility of the doctor and his assistants, usually is carried out by the intensive care unit nursing personnel, who have been trained to recognize the symptoms of excessive tracheal excretion and mucous plugging and can astutely carry out tracheal toileting with sterile suctioning techniques.

Preliminary tracheostomy versus nasal-pharyngeal intubation. Transnasal or transoral tracheal intubation is less than ideal for most patients with head and neck cancers. For facial, frontal, and temporal exposure, sterility precautions are interfered with by the presence of the anesthetic delivery equipment. Monitoring nerve function during surgical dissection is difficult because of the proximity of and coverage by surgical drapes. Both of these considerations might be factors in wound infection and surgically inflicted cosmetic disturbances.

When the location of the cancer requires entrance into the oral-laryngeal-pharyngeal airway in the course of surgical dissection, the presence of the endotracheal tube can interfere with tumor exposure and resection, as well as with reconstruction of the continuity of the surgically transected mucosa. In addition, an exophytic tumor mass might be traumatized by the passage of the endotracheal tube and tumor cells, or actual fragments of the tumor mass may be disseminated into the pulmonary tree.

The decision to use preliminary tracheostomy must be made cooperatively with the anesthesiologist, keeping in mind the location of the primary tumor. The laryngeal lesion with subglottic extension might well mandate that the tracheostomy tube be placed lower than through the first or second tracheal ring. A low-lying tracheal stoma may interfere with postoperative construction of a permanent laryngeal stoma. Ideally, the tracheostomy should be placed so that there is no continuity with the exposed neck structures. Good planning of the type and direction of skin flaps in the neck might prevent this communication. Commonly, the two wounds are in communication; but if care is exercised in placing the postsurgical drains, then complications are minimized.

The particular tracheostomy tube or laryngotomy appliance used depends in great part on the preference and experience of the team of therapists. Intraoperatively and in the early postoperative period, it is essential that the cuffed tube, whether metal, plastic, or glass, be readily adaptable to different adapters and T tubes that may be used by inhalation therapy and other intensive care personnel. Attention is drawn to a recently reported[14] near catastrophe caused by an adapting tube that had an imperfect lumen in one of its adapting arms. Within the past year two other such instances of mechanical deficiencies have been found in commercially available pulmonary ventilation equipment.

Laryngeal stoma care. Postoperative tracheotomy or laryngotomy tubes must be sutured in place during the early postoperative period. It is inadvisable to use a constricting type of strap or elastic band about the neck. The tracheostomy tube should be held in the stoma by sutures placed through the flanges of the tracheostomy tube and to the skin on either side of the stoma. This procedure prevents constricting neck edema and, most important, prevents the inadvertent removal of the stomal tube, an incident that can be catastrophic if not immediately recognized.

It does appear as though the glass[7] and some of the plastic tubes cause less irritation to the stoma than do the more conventionally used tubes. In the laryngectomy patient, one must always be alerted during the long-term convalescence to the development of endotracheal accumulations of precipitated mucus. This can encircle the trachea and, in essence, close off the airway lumen, causing acute respiratory distress. This complication is more prone to develop during a change of seasons or a change of the patient from the hospital to a convalescent care environment or back to his home, because of heat and humidity changes. Often the patients find that they can prevent this life-threatening complication by increasing the humidity of their environment by placing a small moistened gauze pad over their stoma or by wetting the crocheted bib type of pad that many patients use to loosely cover their stoma.

Incisional placement

Although the appearance of the wound and the postoperative appearance of the patient is of real importance to both the patient and the physician, cosmetic considerations are not the first consideration in incisional placement. The incisions must be made so as to offer the patient not only the best opportunity of cure but the least chance of surgical morbidity related to wound breakdown.[3] If the neck has been biopsied previous to definitive surgery, it is mandatory that the biopsy excision tract, both in the skin and the underlying tissues, be excised in continuity with the dissection. This situa-

tion sometimes makes the placement of skin incisions difficult. The principle is to avoid Y or T types of incisions overlying the carotid artery, and the goal is to cross the carotid artery at a "lazy angle" or, preferably, at as much of a right angle as possible. The popularization of Macfee bilateral transverse incisions is well justified, as is the inverted hockey stick or lazy S incision with the exposure coming from the submental area lateral to the postclavicular angle or, in the opposite direction, from the lateral mastoid immediately down to the suprasternal notch.[2,18] The drains must be brought out through separate stab incisions and preferably should be suction type of drains that deflate the wound flaps and obliterate dead space.

Cardiopulmonary depression

The onset of cardiopulmonary complications can be rather accurately identified by careful intraoperative monitoring of central venous pressure changes. The routine use of central venous pressure monitoring is one of the most significant advances made in allowing early recognition of postoperative physiological alterations. This monitoring, however, does not minimize the importance and necessity of trying to avoid intraoperative and subsequent postoperative complications through surgical anesthetic cooperation. The surgeon, for example, should always notify the anesthesiologist that he is manipulating the carotid sinus area or is about to mobilize and resect the tumor in an inaccessible area and that bleeding cannot be controlled until the specimen is removed. Minimizing trauma to the carotid bifurcation can lessen the hypotensive episodes that sometimes occur with manipulation of this area. Intracranial pressure phenomena can similarly be minimized by careful attention to the maintenance of vital signs at the time that jugular vessels are ligated, as well as at the time that carotid vessels are manipulated. Although it is unusual that bilateral jugular ligation is carried out simultaneously, complications of such ligation can be minimized with preoperative Queckenstedt testing. The tendency toward preservation of one jugular vessel on the side of the neck contralateral to the primary tumor, if preserved with judgment and experience, is a consideration that is receiving renewed interest and will reduce the incidence of facial edema.

Wound drainage

Placing the operative suction drains so that they adequately decompress the skin flaps is of critical importance. Usually two drains are necessary in a neck dissection, and they should not lie against any major vessel. Attention must not only be given to their placement, but it must be seen to that they remain patent throughout the postoperative period, when they are in constant suction. Dressings are seldom used to cover a neck wound, because it is necessary to keep the neck visible and to identify any accumulation of blood or serum under the skin flaps.

Carotid artery exposure

Intraoperative bleeding from the carotid artery or its immediate tributaries should seldom be a severe complication of surgery if the anatomy is adequately understood and the surgeon remains fully cognizant of the proximity of the tumor to the carotid vessel. Vessels such as those in the sphenoid palatine pterygoid area may at times cause temporary bleeding while the tumor mass is being mobilized, but packing and sometimes individual ligation or cauterization rapidly controls such bleeding after the tumor mass has been removed. In the neck area it is unusual to encounter alarming operative hemorrhage because of the protection the carotid artery affords itself from tumor invasion. With the exception of carotid body tumors, it is essentially a rare phenomenon for the experienced surgeon to encroach on the continuity of the carotid artery in the case of head and neck surgery. If, however, it does occur and is not caused by a simple laceration that can be primarily repaired but by true tumor invasion or fixation, it is unlikely that primary repair would be successful. Prosthetic replacement should be attempted, but its success depends almost solely on the prevention of postoperative infection, as well as on total tumor resection.

The more usual bleeding complication is associated with fistulization or poor wound healing and occurs usually after the seventh postoperative day. This complication is fortunately becoming a phenomenon of the past. Actual carotid artery erosion by tumor or infection in the postoperative period has come in great part to be prevented by anticipatory measures. If postoperative wound infection can be avoided and the tract of an anticipated or actual fistula can be directed away from the carotid artery itself, then the carotid artery, which may have been essentially debrided of its encompassing protective sheath, will seldom be a postoperative bleeding problem.

The successful protection of the carotid vessel by one of many varied techniques of muscle or dermal flaps primarily depends on the experience of the surgeon. It is recommended that every neck dissection should be accompanied by some type of coverage of the carotid vessel, not so much to protect the carotid artery as part of a routine neck dissection, but to develop expertise on the part of the surgeon in using muscle flaps of scalene, levator, or trapezius muscle or dermal skin grafts to cover it. Then when the situation does arise and it appears that this coverage might be necessary because of the postirradiated nature of the wound and the scope of the surgical dissection, it is less of a cumbersome task to the surgeon. Coverage of the carotid vessel throughout the length of exposure can be a difficult procedure if the surgeon has not become adept and found through experience that there is tissue adjacent laterally or deep in the neck that ordinarily allows good coverage.

Carotid artery precautions. If there is worry concerning the viability of the carotid vessel as indicated by seepage of bright red blood, the neck wound should be immediately opened, the carotid artery exposed, and appropriate measures taken to prevent actual rupture. This procedure ordinarily will require ligation rather than imbricative repair. The proximity of a fistulus tract to the carotid vessel alerts the therapy team to the necessity for carotid artery precaution techniques, and the patient's wound is appropriately irrigated and cleansed at frequent intervals throughout the day. Antibody coverage is maintained. The patient is kept under watchful supervision in the intensive care unit with an indwelling intravenous catheter left in place and blood for transfusion kept in the immediate vicinity.

On those rare instances where carotid artery blowout actually does precipitously occur,[12] the individual who is first on the scene controls bleeding with point pressure rather than gauze or towel pressure and calls for emergency procedures to be activated. The patient is moved to the operating room while point pressure is still being applied to the bleeding site and blood is being transfused. No operative intervention is undertaken until the patient's vital signs are stabilized and adequate pulmonary and cardiac resuscitation have been instituted. Treatment of choice invariably is both high and low ligation of the carotid vessel. It may require removing a portion of the clavical to place ligating sutures in the proximal position of the carotid artery. Both internal and external ramifications of the carotid artery are carefully imbricated high in the neck.

In the past 7 years, the National Cancer Institute has experienced only two carotid vessel ruptures, both of which were recognized before they were precipitous in nature. During the past 16 years, no neurologic changes have been observed in the total of 19 patients with ruptured carotid vessels who have had unilateral carotid artery ligation. There have been two deaths in this series of carotid vessel blowouts, but no deaths have been encountered for over 12 years. Carotid vessel blowouts usually need not be a fatal experience if the team of people involved in patient care are alerted to the precautionary measures that must be taken when a hemorrhage is suspected and to the therapeutic endeavors that are most appropriate when a hemorrhage has occurred.

Subclavicular dissection

Lymph nodes and the scalene fat pad are adjacent to and beneath the clavicle. Their removal is necessary if adequate neck dissection is to be performed. Major vessels lie directly in this deep fossa of the neck, and their inadvertent laceration can be fatal if control is not obtained immediately. Such vessel ligation may often require mobilization of the clavicle in order to get into the upper chest, where these major vessels have been torn.

Pneumothorax. Similarly, the apex of the lung can be lacerated, and a pneumothorax can develop. This situation is often not identified until the postoperative period and is usually handled very adequately by insertion of chest tubes for water seal suction. It need not be a serious complication if it is recognized before pulmonary distress is encountered.

Lymph fistulas. The often overlooked, easily lacerated thoracic duct lying in the subclavicular fossa should always be looked for and carefully ligated by the physician when he is dissecting in the lower left side of the neck. Accumulations of lymph beneath the skin flaps can be a distressing complication to what was otherwise a very clean and uneventful neck dissection. While adequate drainage and pressure over the skin will often bring about closure of the fistula, it is not uncommon that the area must be exposed and the duct itself isolated and ligated. There is a thoracic duct on the right side, although the left side is more often a complicating problem. However, after ligation of the left thoracic duct, the right thoracic vessel rapidly becomes functional, as determined by lymphographic studies and experience at surgery. When performing staged radical neck dissection with the right side of the neck being secondary to the left side, the physician must seriously consider the possibility of right thoracic duct tear.

Nerve trauma

Familiarity with the anatomy of the head and neck area does not always allow preservation of motor and sensory innervation to portions of the head and neck area.[20,21] Proper identification of the facial nerve will avoid transection of its ramifications unless tumor infiltration contradicts conserving the nerve. The mandibular branch of the facial nerve ordinarily courses in a uniform pattern across the lower mandibular margin. Avoidance of this area by superior reflection of the tissue containing the facial vessels as they course through the upper neck may serve to prevent trauma to this small nerve, which could cause temporary or permanent denervation in the muscles of the angle of the mouth. Inadvertent transection of this nerve ordinarily results in permanent cosmetic changes noted particularly with attempts to smile and in resultant asymmetry of one commissure of the mouth. Attempts can be made at plastic reconstruction of the muscle supporting structures of the angle of the mouth. Nerve grafts of the major portion of the facial nerve are always to be considered. The location of the tumor and its metastases determines whether the facial nerve, the spinal accessory nerve, and the recurrent laryngeal nerve, as well as the hypoglossal and lingual nerves, can be avoided. Seldom is it necessary to do anything other than mobilize these functional nerves. The superior laryngeal nerve is sometimes transected by thyroidectomy unless its small size and proximity to the upper pole of the thyroid is kept in mind during ligation of the superior thyroid vascular pedicle. Little can be done if the recurrent laryngeal nerve is cut, although reanastomosis should be attempted. The lingual and hypoglossal nerves seldom need to be sacrificed; but when it is necessary because of tumor invasion, grafting or reanastomosis might serve to prevent permanent tongue disability.

According to many sources, one can now be encouraged to preserve, if the cancer allows, the spinal accessory nerve. If sacrifice is carried out, attempts at great auricular nerve grafting are usually indicated to restore some degree of trapezius function and allow the patient to comfortably raise his hand above his head and shrug his shoulders. The most common complaint noted by these patients is arm elevation and shoulder distress during the winter, when heavy clothing seems to be an excessive burden to the affected shoulder musculature.

The vagus nerve can be inadvertently transected, as can the phrenic nerve, in the course of tumor removal from either side of the neck. Avoidance of these nerves is mandatory unless actual tumor invasion justifies the resultant diagrammatic paralysis, which ensues along with voice and breathing complications as a result of transection of either of these nerves.

Horner's syndrome. The cervical sympathetic chain and its easily identified ganglia lie deep in the midneck, overlying the paravertebal fascia. Inadvertent trauma to the area will be easily identified in the postoperative period with recognition of Horner's syndrome. This complication is avoidable except in the very rare instance when the tumor extends from the pharynx or larynx to the paravertebral area or when retropharyngeal nodal fixation has developed.

SYSTEMIC COMPLICATIONS

A distressing and frustrating complication of head and neck surgery is related to controlling the patient's tendency toward excessive alcohol consumption and tobacco exposure. It is absolutely mandatory that these patients be forbidden to continue such carcinogenic exposure. Psychiatric counseling will often be of assistance in relieving problems related to curtailing such exposure.

Similar guidance from experienced therapists, whether it be psychiatric, social, occupational, or physical, will assist the patient in accepting and accommodating cosmetic alterations, voice changes, chewing and swallowing problems, and prosthetic tolerance, thus facilitating his return to his family and community as a functional citizen. The insidious problems that these patients must face, as well as the obviously distressing ones, are often overlooked by the busy surgeon, who sees the patient only for short intervals in an outpatient status after his discharge from the hospital. The total team effort comes into play here as much as in the management of the surgery or the immediate complications.

Pain

There is little postoperative pain associated with surgical procedures in the head and neck area, yet often these patients have been under rather heavy barbiturate or narcotic medication for a period of time previous to referral for definitive cancer treatment. Postoperative control of their narcotic type of desire is often difficult, as well as usually being

contraindicated, especially in the patient with a tracheostomy or any other type of pulmonary disability. Analgesic medication administered orally or rectally more often than not will satisfy these patients' need for pain relief.

Stress ulcers

Postoperative cosmetic change, functional disability, indwelling feeding tubes, and voice alterations create a stressful situation for even the most stable of patients. The presence of blood in the stool and, less often, pain in the epigastrium may be an indicator of the stress being experienced by some patients during convalescence. The acute peptic ulceration associated with such stress may be insidious in nature but must be constantly kept in mind by the treatment team. Seldom will this bleeding be of a serious nature, yet operative intervention may be the recommended course of therapy when frank bleeding does occur.

RECURRENT DISEASE AND RADIATION

Coexistent with the rather alarming trend toward utilizing radiotherapy for many of the cancers developing in the head and neck area is the increased number of patients with recurrent or residual cancer being referred to the surgeon. These patients present a most formidable problem related to accurate preoperative diagnostic evaluation of the extent of local disease and regional neck disease, as well as the formidable problems that often accompany attempts at aggressive surgical resection. Patients can accept a tremendous insult from one or the other of these two modalities delivered singularly, but a combination of the two in even less magnitude often promotes morbidity that is distressing. Wound healing, fistulization, bone necrosis, dental complications, stricture, brawny neck edema, and induration and facial edema are all complications that are prevalent. Radiotherapy delivered in an attempt to avoid surgery regardless of the indications for one or the other modality seems to be even more prone to causing the development of these problems. In handling the surgical challenge presented by these patients, the surgeon must use all his talents as he delicately handles tissue, meticulously develops tissue planes, and reapproximates transected margins. Preoperative, intraoperative, and short-term postoperative antibiotic coverage, while indicated in most aggressive surgical procedures for cancer, is mandatory in the postradiated patient. Antibiotic coverage, however, must not serve as an excuse to the surgeon for using less than optimum surgical technique.

More often than not, the long-term morbidity associated with an operation or radiation failure can be lessened by the preoperative preparation of full-thickness skin tubes or pedicles[6] with the use of such innovations as the deltopectoral flap, the extended thoracoacromial flap, and the less often used forehead visor flaps. It is recommended that the surgeon who infrequently utilizes skin pedicles for wound closure develop expertise under the watchful guidance of the experienced plastic surgeon or else include the plastic surgeon in the team approach so that he is in part responsible for the wound closure and patient rehabilitation.

SUMMARY

In spite of the multitude of problems that may be associated with aggressive surgery of the head and neck area, these patients are usually free of pain, ambulatory, and able to be nutritionally monitored without intravenous fluid administration during the postoperative period. Pulmonary complications can be minimized by meticulous attention to cleansing the airway, and systemic physiologic complications seldom need to be a problem for the therapy team. Management of these patients, however, requires the expertise of an experienced surgical oncologist who develops the team approach with an attentive resident staff, well-trained and experienced personnel in the operating room and the intensive care unit, and the day-to-day nursing staff, as well as the dental, nutritional, social, and vocational guidance staff. Mortality related to surgery of the head and neck area can be less than 1% and morbidity less than 10%, even in those patients who have been previous treatment failures, if attention is directed to the principles of good extirpative surgery and intense rehabilitation efforts on the part of the treatment team. While it is true that aggressive surgery can promote aggressive complications, this danger can be minimized by the experienced head and neck surgeon.

REFERENCES

1. Artz, C. O., and Hardy, J. D.: Complications in surgery and their management, ed. 2, Philadelphia, 1967, W. B. Saunders Co., pp. 273-305.
2. Babcock, W. W., Jr., and Conley, J.: Neck incision in block dissection, Arch. Otolaryngol. **84**:554-557, 1966.
3. Bakamjian, V. Y. Total reconstruction of pharynx with medially based deltopectoral skin flap, N. Y. State J. Med. **68**:2771-2778, 1968.
4. Ballantyne, A. J., and Guinn, G. A.: Reduction of shoulder disability after neck dissection, Am. J. Surg. **112**:662-665, 1966.
5. Brown, J. B., Fryer, M. P., and Kolliopoulos, P.: Long-term control of cancer of head and neck with planned use of natural survival and healing tendencies, Arch. Surg. **86**:945-954, 1963.
6. Chretien, P. B., Ketcham, A. S., Hoye, R. C., and Gertner, H. R.: Extended shoulder flap and its use in reconstruction of defects of the head and neck, Am. J. Surg. **118**:752-755, 1969.
7. DeKernion, J. B., Ketcham, A. S., and Swerdlow, H.: An improved glass tracheostomy tube, Am. J. Surg. **117**:759-760, 1969.
8. Gowen, G. F., and Desuto-Nagy, G.: The incidence and sites of distant metastases in head and neck carcinoma, Surg. Gynecol. Obstet. **116**:603, 1963.
9. Henkin, R. I., Hoye, R. C., Ketcham, A. S., and Gould, W. J.: Hyposmia following laryngectomy, Lancet **2**:479-481, 1968.
10. Henkin, R. I., Schechter, P. J., Hoye, R. C., and Mattern, C. F. T.: Idiopathic hypogeusia with dysgeusia, hyposmia, and dysosmia; a new syndrome, J.A.M.A. **217**:434-440, 1971.
11. Hoye, R. C., Herrold, K. M., Smith, R. R., and Thomas, L. B.: A clinicopathological study of epidermoid carcinoma of the head and neck, Cancer **15**:741-749, 1962.
12. Ketcham, A. S., and Hoye, R. C.: Spontaneous carotid artery hemorrhage after head and neck surgery, Am. J. Surg. **110**:649-655, 1965.
13. Ketcham, A. S., and Smith, R. R.: Elective esophagostomy, Am. J. Surg. **104**:682-685, 1962.
14. Millar, R. C., and Ketcham, A. S.: Tracheostomy obstruction secondary to a T-adapter, Anesthesiology **38**:494-495, 1973.
15. Mladick, R. A., Horton, C. E., and Adamson, J. E.: Cricopharyngeal myotomy, Arch. Surg. **102**:1-5, 1971.
16. O'Brien, P. H., Carlson, R., Steubner, E. A., Jr., and Staley, C. T.: Distant metastases in epidermoid cell carcinoma of the head and neck, Cancer **27**:304-307, 1971.
17. Royster, H. P., Noone, R. B., Graham, W. P. III, and Theogaraj, S. D.: Cervical pharyngostomy for feeding after maxillofacial surgery, Am. J. Surg. **116**:610-614, 1968.
18. Rush, B. F., Jr.: A standard technique for incontinuity incisions of the head and neck, Surg. Gynecol. Obstet. **121**:353-358, 1965.
19. Scannell, J. B.: The function of the dental specialist in the treatment of cancer of the head and neck, Am. J. Surg. **110**:592-594, 1965.
20. Stewart, G. R., Mountain, J. C., and Colcock, B. P.: Non-recurrent laryngeal nerve, Br. J. Surg. **59**:379-381, 1972.
21. Swift, T. R.: Peripheral nerve trauma in radial neck dissection, Mod. Med.: November 1971.
22. Wyse, E. P., Hill, C. S., and Ibaney, M. L.: Other malignant neoplasms associated with carcinoma of the thyroid, Cancer **24**:701-708, 1969.
23. Yashar, J. J., Guralnick, E., and McAuley, R. L.: Multiple malignant tumors of the oral cavity, respiratory system, and upper digestive system; experience at the Pondville State Hospital from 1949 to 1959, Am. J. Surg. **112**:70-75, 1966.

Chapter 11

Complications and sequelae of radiation therapy in the head and neck

Richard A. Mladick, M.D.
David S. Postlewaite, M.D.
Charles E. Horton, M.D.
Jerome E. Adamson, M.D.
James H. Carraway, M.D.

Roentgen discovered x-rays[14] in 1895, and the adverse effects of radiation were noted as early as 1896.[1] In 1950 a new era of radiotherapy began with the introduction of high-energy radiation sources.[8] Although dental x-rays, fluoroscopy, and certain radioiosotopic studies may produce occasional complications, radiation therapy is responsible for the vast majority of problems in the head and neck region. Accidental exposure is not uncommon, but in these cases the extremities are most frequently injured.

DETERMINATE FACTORS OF RADIATION INJURY

The more common sources of radiation are orthovoltage or conventional x-ray, cobalt 60, electron beams, accelerators, radium or radioisotopes, Grenz or Bucky's rays, and Chaoul voltage or contract therapy. With higher energy sources the radiation is more accurate and effective and causes less damage to normal tissues. For example, orthovoltage damages skin more than cobalt 60. Grenz and Bucky's rays are produced with a low voltage of 5 to 15 kv., and thus emit low-energy x-rays just above ultraviolet on the energy spectrum. These high-intensity but low-voltage x-rays have a superficial effect and lose most of their energy in the first 1 to 2 mm.

of tissue. They are frequently used in dermatologic practice for the treatment of skin lesions. Contact therapy or Chauol voltage is somewhat stronger, with 30 to 50 kv. Orthovoltage, or conventional x-ray, is usually 250 to 400 kv. Megavoltage, or high-energy emissions (such as cobalt), are over 1 million kv.[6] Actinic rays are just below Grenz rays on the energy spectrum and are the most common cause of skin injury, which frequently results in the occurrence of actinic keratosis, basal cell carcinoma, and even squamous cell carcinoma. In addition to the source and type of radiation, other significant factors are:

total dose of irradiation The extent of injury is directly proportional to the dose.

tissue susceptibility Some tissues are able to withstand radiation better than others and recover more rapidly. Traumatized, diseased, poorly vascularized, and fast-growing tissues are generally most susceptible. The following is a list of tissue susceptibility in decreasing order: lymphocyte, granulocyte, epithelial cell, endothelial cell, pleura, peritoneum, blood vessel, connective tissue cell, muscle cell, bone cell, and nerve cell.[2]

tissue absorption A factor that varies with the volume of tissue, density of tissue, and the source.

54

field size A factor that directly affects the amount of scatter. Thus, the greater the field size, the greater the possibility of damage to surrounding tissue.

fractionation Lengthening the course of therapy without altering the total dose allows more time for tissue to recover between treatments.

PATHOPHYSIOLOGY

At the cellular level the nucleus is most sensitive to the effects of irradiation. In general, the irradiation causes ionization of molecules, and the affected molecules react with other molecules. Reversible and irreversible changes are rendered in the cell. The functional result of these changes is delay or inhibition of mitoses, cell death before or after division, chromosome breakage, and functional cell deficits.[15] Some clinical changes, such as erythema, epilation, depression of sebaceous gland function, and pigmentation, may be reversible or irreversible. Acute and chronic radiation dermatitis, ulceration, and cancer are not only irreversible, but progressive.

In skin the early erythema often appears as a pale pink color and disappears about the third day after treatment with approximately 450 R of moderately hard radiation. The late erythema begins about the fifth to the tenth day and slowly becomes deeper in color during the following weeks. By the fourteenth to the sixteenth day it reaches a maximum, even violet color, and begins to subside. About the twelfth day pigmentation appears and may begin to obscure the erythema. A late reaction begins on the thirty-fourth to fortieth day and lasts 2 to 3 weeks.[10]

The early erythema is probably caused by the release of active amines and ionized molecules from the injured epidermis and corium. Capillaries dilate, arterioles enlarge, endothelial permeability increases, and capillary stasis ensues. Later destructive changes in the blood vessels eventually result in obliterative vascular changes with endarteritis and thrombosis of small vessels and, finally, fibrosis. As the number of capillaries decreases, there is an overall reduction in blood flow to the tissue. Skin viability, potential for repair, and susceptibility to trauma are adversely affected.

In the mouth additional clinical changes are caries and mucositis. Mucositis may result from as little as 1,000 R. The etiology of the caries is thought to be either the direct effect of radiation, with softening and discoloration of the dentin, or secondary to xerostomia. The pH of saliva falls to 4 after irradiation, and the character of the saliva changes

with a decrease in quantity and mucin output. Associated factors that may be related to the development of caries are the patient's inherent susceptibility, gingival recession and disease, the status of oral hygiene, and dietary alterations. The salivary glands show destruction of the mucus cells; there is edema and degeneration of serous acini, which proceeds to a fibrous atrophy without regeneration.[16]

CLINICAL PICTURE OF COMMON PROBLEMS

Scalp. Mild secondary changes that result from radiation may be hyperpigmentation or hypopig-

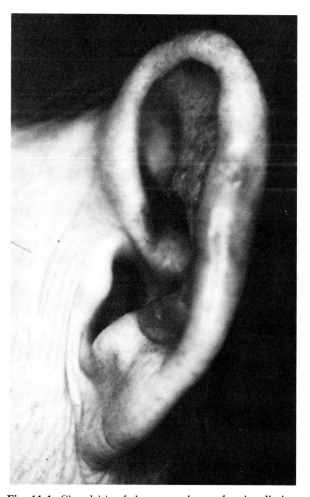

Fig. 11-1. Chondritis of the external ear after irradiation; the ear is erythematous, swollen, and tender. Early breakdown has developed in the anterior scapha. Once the breakdown develops to this stage, the treatment must be surgical. The ear had been treated with high-intensity but low-voltage x-rays that have a superficial effect and that have lost most of their energy in the anterior skin and underlying cartilage.

mentation, alopecia, and atrophy. Severe complications can include ulceration, with or without bone exposure, osteoradionecrosis of the cranium, and carcinoma.

Orbit. Our experience has been that problems in the middle and lateral portions of the free eyelid are rare. However, carcinomas treated by irradiation in or near the medial canthal region have frequently been troublesome and recurrent carcinomas have developed deep in the orbital soft tissues or adjacent bones, resulting in an extremely difficult and sometimes incurable disease.

Cheek, nose, ear. Radiation problems that develop in these regions are generally the result of treatment for skin carcinoma. A number of benign conditions, such as hirsutism, lupus, hemangioma, acne, and keloids are also occasionally treated with radiation. Secondary changes and complications are essentially the same as in the scalp. In addition, a common problem is a mild or moderate degree of radiation scarring or simple atrophy of the skin from some of the low-voltage dermatologic treatments. Some of the severe complications are through-and-through ulcerations of the cheek, rampant chondritis of the ear or nose, and carcinomas (Fig. 11-1). Areas that have been especially troublesome are the base of the ala and the columella. In these regions tumors are frequently penetrating, and the post-irradiation ulcerations and recurrent carcinomas that develop have been especially difficult to treat. In a number of these cases, almost a "field fire" type of reaction follows the radiation. The surrounding adjacent nasolabial areas become indurated, red, thickened, edematous, and painful, and recurrent carcinoma spreads deeply, both subcutaneously and into underlying bone (Fig. 11-2).

Mouth and pharynx. Caries, mucositis, and osteoradionecrosis are the most frequent problems seen in the mouth. Occasionally, rather marked edema of the tongue and epiglottis develop, which contributes to dysphagia. The painful mucositis, trismus, and inability to smell and taste interfere with nutrition. Osteoradionecrosis of the mandible is a dreaded complication (Fig. 11-3). If osteoradioencrosis of the mandible becomes infected from whatever source, there is almost always a rampant, severely painful, virulent, suppurative osteomyelitis. The infection is extensive and progressive, since the compromised blood supply further decreases the already poor resistance of the bone. Sequestration may come slowly or rapidly and may be fragmentary or massive. Repair and remodeling does not take place. The bone

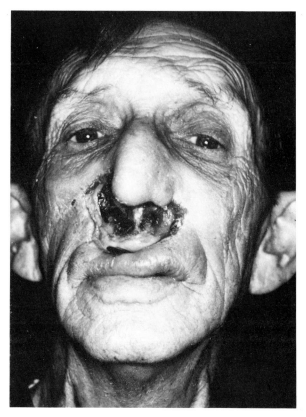

Fig. 11-2. Breakdown and recurrent carcinoma in the upper lip and base of the nose after irradiation of a basal cell carcinoma. In this area recurrence is extremely difficult to treat because the surrounding tissues are indurated, thickened, and edematous; the ulcerated area is especially painful. My clinical experience (R. A. M.) has been that carcinomas recurring after radiation therapy in this area appear to spread deeply and into the underlying bone.

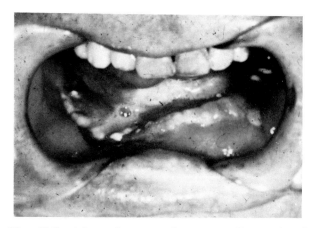

Fig. 11-3. Advanced suppurative osteoradionecrosis of the mandible. This is a very difficult and painful condition that requires thorough débridement of the involved mandible.

becomes progressively moth-eaten.[3,13] *Staphylococcus aureus* and *S. albus* are the organisms usually found in suppurative osteoradionecrosis, but hemolytic streptococci, pneumococci, *Escherichia coli,* and *Pseudomonas* may also be found. The condition is frequently so painful that addiction to alcohol or narcotics, or both, ensues.

TREATMENT

The complications and sequelae of radiation therapy may be mild or severe, may appear immediately or decades later, and may require either no treatment or extensive surgery.

Some of the mild, transient sequelae of radiation therapy need only conservative medical treatment. For example, the mucositis, xerostomia, or dysphagia may respond well to a liquid or soft diet, glycerol gargles, and a topical anesthetic. The acute or early erythema may be uncomfortable but frequently will do quite well with emollient creams and meticulous skin care that avoids external trauma such as shaving nicks. Some of the mild cases of nose or ear chondritis may respond to conservative medical management. Mild laryngeal chondritis can be treated by conservative medical management and a tracheostomy.[17]

Advanced or severe complications, such as radiation ulceration, suppurative osteoradionecrosis, and radiation cancer, are clearly surgical problems and are discussed under the separate regions of the body.

General principles

Certain general principles have evolved in the surgical treatment of radiation problems:

1. Irradiated tissue heals poorly and will not tolerate closure under tension, infection, rough handling, or external trauma.
2. Surgery is contraindicated for an acute radiation burn.
3. Irradiated tissue will generally not accept a skin graft.
4. Ideally, all ulcerated or involved irradiated soft tissue should be resected, and reconstructive flaps should be set into normal surrounding tissue.
5. A flap set into an irradiated area will establish a new blood supply very slowly and should not be detached as soon as a flap set into normal tissue.
6. The nonirradiated flap, which brings new blood supply into an irradiated area, will have a beneficial effect on the surrounding marginally involved tissue.
7. It is wise to protect the carotid artery by a muscle flap or dermal graft in extensive composite resections in irradiated fields.
8. Sutures should be left in irradiated skin longer than in normal skin.
9. Any radiation ulcer or fistula may harbor persistent or recurrent carcinoma.

Indications for surgical treatment

In most cases the indication is an actual or potential breakdown of the irradiated tissue, which if not treated would progress to ulceration, infection, or carcinoma. In some cases the complete resection of the ulceration and involved area is the only way to rule out a malignancy. In an area such as the mandible or ear, surgical resection of the osteoradionecrosis or chondritis may be necessary to relieve severe pain.

Treatment of regional problems

Scalp. In superficial burns, it is possible to carry out dermabrasion or shaving, with or without split-thickness skin grafts.[7] When ulceration extends to bone tissue, the most expedient procedure is resection of all irradiated tissue and reconstruction with local flaps. When an area of exposed bone is too large to be covered with local flaps, it can be treated by drilling the bone and expectantly waiting for granulation tissue[5] or excising the bone down to dura and covering with a split-thickness skin graft. Distant flaps are difficult to carry to the skull without multiple procedures utilizing an arm as a carrier. The alternative is the direct jump flap using the skin of the medial aspect of the upper arm.

Orbital region. Because of the danger of deeply penetrating recurrences in the orbital region, a high index of suspicion and frequent examinations and biopsies are necessary. Resections may need to be deep, with removal of involved bone tissue. Reconstruction can be performed with forehead flaps for the medial canthal region, or if total eyelid reconstruction is needed, the Mustarde flap can generally bring in nonirradiated cheek skin. With the far-advanced cases with orbital cancer recurrences, orbital exenteration and skin grafting is necessary.

Cheek, nose, ears. Wide resection of the involved area with reconstruction by local flaps is the first choice of treatment. Bilobed postauricular and cervical flaps from nonirradiated areas are frequently ideal for cheek reconstruction. Forehead and nasolabial flaps are preferred for nasal reconstruction

(Fig. 11-4). Cervical tubes may also bring in non-irradiated skin when the entire face has been exposed to radiation. Necrosis of nasal cartilage or bone, or necrosis of ear cartilage, will require removal of involved tissue (Fig. 11-5, *A*). Reconstruction must await resurfacing by nonirradiated flaps (Fig. 11-5, *B*). Small partial ear defects are best reconstructed by using nonirradiated postauricular skin flaps. Total ear reconstruction is rarely indicated. A prosthesis can be used if the irradiated skin in the region will withstand the glue. In the cheek affected by mild irradiation dermatitis, atrophy, or superficial scarring, a skin graft may succeed if the resection is carried down to healthy, bleeding tissue. The skin graft is,

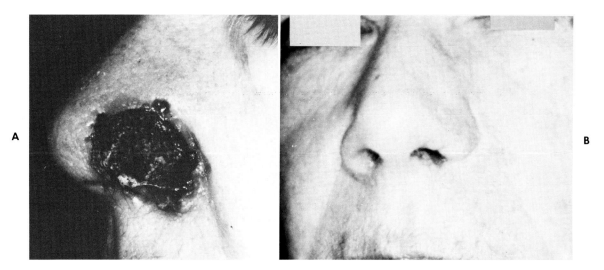

Fig. 11-4. A, Result of accidental overdosage to the left ala. **B,** This radionecrotic ulcer was allowed to heal, the defect was excised, and a nasolabial flap was shifted in to reconstruct the ala.

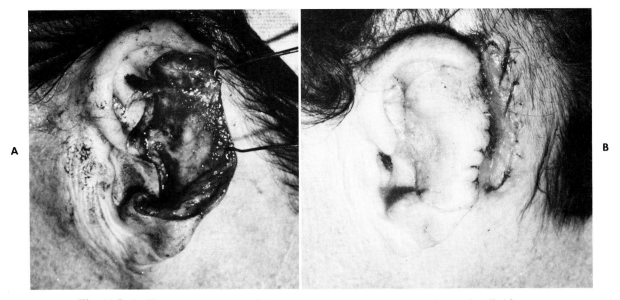

Fig. 11-5. A, This chondritis, caused by irradiation, was treated with thorough débridement of the involved cartilage; the less-injured postauricular skin was spared. **B,** Reconstruction of the ear was done with a nonirradiated postauricular flap.

however, contraindicated in acute necrosis or deep, penetrating burns. Large through-and-through cheek defects may require two flaps: a forehead flap for lining and a deltopectoral flap for external coverage. Other ways of handling these large cheek defects can be the use of the Mutter (nape of the neck) flap or the acromiothoracic tube with a prelined pancake or prefolded marsupialized end.

Mouth and mandible. Osteoradionecrosis is the big problem in the mouth and mandible region. It has been treated in many ways over the years, and there is still no unanimity of opinion. Conservative drilling of dead bone was advocated by Hahn and Corgill,[5] who felt that this drilling should be done through the dead cortex to allow granulation from bleeding bone or soft tissue to grow up and slowly sequester off the dead bone. The remodeling by this technique could take as long as a year, but they felt that even if it failed, a larger resection could be done at a later date. Nickell[12] advocated a moderately conservative resection and immediate resurfacing with an island flap. This method has achieved some very excellent results based on biologic excision.[9] That is, the new healthy tissue with adequate blood supply helps in the sequestration and the remodeling of the bone. Gaisford and Rueckert[4] felt that extensive and thorough cleanout of all involved

bone was indicated. Almost all have agreed that the intraoral approach is preferable, for it avoids having to go through the overlying irradiated skin, which, in most cases, will have some degree of involvement. Once the patient has been cured of his osteoradionecrosis by resection, reconstruction is rarely indicated or successful unless the soft tissue covering has been resurfaced with healthy flaps. It should be noted that the maxilla is rarely involved, since it has an excellent blood supply and tolerates x-ray therapy much better than the mandible.

Pharynx, larynx, and neck. The major problems in the pharynx, larynx, and neck region are postoperative complications that follow extensive surgical resections. Although the most severe complications generally occur in patients who have been treated with curative doses ranging from 5,000 to 7,000 R, severe complications may also follow the smaller planned preoperative doses (2,000 to 4,000 R) that are frequently advocated. The most serious postoperative complication is a breakdown or leakage of the intraoral closure, which may lead to contamination of the irradiated neck tissues. Saliva dissecting under skin flaps produces a necrotizing infection and skin slough, which may cause a carotid artery blowout.

Because of the reaction and inflammation from

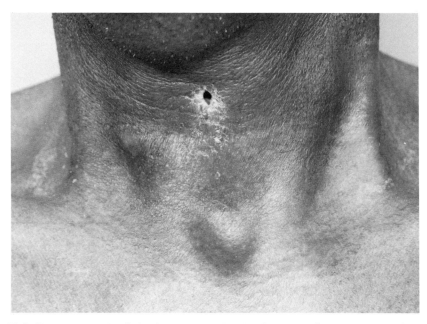

Fig. 11-6. Severe necrosis of the larynx and the development of a spontaneous laryngeal cutaneous fistula as a result of irradiation. Such advanced chondritis will require a laryngectomy.

the recent surgery, it may be difficult to transfer a muscle flap to cover the carotid arteries. Although an adjacent skin flap may be used for cover once the carotid arteries are clean enough, it is a mistake to try to cover the inflamed, infected adventitia or carotid sheath. Purulence will develop under the flap, and a carotid artery blowout may still occur. Once the proper dressing routine is instituted with frequent changes of saline compresses, the neck tissue will improve rapidly, and the carotid arteries may then be safely covered with a homograft or split-thickness skin graft as a temporary biologic dressing. As soon as the skin grafts have provided satisfactory coverage, the safety of the carotid artery is established, and the fistula or pharyngotomy can be closed electively by a flap from the nape of the neck or some other adjacent region. If a carotid artery blowout occurs, the artery must be ligated well, proximally and distally, and covered with normal tissue.[11]

Severe radiation necrosis of the larynx with oral fetor requires a laryngectomy and resection of the overlying skin[5] (Fig. 11-6).

If cervical esophageal obstruction develops from radiation fibrosis, the involved area may be dilated, or the area may be resected and reconstructed with a deltopectoral flap. Radiation neuritis may be relieved by alcohol injections or a resection of the nerve.

The surgical treatment of radiation sequelae is one of the most difficult undertakings in plastic surgery. Possibly because of the poor blood supply and possibly because these lesions are frequently infected when the surgery is undertaken, there is a very high incidence of failure of the skin graft or flap.

RADIATION CANCER

Carcinoma can develop in the site of any chronic scar tissue, whether it be from a thermal burn, osteomyelitis, or a radiation burn. The incidence of cancer developing in radiation burns is clearly higher than in any other type of scar. Although the exact dose of radiation therapy necessary to cause this cancer has not been established, it is most commonly a dose that has exceeded 3,000 R. Radiation cancer is not necessarily correlated only with burns caused by short-term high doses; it has been noted just as frequently in burns from low doses used over a long period of time. In many cases of radiation cancer there was never a history of any acute problem developing from the radiation. The latent period from the initiation of radiation exposure to the appearance of malignancy has been from 3 to 50 years, averaging approximately 20 to 30 years.[15]

Because there has been a high incidence of carcinomatous changes in patients radiated for benign disease, there is a tendency to severely limit the indications for radiation therapy.

The treatment of radiation cancer is the wide local resection of not only the actual neoplastic area, but all of the irradiated tissue, with appropriate reconstruction. The incidence of nodal metastases from this type of carcinoma is generally low and a regional lymph node dissection is generally not indicated. However, nodes are frequently palpable because of the associated infection in the radiation ulceration. In many cases, the radiation problem occurs in the midst of a regional group of lymph nodes, and it is anatomically easier to resect the entire lymph node region in continuity than it is to resect just a portion of it.

PREVENTION

Because radiation sequelae are so difficult to treat, it is quite obvious that their prevention is especially important. Having a well-qualified radiotherapist administering radiotherapy is most important. The patient should be instructed in good skin care before and after radiation therapy. When treatment is planned for intraoral lesions, a completed dental examination should be carried out. Carious teeth should be removed or repaired, and the teeth should be treated with fluorides. All of the proper measures should be taken to ensure optimum oral hygiene. At least 14 to 17 days should be allowed after the extraction of teeth before radiotherapy is begun.

It would appear that with qualified radiotherapists undertaking or supervising practically all radiotherapy, the incidence of complications will dramatically decrease. The severe problems seen too frequently in the past will, hopefully, be eliminated in the future.

REFERENCES

1. Daniel, J.: The x-rays, Science, **3**:562, 1896.
2. Desjardins, A. U.: Radiosensitiveness of cells and tissues and some medical implications, Arch. Surg. **25**:926, 1932.
3. Ewing, J.: Radiation osteitis, Acta Radiol. **61**:339, 1926.
4. Gaisford, J., and Rueckert, F.: Osteoradionecrosis of the mandible, Plast. Reconstr. Surg. **18**(6):436, 1956.
5. Hahn, G., and Corgill, D. A.: Conservative treatment of radionecrosis of the mandible, Oral Surg. **24**:707, 1967.
6. Hendee, W. R.: Medical radiation physics, Chicago, 1970, Year Book Medical Publishers, Inc.
7. Hynes, W.: Shaving in plastic surgery with special

reference to the treatment of chronic radiodermatitis, Br. J. Plast. Surg. **12:**43, 1959.

8. Lederman, M.: Megavoltage advances vs. the orthovoltage era, J.A.M.A. **22:**17, 1972.

9. Marino, H.: Biologic excision; its value in the treatment of radionecrotic lesions, Plast. Reconstr. Surg. **40:**180, 1967.

10. Martin, H., Strong, E., and Spiro, R. H.: Radiation-induced skin cancer of the head and neck, Cancer **25:**61, 1970.

11. Mladick, R. A., Horton, C. E., Adamson, J. E., and Cohen, B. I.: Management of catastrophic postoperative breakdown after massive oropharyngeal cancer surgery, Plast. Reconstr. Surg. **49:**316, 1972.

12. Nickell, W. B., Vasconez, L. O., Jurkiewicz, M. J., and Salyer, K. E.: One stage surgical repair of mandibular osteoradionecrosis with jaw preservation, Am. J. Surg. **126:**502, 1973.

13. Regaud, C.: Sur la sensibilite du tissue osseux normal vis-a-vis des radiations x and y et sur le mecanisme de l'osteoradio-necrose, Compt. reud, Soc. de biol., Paris **37:**629, 1922.

14. Reynolds, R. J.: The early history of radiology in Britain, Clin. Radiol. **12:**136, 1961.

15. Rintala, A.: Local radiation burns, Acta Chir. Scand. Suppl. **376:**1, 1967.

16. Stein, J.: Management of bone in the patient before, during, and after treatment for oral cancer, Cancer **18:**269, 1968.

17. Stell, P. M., and Morrison, M. D.: Radiation necroses of the larynx; etiology and management, Arch. Otolaryngol. **98:**111, 1973.

Chapter 12

Combined therapy in the treatment of intraoral cancer

Robert G. Chambers, M.D.

Cancer of the intraoral mucosa continues to be a devastating disease; in its more advanced stages, it is a poor responder to any single modality of therapy. By 1940 both radiation and surgery obviously left much to be desired in the treatment of primary lesions in this region, as well as in the cervical metastases.[4] In 1946 planned combined therapy was instituted; that is, heavy local irradiation given to the primary growth and external irradiation to the nodes was followed in 4 to 6 weeks by radical neck dissection and resection incontinuity of the primary growth. Of this original trial series of 14 patients, 12 (80%) were living and well 3 years later.

It is in the area of the oral mucosa that preoperative irradiation can have the most benefit. Preoperative irradiation seems to add the following advantages: reduction in the size of the primary tumor, diminution of the vitality of the tumor, decrease in the surrounding tissue reaction, and some sealing of the lymphatic channels.[24] The irradiation dosage is a full tumor dose; 5,000 to 6,000 R. In other words, radical radiotherapy is used prior to radical surgery.

Before radiotherapy is instituted, dental hygiene is corrected if necessary, but healthy viable teeth are not sacrificed; radionecrosis should not be a problem if proper care is taken.

Because marked changes in the tumor and adjacent anatomy are produced by the preoperative radiation therapy, the original tumor anatomy and appearance is carefully recorded by photographs, drawings, and detailed description before therapy is started. The subsequent surgical procedure to be performed is planned before therapy starts, and the planned procedure is adhered to in spite of excellent clinical response to irradiation. Irradiation is never given in the hope of making the subsequent operation less radical.

As a rule, tumors vary in their reaction to irradiation according to their cell differentiation.[4] The small- to moderate-sized well-differentiated cancer often is best operated on immediately.[3] Lesions in alcoholics who are heavy smokers are preferably treated whenever possible with surgery because of these individuals' poor tolerance for irradiation. The very old patient with a moderate-sized lesion, usually well differentiated, tolerates a resection far better than a prolonged course of irradiation.[1]

I have personally examined and followed through to death or a tumor-free 5-year survival, 500 private patients between 1947 and 1965 who had carcinoma of the oral cavity. In 1965 all patients having combined therapy received concomitant hydroxyurea therapy. These cases have been reported elsewhere. This therapy seems to be an excellent adjunct, and the study is continuing with gratifying results.

Of the 500 patients studied between 1947 and 1965, 300 had combined therapy and formed the basis of this report. Each patient was evaluated for response to combined therapy by the following criteria.

Location. The primary site of the tumor was listed. The oral mucosa is identified as encompassed in that area between the anterior gingiva and the circumvallate papillae of the tongue. Areas posterior to and including the anterior tonsillar pillar and the base of the tongue are considered pharyngeal cancer.

Lesions of the labial mucosa of the lips are more appropriately discussed as primary lip cancer.

Clinical staging. Clinical staging was based on the clinical staging system for carcinoma of the oral cavity established by the American Joint Committee for Cancer Staging and End Results Reporting.

T   *Primary tumor*
TIS Carcinoma in situ
T1   Tumor 2 cm. or less in greatest diameter
T2   Tumor greater than 2 cm. but not greater than 4 cm. in greatest diameter
T3   Tumor greater than 4 cm. in greatest diameter
N   *Regional lymph nodes*
N0 No clinically palpable cervical lymph node(s); or palpable node(s) but metastasis not suspected
N1 Clinically palpable homolateral cervical lymph node(s) that are not fixed; metastasis suspected
N2 Clinically palpable contralateral or bilateral cervical lymph node(s) that are not fixed; metastasis suspected
M   *Distant metastasis*
M0 No distant metastasis
M1 Clinical and/or radiographic evidence of metastasis other than to cervical lymph nodes

Radiation therapy. All patients received time dose-related cancericidal therapy. The fields were designed to include the primary site of involvement and any regional involvement. Before the availability of cobalt 60 orthovoltage, combined external and intraoral portals were used.

Surgery. Surgical procedures consisted of all varieties of operation, each designed to fit the individual case and staging and meticulously decided on before radiation was started. T1 lesions, unless histologically undifferentiated, were operated on without benefit of preoperative irradiation. Among the 500 patients there were 150 T1 well-differentiated carcinomas and 50 T1 undifferentiated tumors.

Results. Of the 300 patients studied who had combined therapy 150 (50%) survived 5 years or more without tumor recurrence. These figures are absolute and represent unselected cases.

LOCATION OF PRIMARY TUMOR

The locations of the primary tumor as related to survival rates were as follows:

Tongue	50%	(75/150)
Floor of the mouth	70%	(45/55)
Gingiva	65%	(20/30)
Buccal mucosa	50%	(5/9)
Soft palate	38%	(16/41)
Hard palate	40%	(6/15)

Although in some locations the total number of patients is small, each patient had a lesion greater than 2 cm. In other words, each of the 300 patients had a T2 or T3 primary cancer.

If each anatomical site is examined in more detail, the value of combined therapy in more extensive cancers seems more definite.

Tongue. There were 150 patients with primary cancer of the tongue who underwent combined therapy; 75 of these were living and well 5 years later. Survival rates were as follows:

Overall	50%	(75/150)
With clinically palpable nodes	38%	(34/90)
Without clinically palpable nodes	68%	(41/60)

Floor of mouth. In the series of 55 patients with cancer of the floor of the mouth, the results of the original pilot studies were reaffirmed. Survival rates were as follows:

Overall	70%	(40/55)
With palpable nodes	40%	(12/30)
Without palpable nodes	75%	(18/25)

When hydroxyurea is administered concomitantly with the preoperative irradiation, the 5-year overall survival rate increases to 80%.

Gingiva. Thirty patients with true gingival carcinoma were followed; 20 of these (65%) survived 5 years without disease. Survival rates were as follows:

Overall	65%	(20/30)
With palpable nodes	52%	(9/17)
Without palpable nodes	80%	(11/13)

Buccal mucosa. There were only 9 cancers primary to the buccal mucous membrane that were treated by combined therapy. All 9 patients had advanced local disease, and 4 had clinical metastases. Survival rates were as follows:

Overall	50%	(5/9)
With palpable nodes	50%	(2/4)
Without palpable nodes	60%	(3/5)

Palate. A total of 56 patients had a primary palatine carcinoma; 22 of these patients were tumor free 5 years later. Survival rates were as follows:

Overall	38%	(22/56)
Soft palate	38%	(16/41)
With palpable nodes	22%	(2/9)
Without palpable nodes	47%	(14/32)
Hard palate	40%	(6/15)
With palpable nodes	25%	(1/4)
Without palpable nodes	45%	(5/11)

The soft palate is usually treated with irradiation because of the decreased accessibility of this area in the more advanced cases. Both hard and soft palatine cancers in their advanced stages are difficult to encompass adequately with an extirpative operation.

DISCUSSION

It must be realized that no single therapeutic approach is applicable to all forms of cancer in the oral cavity. Several potent agents are at our disposal, which, when properly selected and applied (often concomitantly), can yield a surprising number of good results in many cases. The choice of treatment for any given cancer must depend on the histologic structure of the growth, its situation, and its stage of progress. The intangibles that are often discussed at great length and in an abstract manner—biologic resistance to tumor and biologic response to tumor—can often be surmised with experience. It is most important to consider these intangibles when choosing the appropriate therapy for a patient. It must be remembered that it is of little use to eradicate a patient's cancer if he dies as a result of our therapeutic zeal or is of no use to himself, his family, or society.

Examples of these biologic intangibles are not hard to find. The patient with cancer of the tongue involving the floor of the mouth and mandible and pterygoid fossa of many months' duration but with no evidence of distant spread should be considered to have some resistance to his tumor. He can be expected to respond to practical attempts to eradicate his disease. On the other hand, at times we are confronted with the necessity of choosing proper treatment for the thin-skinned, elderly, light-complected patient. Such a patient too frequently deteriorates rapidly during a course of irradiation, but he would recover quite satisfactorily with a well-planned operative procedure if feasible.

SUMMARY

Survival rates of patients with cancer of the oral cavity who were treated with radiation therapy and surgery have been presented. Combined therapy is of benefit for the advanced lesion. A small, confined cancer in the mouth can easily be eradicated with combined therapy.

REFERENCES

1. Maccomb, W. S., and Fletcher, G. H.: Cancer of the head and neck, Baltimore, 1967, The Williams & Wilkins Co.
2. Powers, W. E., and Palmer, L. A.: Biologic basis of preoperative radiation treatment, Am. J. Roentgenol. Radium Ther. Nucl. Med. **102**(1):176, 1968.
3. Southwick, H. W.: Cancer of the tongue, Surg. Clin. North Am. **53**:(1):147, 1973.
4. Ward, G. E., and Hendrick, J. W.: Tumors of the head and neck, Baltimore, 1950, The Williams & Wilkins Co.

Chapter 13

Tumors of the lip

Tolbert S. Wilkinson, M.D.

Although it is generally understood that squamous cell carcinoma is the most common malignancy of the lip, a number of less well known discrete benign and malignant tumors occur on the lip. Resection and reconstructive principles apply equally to benign and malignant tumors. Resection is indicated for cure in the malignancies and for diagnosis in certain benign lesions since they may closely resemble lip cancer. Certain benign tumors, such as the hemangiomas, must be resected to prevent distortion and destruction of the lip.

SIGNIFICANT TUMORS OF THE LIP
Granular cell myoblastoma

Granular cell myoblastomas are red, pedunculated, smooth-surfaced lesions that occur both on the upper and lower lip.[12,17,18,45] Microscopic examination reveals typical uniform polyhedral, cytophilic granular cells. Myelin figures and granules are similar to those of mast cells.[34] The presence of unmyelinated nerve fibers, virallike particles, and structures resembling degenerated axons lend credence to the theory that these benign neoplasms originate in Schwann cells rather than in mesenchymal elements. Simple excision is curative.

Lipoma

Because of its rarity in the lip, lipoma is seldom considered in differential diagnoses. Intraoral lipomas grow slowly and are usually superficial. In a series of 68 oral lipomas, the majority had been present for over 5 years prior to excision.[39] Although only one case was confined to the central lip, the majority of the intraoral lipomas occur in the buccal mucosa adjacent to the commissure. Simple excision is adequate.

Rhabdomyoma

Rhabdomyomas of the lip are benign, soft, discrete lesions that occur in both the upper and the lower lip. They are extremely rare: only 21 cases have been reported.[46] Simple excision with limited margins is adequate therapy.

Vascular tumors

Capillary and cavernous hemangiomas occur on the upper and the lower lip. They characteristically appear in infancy and grow rapidly. Since the lip is a cosmetically and functionally vital area, early surgical intervention is imperative. Even pure capillary hemangiomas grow to massive size (Fig. 13-1), destroying essential portions of the facial features before regressing. Unlike many capillary tumors, cavernous hemangiomas (Fig. 13-2) rarely regress. The results of steroids administered orally to our patients have been disappointing. Carbon dioxide snow, pinpoint or subcutaneous needle cautery, intralesional sclerosing injections, or staged minor excisions should be initiated in the rapid growth stage. Total resections of less than one fourth of the lip have little morbidity. Staged excisions are preferable for large lesions in children. Excision for diagnosis is occasionally indicated, since malignant hemangioendotheliomas may be mistaken for benign vascular lip tumors.

Hemangiopericytomas are also exceedingly rare in the oral cavity. Only two have been reported in the lip.[25] Hemangiopericytomas are benign, discrete, nodular lesions with a pseudocapsule infiltrated by tumor cells. Local excision is curative.

Sixteen cases of oral vascular leiomyomas have been described in the literature. Three occurred in the lip.[29] Microscopically, irregularly distributed, thick-walled blood vessels with small lumens are

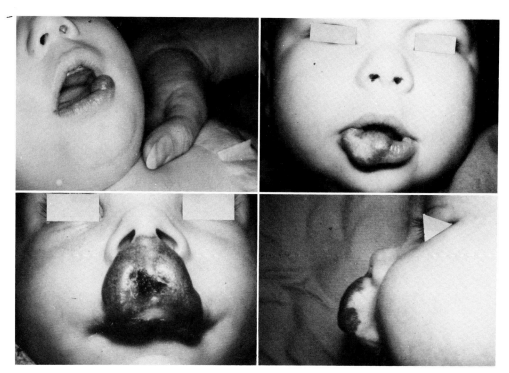

Fig. 13-1. Hemangiomas of the lip, capillary type.

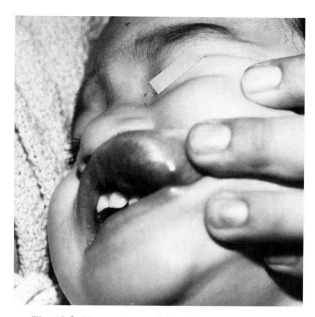

Fig. 13-2. Hemangioma of the lip, cavernous type.

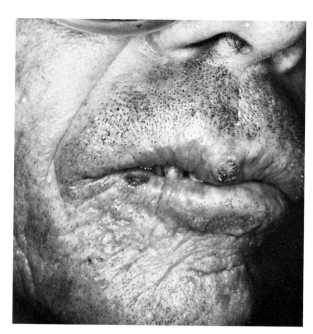

Fig. 13-3. Keratoacanthoma of the upper lip.

characteristic. The muscularis layers are irregularly hypertrophied and hyperplastic. These lesions grow quite slowly and characteristically shrink with exposure to cold. Simple excision is curative.

Odontogenic tumors

Nine cases of "calcifying epithelial odontogenic tumors" have been reported, including a single primary lip tumor.[10] These tumors are believed to be epithelial, arising from the enamel organ of an unerupted tooth. They are characteristically soft and well circumscribed and contain calcium deposits and stromal material that is identified histochemically as amyloid. In the lip the tumor arises from multipotential oral mucosal cells, as have the occasional ameloblastomas found in oral mucosa remote from the teeth. Odontogenic tumors of this type require only simple excision.

Keratoacanthoma

Like squamous carcinoma, keratoacanthomas almost always occur on surfaces constantly exposed to sunlight. Clinically and microscopically, these rapidly growing lesions are initially indistinguishable from squamous carcinoma. As keratinization proceeds, the characteristic central crater forms (Fig. 13-3). Verrucas of the lip may have a similar appearance in early stages (Fig. 13-4). Like squamous carcinoma, keratoacanthoma is three times more common in males.

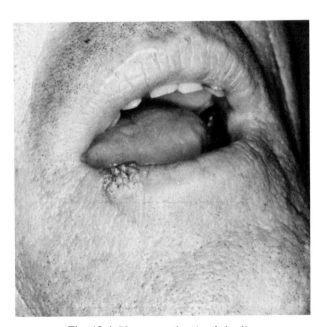

Fig. 13-4. Verruca vulgaris of the lip.

The age group affected is younger than in patients with squamous carcinoma, and keratoacanthoma occurs only one third to one fourth as often as carcinoma. Twelve percent of keratoacanthomas occur on the lip, arising from pilosebaceous follicles at the white roll line.[20] Excisional biopsy is required for diagnosis even in late lesions less likely to be misdiagnosed.

Lymphangioma

Lymphangioma simplex may occur as a single nodule on the lip or as a group of nodules or excrescences. Macrocheilia may result from continuous, untreated growth. Microscopically, there is a profusion of endothelial-lined spaces with loose connective tissue. Simple excision of smaller lesions is curative, but multifocal lesions may require staged excisions and total or subtotal lip reconstruction.

Neurofibroma

Neurofibromas are benign subcutaneous tumors that may occur along peripheral nerves. They originate from Schwann cells and may occur singly or multiply in von Recklinghausen's disease.

The clinical diagnosis of neurofibroma is rarely in doubt, since these lesions are usually multiple and occur in many parts of the body. Lipomas, nevi, and cafe-au-lait spots identify the syndrome. Microscopically, there are interlacing strands of spindle cells with a moderate amount of intercellular collagen and included nerve fibers. Isolated lip neurofibromas seldom require treatment other than simple excision and closure (Fig. 13-5).

Plexiform neurofibromas may involve the lip as part of facial hemihypertrophy (Fig. 13-6) and will require more complex reconstruction and cosmetic procedures.

Pigmented lesions and melanoma

Malignant melanoma of the lip comprises only 0.4% to 1.3% of melanomas.[9,33] The majority of mucosal pigment lesions (junctional, compound, intramucosal, blue nevi, pigmented ephelis, and lentigo) are benign but frequently indistinguishable from early melanoma. In a series of 155 melanotic mucosal lesions, 42 were melanoma. Sixty-five percent of the benign lesions occurred on the lip, whereas only 16.7% of the melanomas were on the lip.[47] One fourth of the malignancies were clinically so benign in appearance that melanoma was not suspected. Oral melanoma is twice as common in men as in women, in contrast to the nearly equal distribution of cutaneous

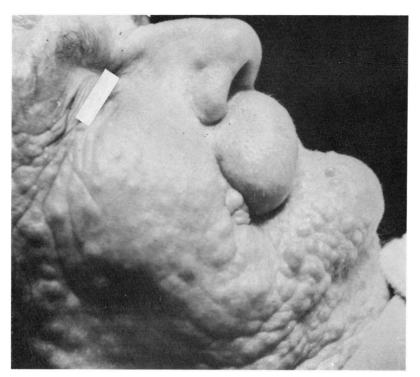

Fig. 13-5. Isolated, enlarging neurofibroma of the lip.

melanoma. Less than one fourth of the malignancies are found in non-Caucasians.[9] Both melanoma and benign pigmented lesions are painless and nonelevated. The benign lesions tend to occur in a younger population, peaking at the third decade, while the melanomas are most frequent in the fifth decade. All pigmented lesions should be excised for pathologic examination and because of the malignant potential of junctional, compound, and blue nevi.[8]

Melanomas of the oral cavity and lips have a marked tendency toward regional and distant spread. Over 50% of the 93 cases reported by Chaudhry[9] metastasized to regional nodes, and 20% exhibited distant metastases. Only 2 of 29 cases followed by Trodahl[47] were free of disease at 5 years, and 22 had died of their disease. Radical surgical excision with en bloc incontinuity elective neck dissection is required.

Minor salivary gland tumors

Salivary gland tumors occur in the minor glands only one tenth to one fifth as often as in the major glands. Both the upper and the lower lip are abundantly supplied with minor salivary glands, primarily

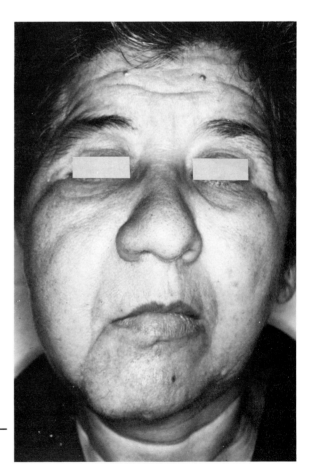

Fig. 13-6. Plexiform neurofibroma with facial hemihypertrophy.

of the mucous-secreting type. The majority of tumors of minor glands are in the palate and cheek, however. All types of salivary tumors are encountered in the minor glands: benign mixed, adenoid cystic, mucoepidermoid, Warthins', adenocarcinoma, and so forth. Some authors reported a preponderance of malignancies,[42,44] and others reported a preponderance of benign tumors.[14,19] From a survey of the literature, Batsakis concluded that benign tumors are as common as malignant ones.[5] Color varies from tan and gray to white. Benign tumors are usually well circumscribed (Fig. 13-7). In a series of 73 primaries reported by Frable and Elzay,[14] only 4 were of lip origin, and all were benign mixed tumors. Hendricks[21] found 1 benign and 1 malignant primary tumor of the lip in a series of 44. The upper lip and buccal mucosa are the second most common sites for benign minor salivary mixed tumors. They rarely occur in the lower lip.

All authors agree that no conclusions as to cell type can be drawn from gross characteristics and that malignancies respond poorly to irradiation. Minor gland masses should be excised with 1- to 2-cm. mucosal margins. Local mucosal rotation flaps may be required for closure.

Overall survival rates for malignant tumors range from 21% to 68%. The adenoid cystic type appears to be most lethal. The decision for elective neck dissection in the absence of palpable nodes should be based on primary lesion size, duration, and cell type. High-grade mucoepidermoid, adenoid cystic, squamous cell, and undifferentiated types are more likely to have metastasized by the time medical consultation is obtained.

Basal cell carcinoma

Basal cell carcinoma accounts for 65% to 75% of cutaneous carcinomas and rarely metastasizes. The majority of metastasizing basal cell carcinomas, however, originate in the head and neck region.[11] Basal cell carcinomas of the lip are almost exclusively found in the upper lip above the vermilion. The male to female ratio for the occurrence of squamous carcinoma of the upper lip is 2:1, compared with 5:1 ratio for the occurrence of squamous carcinoma of the upper lip.[26] All forms of basal cell lesions may be found, from the typical round, pearly bordered lesion to the diffuse, infiltrating morphea type (Fig. 13-8). The characteristic microscopic picture is of nests or lobules of uniform, darkly staining tumor cells with peripheral cells arranged in rows with perpendicular long axes. Mitotic figures are rare.

Superficial lesions may be controlled in over 95% of cases by limited excision or electrodessication and curettage. Response to topical 5-fluorouracil cream has generally been disappointing because of frequent recurrences. Simple excision along facial lines is effective and efficient. Recurrent basal cell carcinomas require lip wedge or further radical excision and frequently require major lip reconstructive procedures.

Metastases from basal cell carcinoma of the upper lip are quite rare, despite the fact that squamous carcinomas of the upper lip metastasize more frequently than squamous carcinomas from the lower

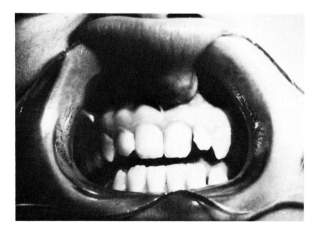

Fig. 13-7. Benign mixed tumor of minor salivary gland.

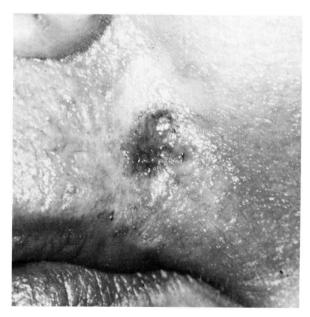

Fig. 13-8. Morpheaform sclerosing basal cell carcinoma.

lip. Only 76 acceptable cases of metastasizing basal cell carcinoma are in the literature.[49] Eighty-five percent of these primary carcinomas were located in the head and neck. Only one case originated in the upper lip. Causative factors are unknown, but only 12 of 47 cases with metastases reported by Conway and Hugo[11] were not originally treated by irradiation, and 3 of these 12 were basal cell carcinomas arising in irradiated skin. Long duration of the primary carcinoma was also characteristic. Surprisingly, 32% of the cases developed distant metastases. In the absence of evidence of distant metastases, therapeutic radical neck dissection can be expected to improve the survival rate.

Adenoid–squamous cell carcinoma

Adenoid–squamous cell carcinoma is a rare and less malignant variety of squamous cell carcinoma. In a series of 213 of these lesions, 144 occurred in the head and neck region. Only 3 cases developed metastases.[23] In a group of 15 adenoid–squamous cell carcinomas confined to the lip, only 3 occurred on the upper lip. The remainder were in the more solar-exposed lower lip. All were preceded by senile keratoses, and none developed metastases.[22] Grossly, these are ulcerative or exophytic growths, varying in color from pink to red or brown. Microscopically, there are characteristic ductlike epithelial islands whose lumens are lined by cuboidal cells and filled with dyskeratotic cells. Age and sex distribution are similar to squamous cell carcinoma, and the majority of patients are light complected. Excision with margins that are wider than usual seems indicated by the report of a 38% recurrence rate in lip primary carcinomas.[22] Elective neck dissections are not required.

Squamous cell carcinoma

Squamous cell carcinoma is the most common "true" vermilion carcinoma. It is primarily a disease of the lower lip of elderly men but may occur at any age (Fig. 13-9). In a review of 3,166 cases, Mackay[26] found a 79:1 male to female ratio for the occurrence of lower lip primary carcinomas. Upper lip primary carcinomas tend to grow more rapidly and metastasize earlier, but only 3% of carcinomas found in men occurred on the upper lip. By contrast, 28% of primary carcinomas found in women were on the upper lip. Only 0.4% to 2% of patients have primary carcinomas on both lips.[6]

Carcinoma is frequently preceded by the development of leukoplakia or hyperplastic cheilitis (Fig.

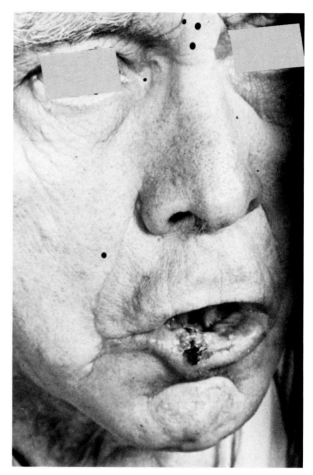

Fig. 13-9. Typical exophytic squamous cell carcinoma.

13-10). In Caucasians, lip carcinoma occurs most often in light-complected individuals with a history of long sunlight exposure. The fact that leukoplakia and squamous cell carcinoma occur infrequently in blacks is attributed to the thicker, more opaque stratum corneum and more pigmented mucosal stratum germinativum. Only 4 of 835 cases investigated by Bernier and Mardelle[6] were non-Caucasian.

The cancer-producing spectrum of solar irradiation, 2,900°-3,400°, is filtered by a combination of keratin layer thickness and pigmentation. Albinos have normal-thickness stratum corneum yet have a high incidence of skin carcinomas. Sunlight is not the only etiologic agent implicated, however.[22,15] Chronic chelitis, hyperkeratosis, leukoplakia, and Bowenoid hyperplasia are mucosal responses to a number of irritative agents, including tobacco, local heat, and local trauma. All should be considered

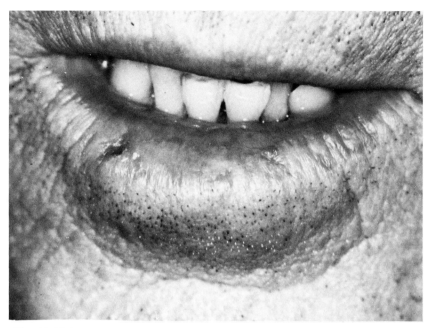

Fig. 13-10. Infiltrating squamous cell carcinoma in leukoplakia of the lower lip.

manifestations of a tendency toward malignant degeneration of the entire exposed vermilion. Approximately 50% of patients with frank carcinoma have evidence of leukoplakia in adjacent or distant mucosa, and an average of 30% of patients with leukoplakia develop carcinoma.[24,43] Successive primary carcinomas develop in 5% to 13.8% of patients who have had simple excision of lip carcinomas.[26,37] The entire lip should be resurfaced at the time that a primary tumor of the lip is excised.[4]

Histologically, squamous cell carcinomas may present all grades of dyskeratosis, from leukoplakia to Broder's Grade IV anaplasia. In the majority of series, one half are Grade II, and less than 2% are Grade III and IV. Mitotic figures, epithelial pearl formations, and keratinization of individual cells are hallmarks (Figs. 13-11 and 13-12).

There are three classic types of squamous cell carcinoma: the exophytic, the ulcerating, and the infiltrating. Superficial surface spread is found more often than deep invasion. Over 90% are Broder's Grade I and II.[13]

Less common are the giant verrucous carcinomas (Fig. 13-13) and diffuse carcinomas of the lip. The former are more indolent and respond more favorably to irradiation. The latter, comprising 2% of Ashley's series,[1] metastasize frequently and have a poorer prognosis.

The lip mucosa is a transitional tissue, intermediate between true epithelium and true squamous cell mucosa. It is especially important to distinguish lesions at the commissures as "lip" or "oral" since the behavior of lip tumors also reflects the transitional nature of their origin. Lip carcinomas metastasize less frequently than intraoral squamous cancers but more frequently than cutaneous squamous cell cancers.

In 2,696 patients with carcinoma of the lip reported by Mahoney,[27] 14% were considered to have cervical metastases at some time during their treatment. Forty-eight percent of these metastases were operable. Other authors report an incidence of positive nodes of 6% to 15.5%[1,2] at the time of initial examination. The size of the primary carcinoma may influence the rate of metastasis. Primary carcinomas less than 1 cm. in diameter have had a 3% metastasis rate, compared with 8% for 2- to 3-cm. lesions and 16% for lesions larger than 3 cm.[28] Progression to Stage III is uncommon. Backus and DeFelice reviewed 6 authors' reports of 2,335 patients with negative lymph nodes at the time of initial examination. Delayed metastases occurred in only 4% to 9% of the patients.[2]

There are no truly reliable guidelines for elective neck dissection. Elective neck dissection in the absence of palpable nodes is not indicated, since only

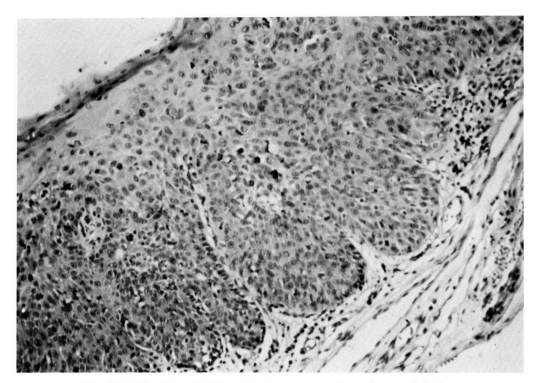

Fig. 13-11. Typical well-differentiated squamous cell carcinoma of the lip.

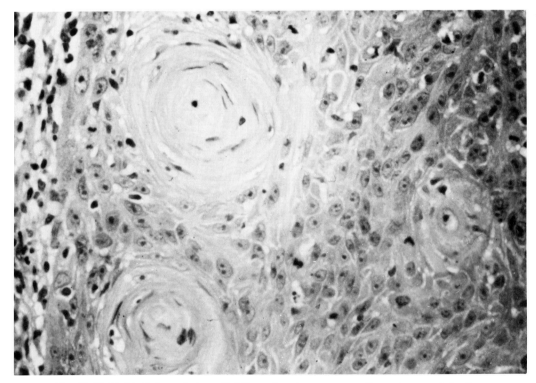

Fig. 13-12. Epithelial pearls in well-differentiated squamous cell carcinoma of the lip.

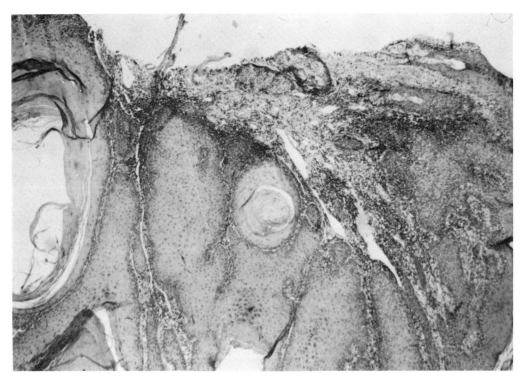

Fig. 13-13. Verrucous squamous cell carcinoma of the lip.

about 1 out of 16 patients would benefit. Poorly differentiated tumors, diffuse infiltrating tumors, and large tumors tend to metastasize more frequently, as do lesions that have been present for many years. Overall, only around 6% of patients develop metastasis after control of the primary tumor, and even at this point there is a high survival rate. Mackay[26] found that local excision controlled the primary tumor effectively in 84% of 3,166 patients.

Clinically positive nodes are present at the time of initial examination in 6% to 16% of patients. Five-year survival rates in the presence of involved nodes are reported in the range of 31% to 58%.[1,2,26] Recurrence following neck dissection in Mahoney's series occurred after both upper cervical and complete neck dissections, although only one half as frequently in the latter.[27] Recurrences after complete neck dissection were in the contralateral superior cervical nodes only. Ashley reported a 90% 5-year survival rate by surgery of patients with postsurgical recurrences and a 60% survival rate of patients with postirradiation recurrences.[1]

Surgery is preferable to irradiation of primary lesions for a number of reasons other than survival rates. Practically identical cure rates in the range of 95% are obtained by both methods when primary lesions are small and superficial. Larger lesions respond less favorably. Ashley reported that 87% of surgically treated patients were free of disease at 5 years, compared with 77% of the irradiated group.[1] When irradiation is applied to larger lesions, the resultant defect requires operative reconstruction. One sacrifices the security of pathologic confirmation of margins and the opportunity of discarding the remaining damaged and precancerous mucosa. Continued solar irradiation to an irradiated lip leads to development of secondary and multiple primary tumors in the region. There are no reports of new primary tumors in resurfaced lips. An additional consideration is the effect of a postirradiation scar on lip mobility. Pain, immobility, and scar breakdown are significant complications.

In summary, neck dissection in the absence of clinically positive nodes is seldom indicated. Each course of therapy should be planned according to the individual case, with size, duration, and degree of anaplasia of the primary lesion, as well as its relation to the midline, taken into account.

RECONSTRUCTION OF THE LIP

The techniques used for lip reconstruction today are distillates of centuries of experience in lip surgery. Three thousand years ago the "Indian" forehead flap was devised for lip reconstruction. The V excision was performed at the time of Celsus in 25 b.c. The "Italian," or Tagliocozzi, method of arm pedicle flaps to the lip was in common usage in 1579. Blasius, Lisfranc, Sedillot, Lexer, and Burow all contributed innovations in upper lip reconstruction in the 1800's. Zeiss, Adelmann, Serre, Nelaton, Ombredanne, Dieffenback, and others devised methods for lower lip reconstruction during this period. The early reconstructions supplied skin and subcutaneous tissue but omitted mucosal lining. In 1785 Chopart advanced cheek flaps of this type, but it was not until 1855 that Alquie modified this procedure by adding mucosal flaps, beginning the present era of surgical techniques. Modern reconstructive techniques are designed to restore contour, color, and function by transfer of skin, muscle, and mucosa.

Generally, most lip losses can be reconstructed with local flaps of skin and muscle of the cheek and mucosa or tongue for lining. Larger losses are rebuilt with distant tissue, with the use of forehead, deltopectoral, or other pedicled flaps with fascial slings or other supports to counteract the effect of gravity on the new lower lip.

Basic flap techniques

Mucosal flaps. The majority of mucosal defects are a result of lip shave procedures and can be remedied by sulcal undermining and mucosal advancement. Local lateral or inferior advancement or rotation flaps suffice for small deficits. When greater bulk is required, the Joseph sulcal rotation flap or the Shutten bipedicled flap of the wet mucosa and submucosa from the opposite lip may be employed. Single pedicle Abbe mucosal and the Millard fleur-de-lis cross lip flaps[31] are useful modifications of the limited lip switch type. Donor sites of the mucosal flaps are closed by local mobilization or inlay split skin grafts.

Abbe-Estlander flaps. The composite pedicle Abbe-Estlander lip switch flap and its several modifications are improvements of the procedure first described by Sabattini in 1838. A V flap of vermillion, skin, white roll, and muscle were transferred on a labial artery pedicle. In 1863 Buck expanded the applications of the lip switch flap and refined the technique. Estlander devised the commissure rotation flap in 1877, and in 1898 Abbe popularized his lip switch flap for cleft lip repairs. Today all of these modifications, either from upper to lower or lower to upper, are referred to as Abbe (midlip) or Estlander

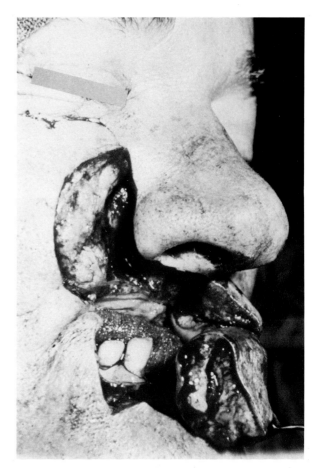

Fig. 13-14. Reconstruction of the upper lip with a W Abbe-Estlander flap after excision of recurrent basal cell carcinoma.

(commissure) or as Abbe-Estlander flaps for convenience (see Figs. 13-17, *C* and *D*, and 13-18, *C*). The original V flap should be designed as a W when the lower lip is used to rebuild the upper one so that the donor scar may be easily hidden in the dental lines (Fig. 13-14).

Cosmetically, there is no better way of rebuilding lip losses if over 2 cm. of lip remain after excisions. Transferring one fourth or even one third of the donor lip in two stages to repair a defect does not leave a debilitating microstomia. The single-stage Estlander corner rotation flap is actually also a two-staged procedure, since the rounded shortened commissure that results must be enlarged to restore symmetry of the lips. Double Abbe flaps that balance the resections of the donor lip were described by Stein in 1848 and modified by Kazanjian. Bowers[7] carried the Stein-Kazanjian concept one step further by using double quadrangular flaps taken from the

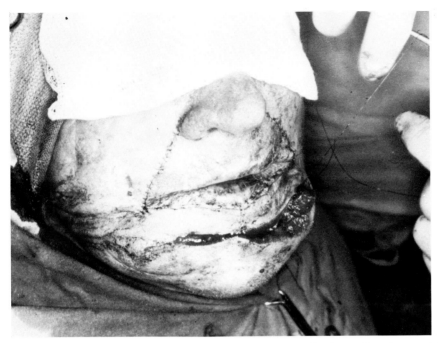

Fig. 13-15. Bilateral nasolabial flaps used to reconstruct the lower lip after excision of a large but superficial subvermilion basal cell carcinoma.

philtral lines (see Fig. 13-18, *C*). This method prevents disruption of lateral nerve and blood supply to the major portion of the remaining upper lip and is cosmetically superior by virtue oft he two vertical philtral line scars.

Transplanted lip flaps regain motor and sensory innervation. Muscle contraction and sweating are reestablished, and the sensations of pain, touch, and temperature differentiation are regained to nearly normal levels in 12 months.[40,41]

Nasolabial flaps. Single or bilateral skin, subcutaneous tissue, muscle, and mucosal flaps may be based inferiorly or superiorly along the nasolabial line for reconstruction of the upper or lower lip (Figs. 13-15 and 13-17, *B*). When mucosa of the lip has not been totally sacrificed, these flaps carry sufficient buccal mucosa to supply most deficits.[38] The cosmetic aspect of the donor site scar makes these flaps quite acceptable, but facial nerve branches and blood supply to the philtral area are divided. Reinnervation occurs rapidly with reestablishment of the oral sphincteric action, and the abundant vascularity of the subnasal area compensates for the interruption

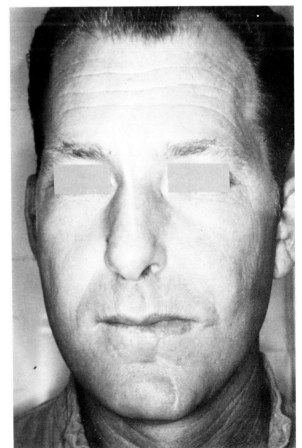

Fig. 13-16. Reconstruction of the lower lip by a modification of the Camille-Bernard method.

of the blood supply. When there is a paucity of mucosa or of bulk in the reconstructed vermilion, nasolabial flaps may be augmented by tongue flaps. Bilateral nasolabial flaps may be so designed that one supplies internal lining for the opposite flap, which supplies external cover (see Fig. 13-18). In 1942 Ferris Smith described a widely based nasolabial flap that has limited applications but may be of value in certain deformities. A delayed flap is turned on itself for lining and is covered by the necessarily widely based nasolabial flap. Because of hair growth, neither

the Ferris Smith nor the double inside-outside nasolabial flaps should be used in men.

Quadrilateral cheek flaps. Sedillot in 1848 and Denonvilliers in 1863 designed square cheek rotation flaps for upper lip reconstruction. Similar flaps for the lower lip were designed by Blasius in 1839 and by Von Bruns in 1859. The Gillies "fan" flap of 1957 is a direct descendant of these earlier ones, modified by elongation of the lateral superior corner and incorporation of a Z-plasty in the inferior closure. Large rectangular flaps of the Dieffenbach (1834) type

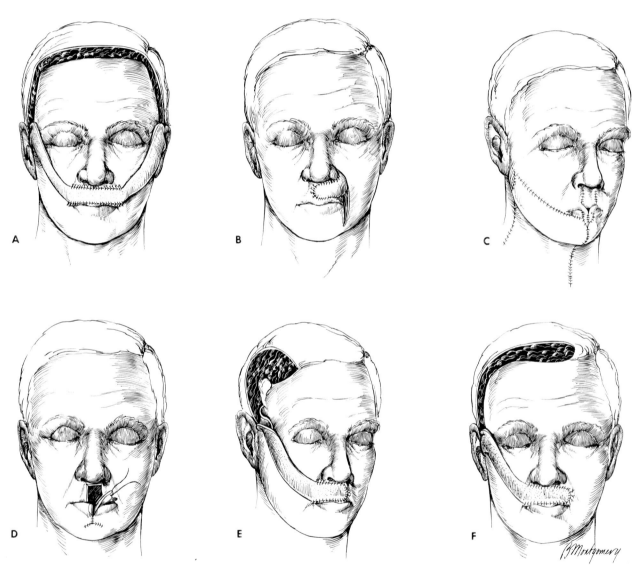

Fig. 13-17. **A,** Double pedicle forehead flap for upper lip reconstruction of skin and vermilion edge. **B,** Superiorly based nasolabial flap. **C,** Converse modification of Dieffenbach cheek flaps utilizing Stein lip flaps centrally. **D, W** Abbe flap for repair of central defects of the upper lip. **E,** Sickle-type scalp and forehead flap for reconstruction of the upper lip. **F,** Temporal artery scalp and forehead flap for reconstruction of the upper lip.

have been modified by May (1941) and Padget (1941). These flaps are based on the facial artery and vein. The defect left by their medial rotation can be filled by mobilization of a masseter muscle flap. Lip switch flaps, single or double, can be added to fill the central portion of the lower lip (see Fig. 13-17, *C*). All of these flaps function poorly and are cosmetically inferior to other methods of lower lip reconstruction.

Camille-Bernard flaps. The Camille-Bernard lateral advancement flap of 1881 was an improvement

of Burow's 1855 technique of lateral advancement. Both methods utilized buccal mucosal flaps to cover the lateral portion of the new lower lip. Modifications by Webster[48] and Freeman[16] have resulted in the most acceptable method in use today for reconstruction of subtotal losses of the lower lip (Fig. 13-16).

Lateral advancement flaps are developed by incisions from each commissure to a junction with a line paralleling the curve of the nasolabial groove. Tissue between this line and the groove is excised to

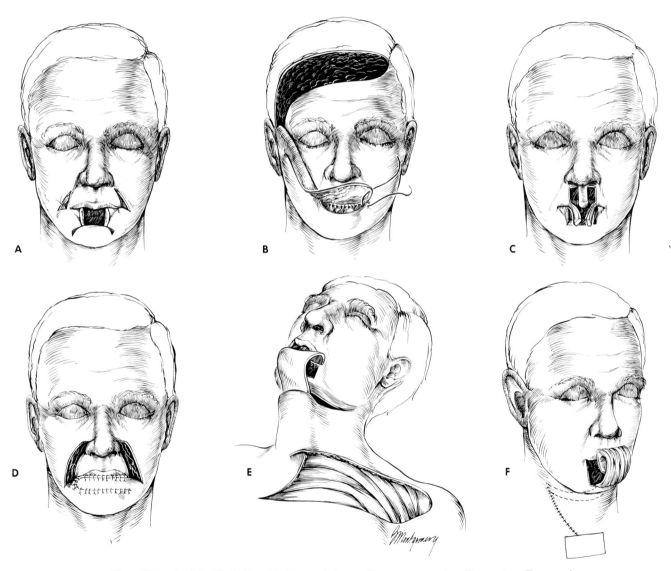

Fig. 13-18. A, Modified Camille-Bernard lower lip reconstruction illustrating Freeman's myoplastic technique (right commissure). **B,** Temporal artery scalp and forehead flap for reconstruction of the lining and external cover of the upper lip. **C,** Double Abbe flaps in philtral lines.[7] **D,** Inside-outside inferiorly based nasolabial flaps. **E,** Deltopectoral flap for lip and mandible reconstruction.[3] **F,** Skin-sternomastoid flap for reconstruction of the oral lining and lip bulk.[35]

allow advancement of the lip flaps. The lower edge of the flaps are formed by incisions that curve from the edge of the defect below the mandible and are parallel to the body of the mandible, including the ramus mandibularis branch of the facial nerve in the flap. The commissure may be re-created by Freeman's myoplastic technique of mobilizing and incorporating orbicularis oris and buccal musculature into a bundle (see Fig. 13-18, *A*). Mucosa for the lateral new lower lip can be obtained by the classic inferiorly based buccal mucosal flaps or by tongue flaps.[30]

Distant pedicle flaps. Local flaps are generally preferable to distant tissue flaps with various pedicles, but these more complex methods of lip reconstruction may be necessary in certain instances.

The various *forehead flaps* may be designed with single or double pedicles for rebuilding the upper or the lower lip. Generally, these flaps are narrower than the usual forehead flap and are tubed at the time of transfer. Flaps taken from the edge of the hairline (Figs. 13-17, *A*, and 13-18, *B*) reconstruct bearded areas and hairless skin adjacent to the vermillion. This is particularly useful when the flap is used for lining as well as external cover. Mucosal grafts or skin grafts may be substituted for oral lining prior to or at the time of transfer. Scalp flaps based on the superficial temporal vessels may be similarly designed (Figs. 13-17, *E* and *F*, and 13-18, *B*).

Advancement flaps from the cervical area are attached to the lower lip, with the neck in flexion. When the flap is released horizontally below the mandible, a split graft is applied to fill the defect transferred from the lip to the neck.

Sternomastoid-skin neck flaps may be employed as in Owen's design[36] or as a muscular island as described by O'Brien.[35] The former is a skin-lined flap incorporating the muscle, which is rotated externally to cover buccal and lateral lip defects. The latter is a true muscle island that is passed subcutaneously with its distal island of skin to form the anterior lower lip (Fig. 13-18, *F*).

For massive skin and soft tissue losses of the face that include lip losses, larger distant flaps must be utilized. One of the more reliable of these flaps is the *deltopectoral flap,* which Bakamjian[3] has utilized to cover many areas of the head and neck. Folded upon itself, the deltopectoral flap is ideal for supplying oral and external surfaces of a lower lip, including a reconstructed mandible if necessary.[32] (Fig. 13-18, *E*).

Other distant pedicle flaps incorporating cervical, pectoral, thoracoepigastric, or other tubed flaps are seldom preferable to the methods previously outlined.

REFERENCES

1. Ashley, F. L., McConnell, D. V., Machida, R., Sterling, H. E., Galloway, D., and Grazer, F.: Carcinoma of the lip; a comparison of five year results after irradiation and surgical therapy, Am. J. Surg. **110:** 549-551, 1965.
2. Backus, L. H., and Defelice, C. A.: Five year end results in epidermoid carcinoma of the lip with indications for neck dissection, Plast. Reconstr. Surg. **17:** 58-63, 1956.
3. Bakamjian, V.: A technique for primary reconstruction of the palate, Plast. Reconstr. Surg. **31:**103-117, 1963.
4. Barton, M., Spira, M., and Hardy, S. B.: An improved method for "V" excision of the lip combined with vermillionectomy, Plast. Reconstr. Surg. **33:**471-473, 1964.
5. Batsakis, J. G.: Neoplasms of the minor and lesser major salivary glands, Surg. Gynecol. Obstet. **135:** 289-298, 1972.
6. Bernier, J. L., and Mardelle, L. C.: Squamous cell carcinoma of the lip, Milit. Surg. **109:**379-405, 1951.
7. Bowers, D. G.: Double cross lip flap for lower lip reconstruction, Plast. Reconstr. Surg. **47:**209-214, 1971.
8. Brenner, M. D., and Harrison, B. D.: Intraoral blue nevus, Oral Surg. **28:**326-330, 1969.
9. Chaudhry, A. P., Hampel, A., and Gorlin, R. J.: Primary malignant melanoma of the oral cavity, Cancer **11:**923-928, 1958.
10. Cole, F. M., and Jones, A. W.: Odontogenic tumors of the lip, J. Clin. Pathol. **20:**585-588, 1967.
11. Conway, H., and Hugo, N. E: Metastatic basal cell carcinoma, Am. J. Surg. **110:**620-624, 1965.
12. Eversoles, L. R., and Sabes, W R.: Granular sheath cell lesions, Oral Surg. **29:**867-871, 1971.
13. Figi, F. A.: Epithelioma of the lower lip, Surg. Gynecol. Obstet. **59:**810-819, 1934.
14. Frable, W. J., and Elzay, R. P.: Tumors of minor salivary glands; a report of 73 cases, Cancer **25:**932-941, 1970.
15. Freeman, B. S.: Early recognition and surgical treatment of carcinoma of the lip, Am. Surg. **21:**962-968, 1955.
16. Freeman, B. S.: Myoplastic modification of the Bernard cheiloplasty, Plast. Reconstr. Surg. **21:**453-460, 1958.
17. Gerancis, J. C., Komorowski, R. A., and Kuzma, J. F.: Granular cell myoblastoma, Cancer **25:**542-550, 1970.
18. Goldberg, A. F.: Granular cell myoblastomas, Oral Surg. **29:**291-293, 1971.
19. Gore, D. O., Annamunthodo, H., and Harland, A.: Tumors of salivary gland origin, Surg. Gynecol. Obstet. **119:**1290-1296, 1964.
20. Hardman, F. G.: Keratocanthoma of the lips, Br. J. Oral Surg. **9:**46-53, 1971.
21. Hendricks, J. W.: The treatment of tumors of minor salivary glands, Surg. Gynecol. Obstet. **118:**101-114, 1964.
22. Jacoway, J. R., Nelson, J. F., and Boywers, R. C.: Adenoid squamous cell carcinoma of the oral labial

processes; a clinicopathologic study of 15 cases, Oral Surg. **32**:444-449, 1971.

23. Johnson, W. C., and Helwig, E. B.: Adenoid squamous cell carcinoma, a clinicopathologic study of 155 patients, Cancer **19**:1639-1650, 1966.

24. Klutsch, W. P., and Tarico, A.: Cancer and leukoplakia of the lip, Nebr. Med. J. **54**:458-470, 1969.

25. Kopp, W. K., and Kresburg, H.: Hemangiopericytoma of the lip, N. Y. State J. Med. **36**:409-410, 1970.

26. Mackay, E. N., and Sellars, A. H.: A statistical review of carcinoma of the lip, Can. Med. Assoc. J. **90**:670-672, 1964.

27. Mahoney, L. J.: Resection of cervical lymph nodes in cancer of the lip, Can. J. Surg. **12**:40-43, 1969.

28. Martin, H. E., McComb, W. S., and Blady, J. V.: Cancer of the lip, Ann. Surg. **114**:226-242, 1941.

29. McGowan, D. A., and Jones, J. H.: Vascular leiomyoma of the oral cavity, Oral Surg. **27**:649-652, 1969.

30. McGregor, I. A.: The tongue flap in lip surgery, Br. J. Plast. Surg. **19**:253-263, 1966.

31. Millard, D. R.: A lip fleur-de-lis flap. Plast. Reconstr. Surg. **34**:34-35, 1964.

32. Mladick, R. A., Georgiade, N. G., and Royer, J.: Immediate flap reconstruction for massive shotgun wound of the face, Plast. Reconstr. Surg. **45**:186-188, 1970.

33. Moore, E. S., and Martin, H.: Melanoma of the upper respiratory tract and oral cavity, Cancer **8**:1167-1176, 1955.

34. Moskovic, E. A., and Azar, H. A.: Multiple granular cell tumors, Cancer **20**:2032-2047, 1967.

35. O'Brien, B.: A muscle-skin pedicle for total reconstruction of the lower lip, Plast. Reconstr. Surg. **45**:395-399, 1970.

36. Owens, N.: A compound neck pedicle designed for the repair of massive facial defects, Plast. Reconstr. Surg. **15**:369-398, 1955.

37. Paletta, F. X., Coldwater, K., and Booth, F.: The treatment of leukoplakia and carcinoma in setic of the lower lip, Ann. Surg. **145**:74-80, 1957.

38. Pierce, G. W., and O'Connor, G. B.: A new method of reconstruction of the lip, Arch. Surg. **28**:317-334, 1934.

39. Shapiro, D. N.: Lipoma of the oral cavity, Oral Surg. **27**:571-576, 1969.

40. Smith, J. W.: The anatomic and physiologic acclimatization of tissue transplanted by the lip switch technique, Plast. Reconstr. Surg. **26**:40-45, 1960.

41. Smith, J. W: Clinical experience with the vermillion bordered lip flap, Plast. Reconstr. Surg **27**:527-543, 1961.

42. Smith, L. C., Lane, N., and Rankow, R. M.: Cylindroma (adenoid cystic carcinoma); a Report of 58 Cases, Am. J. Surg. **110**:519-526, 1965.

43. Spira, M., and Hardy, S. B.: Vermillionectomy—review of cases with variations in technique, Plast. Reconstr. Surg. **33**:39-46, 1964.

44. Stuteville, O. H., and Corley, R. D.: Surgical management of tumors of intraoral minor salivary glands, Cancer **18**:1578-1586, 1967.

45. Syers, C. S., and Keen, R. R.: Granular cell myoblastoma occurring on the upper lip, Oral Surg. **27**:143-144, 1969.

46. Tandler, B., Rossi, E. P., Stein, M., and Matt, M. M.: Rhabdomyoma of the lip; light and electron microscopic observations, Arch. Pathol. **89**:118-127, 1970.

47. Trodahl, J. N., and Sprague, W. G.: Benign and malignant melanocytic lesions of the oral mucosa, Cancer **25**:812-823, 1970.

48. Webster, R. C., Coffey R. J., and Kelleher, K. E.: Total and partial reconstruction of the lower lip with innervated muscle bearing flaps, Plast. Reconstr. Surg. **25**:360-371, 1960.

49. Wermuth, B. M., and Fajardo, L. F.: Metastatic basal cell carcinoma. Arch. Pathol. **90**:458-462, 1970.

Chapter 14

Reconstruction of the nose after surgery for cancer

Ray A. Elliott, Jr., M.D.

The loss of nasal tissue for which reconstructive surgery is required may be caused by congenital malformation, infection, trauma, or neoplasm. This chapter deals with the repair of defects created by the surgical treatment of cancer, but many of the principles and techniques discussed have a more general application.

Most of the malignancies of the nose arise in the skin. They are predominantly basal cell cancers, but there is an incidence of squamous cell cancer as well.[8] Metastasis to regional lymph nodes is rare. Wide local excision affords an excellent prognosis; therefore, reconstruction of the defect is seldom delayed.

Squamous cell cancer occasionally arises in the nasal and paranasal cavities. The prognosis is less favorable than that of similar lesions of cutaneous origin. These lesions are often poorly differentiated, are frequently far advanced when first diagnosed, and show a greater tendency to metastasize to regional lymph nodes.[11] In this small group it is advisable to delay any major reconstruction for at least 6 months to a year.

SELECTION OF REPAIR METHOD

The primary objective in a surgical plan for treatment of a patient with cancer is complete excision of the tumor with a wide margin of normal tissue. The position and function of the nose requires additional objectives of cosmetic and functional rehabilitation. Results are likely to be better if one surgeon is qualified to plan as well as perform the tumor excision and the reconstruction. The surgeon's armamentarium of reconstructive techniques must be broad enough to eliminate any compromise with tumor margins.

General factors

The surgeon must consider the patient's age, general health, social motivation, and desire to be rehabilitated. The patient's economic situation and the amount of time he can allow for reconstruction are also important.

Specific factors

The extent and type of tissue loss, the condition of remaining tissue, and the characteristics of available donor sites will affect the selection of the repair method. Scars from previous injury, surgery, or radiation may prevent the safe use of remaining tissues or usual donor sites. The donor site must yield sufficient material to restore the defect, and the plan for its transfer must be safe, yet expeditious. The reconstructed nasal cover must be free of hair, and it should afford a reasonable match of skin color and texture. Furthermore, if the thickness of transferred tissue approximates that of the defect, the necessity for additional defatting operations will be avoided.

Principles of reconstruction

The principle of restoring tissue defects with tissue similar to that which was lost is generally sound. However, there are exceptions. A defect in the nasal lining, for example, may be more readily repaired by a free graft or pedicle of skin than by a mucous membrane transplant.[1] Properly selected soft tissues

80

may give a satisfactory cosmetic and functional result in some cases of deep loss involving the supporting structures, thus obviating the discomfort, increased operating time, and potential problems inherent in the use of autogenous grafts of bone or cartilage.

It is generally accepted that the nearer the donor site is to the defect, the better the cosmetic and functional effect will be.[10] When the reconstruction requires a pedicle graft or flap, much time may be saved by the proximity of acceptable tissue.

The deformity of exposed donor sites must be minimal. The very best nasal reconstruction will not be acceptable to the patient if it has created a new gross deformity in an exposed area. The prominence of the nose as a central feature and the superiority of adjacent donor sites may justify the use of tissue

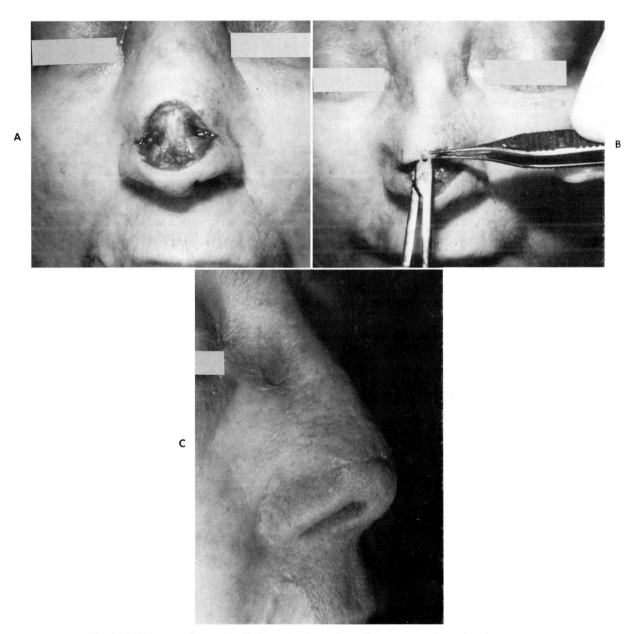

Fig. 14-1. Primary closure. **A,** Defect after lateral cartilages were trimmed and mucosa was closed. **B,** Extensive undermining. **C,** One month after primary closure and tip elevation.

from exposed areas, but the advantages and disadvantages must be carefully weighed and the anticipated deformity explained to the patient before the operation.

PRIMARY CLOSURE

The thickness and relative immobility of the skin over the lower one half of the nose sharply limits the use of primary closure in the alar region to repair defects resulting from the excision of small lesions. Occasionally in older patients a large midline defect of the tip can be closed primarily by mobilization of the remaining nasal cover and elevation of the tip (Fig. 14-1). When the malignancy involves the thin, mobile skin overlying the nasal bones or lateral cartilages, defects measuring up to a centimeter in diameter can sometimes be closed primarily without appreciable deformity; however, flaps of nasal tissue are used for the repair of the majority of these defects.

Planned incisions and lines of closure should follow the dynamic "wrinkle lines" of the skin whenever possible.[7] Most primary closures are accomplished

without undermining, and wounds are closed with a single layer of fine, interrupted sutures. Tumor margins must never be compromised to obtain a primary closure.

FREE GRAFTS

The defect created by the excision of a superficial lesion on the upper portion of the nose may be repaired satisfactorily with a free skin graft, preferably a full-thickness graft. Composite grafts of skin and fat, skin and cartilage, or skin, fat, and cartilage have been more popular for the repair of defects on the lower portion of the nose.

Split-thickness grafts

Skin grafts from remote donor sites seldom afford a good color match, and some shrinkage of these grafts is routine. They are preferred for secondary closure of granulating wounds and for a temporary cover when the adequacy of tumor excision is in question or the definitive reconstruction is delayed. Split grafts also serve well for the repair of some defects in the nasal lining, where color match is of no

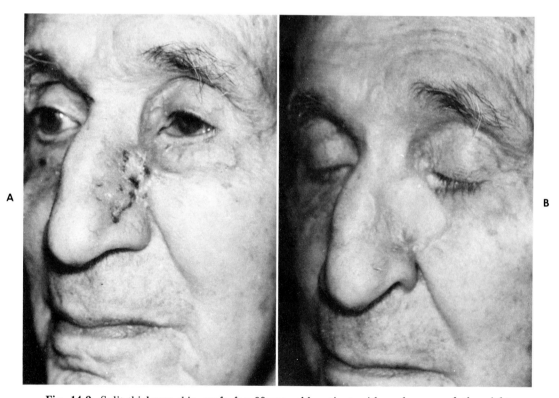

Fig. 14-2. Split-thickness skin graft for 88-year-old patient with melanoma of the right cheek and basal cell cancer of the nose and left cheek. **A,** Extensive superficial cancer. **B,** Four months after expedious graft coverage; color match was poor.

consequence. In unhealthy elderly patients with extensive defects of the nasal cover, their selection over full-thickness grafts or flaps may be justified for expeditious simplicity (Fig. 14-2).

Full-thickness skin grafts

For the repair of larger defects of the thin cover overlying the lateral cartilages and nasal bones, full-thickness grafts are often chosen if conditions are suitable for their survival. They will not survive over bare bone or cartilage.

These grafts are cut from the upper eyelid, post-auricular, or supraclavicular donor sites to afford the best match of color, texture, and thickness (Fig. 14-3). The quantity of available skin, which varies with the age of the patient, will often dictate the final choice. Surprising amounts of skin may be obtained from these donor sites in older patients.

Full-thickness grafts are seldom used on the lower portion of the nose, because they do not provide sufficient thickness or satisfactory texture for replacement of the thicker, sebaceous skin of this region.

Composite grafts

The use of free composite grafts from the ear has been advocated for the repair of small, deep losses about the ala, tip of the nose, and columella.[4] When the repair requires a cover, supporting structure, and lining, grafts with two surfaces of skin and intervening cartilage or fat are used. Flat grafts consisting of a single layer of skin and fat may be used to restore deep cover defects, but their patchlike appearance is a disadvantage (Fig. 14-4).

The composite graft must be brought into contact with a good, minute blood supply, and no portion of the graft should be farther than 1.0 cm. from the nearest blood supply. The technical suggestions of Davenport and Bernard[3] may improve the take of these grafts, but loss of volume, morbidity, and total loss still occur.

FLAPS OF NASAL TISSUE

Flaps of nasal tissue are chosen for the repair of nasal defects whenever the donor site can be closed primarily without a conspicuous deformity. Well-designed flaps will carry an adequate blood supply for their survival over bare bone and cartilage, and they afford an ideal match of color, texture, and thickness.[5]

Banner and bilobed flaps

The banner flap can be used on all areas of the dorsal nasal cover, even for repair of defects on the troublesome thick sebaceous lower portion (Fig. 14-5). A vertical banner flap from the border of the columella may be sufficient for the reconstruction of

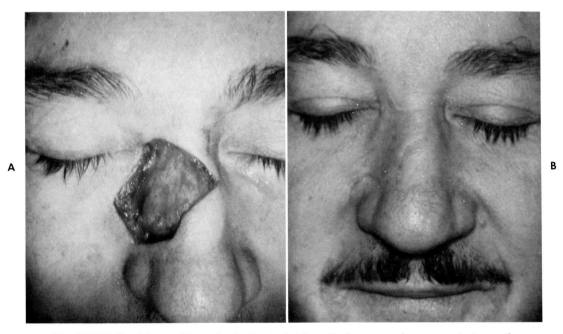

Fig. 14-3. Full-thickness skin graft. **A,** Surgical defect. **B,** One year after postauricular graft.

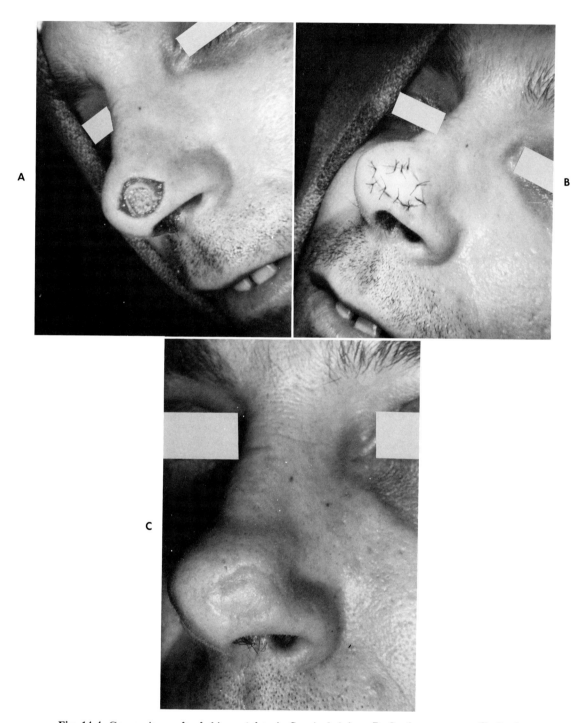

Fig. 14-4. Composite graft of skin and fat. **A,** Surgical defect. **B,** Graft at surgery. **C,** Graft has patch appearance 8 months after procedure.

an alar rim. The bilobed flap is useful for larger defects and for the delivery of tissue to the nasal tip, where use of a single flap might cause elevation of an alar rim (Fig. 14-6). In borderline cases the decision to rotate the second flap need not be made until it is apparent that primary closure of the donor site of a banner flap will lead to distortion of the ala. I have used the banner and bilobed flaps for the repair of more than 150 defects. One flap was partially lost, but it was of interest to find in this case that the small resulting defect healed with a very satisfactory cosmetic result.

Other flap designs

A variety of other rotation flaps of nasal cover have been described, but my experience with these flaps has been limited. I have found that local flaps not utilizing the principles of the banner flap are more difficult to rotate, and when these flaps are used to repair defects on the lower nose, there is some distortion of the alae.

REGIONAL FLAPS

Large, deep defects that expose or sacrifice cartilage and bone and major through-and-through defects require flap reconstruction. Sizeable flaps of good quality are readily obtained from the adjacent area of the forehead or cheek. The upper eyelid may yield suitable tissue for selected small repairs.

Forehead flaps

My first choice for the repair of total or large subtotal defects is tissue from the forehead. The color match is good, and the flaps are thin enough to per-

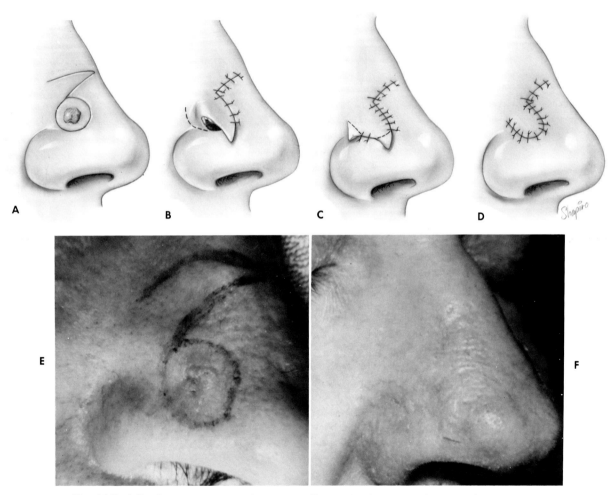

Fig. 14-5. **A-D,** One-stage banner flap repair. **E,** Basal cell cancer of thick sebaceous skin with flap design. **F,** Six months after the operation. (From Elliott, R. A.: Plast. Reconstr. Surg. **44:**148. © 1969, The Williams and Wilkins Co., Baltimore.)

mit shaping yet rigid enough to maintain their new form. I prefer the transverse flap design for major repairs. To repair a unilateral defect, tissue from the ipsilateral forehead is used for the graft, and the pedicle is based above the opposite eyebrow to include the supraorbital artery and the frontal branch of the superficial temporal artery (Fig. 14-7). To repair a midline or total defect, the graft can be obtained from either side (Fig. 14-8).

Transverse flaps can be transferred safely without a delay procedure. The flap may be folded at the time of transfer to repair an alar or columellar loss. Nasal lining is also completed at the time of transfer by folding in skin flaps hinged on the margins of a mature defect or by applying a split-thickness skin graft to the undersurface of the flap. At the time of transfer the forehead defect is covered with a split-thickness skin graft, and any unsatisfied pedicle

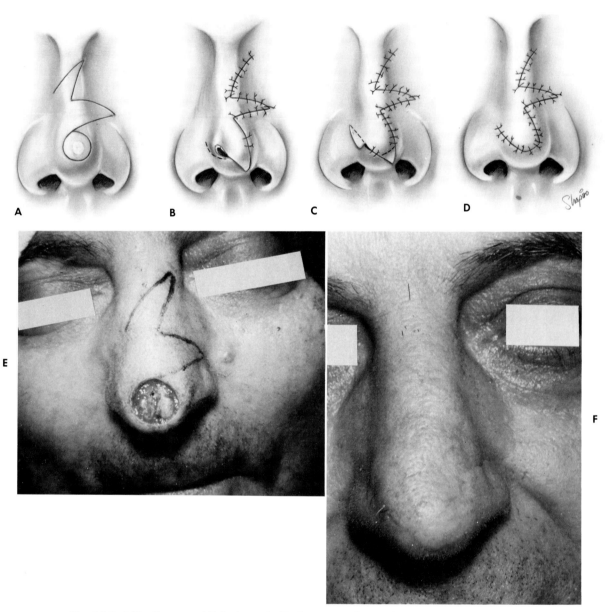

Fig. 14-6. A-D, One-stage bilobed repair. E, Surgical defect and flap design. F, Two years after the operation. (A-D From Elliott, R. A.: Plast. Reconstr. Surg. 44:148. © 1969, The Williams & Wilkins Co., Baltimore.)

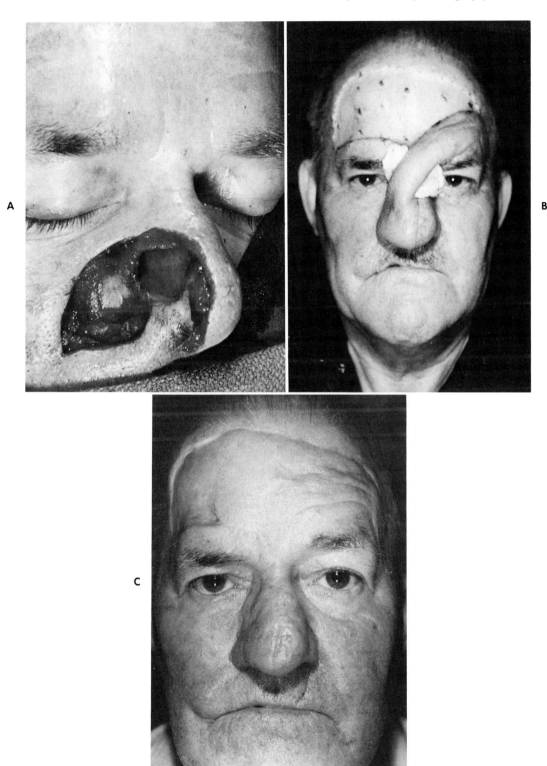

Fig. 14-7. Forehead flap, transverse design, for repair of unilateral defect. **A,** Surgical defect; right half of the nose was amputated. **B,** Transfer of undelayed tubed flap with split-thickness grafts for lining of the flap and coverage of the forehead. Cheek was closed primarily. Patient 3 weeks after the excision and first stage of repair. **C,** Postoperative result 3 months after the pedicle was returned to the forehead.

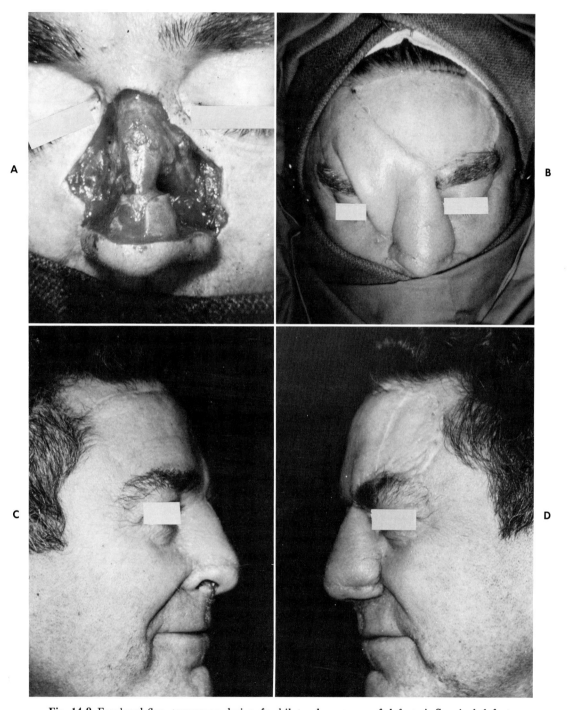

Fig. 14-8. Forehead flap, transverse design, for bilateral coverage of defect. A, Surgical defect. B, Transfer of unlined, undelayed flap with folded pedicle and skin graft to the forehead; shown 3 weeks after the operation. C, Flap 4 months after the pedicle was divided and returned to the forehead. D, Split-thickness skin graft on donor defect 4 months after the operation.

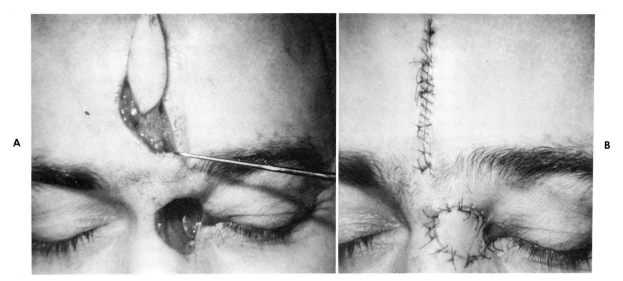

Fig. 14-9. Forehead island flap. **A,** Defect of the nose; island flap is mobilized on sub-cutaneous pedicle and is ready to be tunneled to the defect. **B,** Closure has been completed without distortion of the brows.

is folded upon itself or tubed. Temporary coverage with a biologic dressing requires more care and is not advocated. Later, when the pedicle is divided, the unused portion is returned to the forehead. The permanent donor defect is thus limited to that portion of the forehead actually used for the reconstruction. Replacing the split graft with a full-thickness graft will lessen this deformity. When used for subtotal reconstruction, a forehead flap seldom requires a bone or cartilage graft for support; but when needed for total nose reconstruction, the graft is inserted several months after the soft-tissue nose has been completed. A minor operation is frequently needed to defat reconstructed nostrils and ensure an adequate airway.

The sickle flap design described by Gordon New[9] and the scalping flap popularized by Converse and Wood-Smith[2] can also be used to deliver forehead tissue to the nose. The sickle flap must be delayed; the scalping flap is transferred without a preliminary delay procedure.

For a limited nasal repair the median forehead flap may afford sufficient tissue (Fig. 14-13). The indications and limitations of this flap design were reviewed by Figi and Moorman.[6] Primary closure of the donor site is desirable but it defines a limitation on the size of the flap that can be obtained. The linear scar in the midline of the forehead tends to blend well and does not spread. An oblique forehead flap affords a longer pedicle, but the oblique

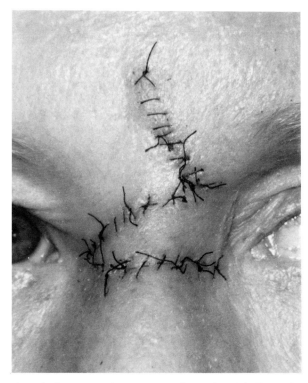

Fig. 14-10. Forehead banner flap from the glabella to the nose.

scars cross the wrinkle lines and are not esthetic. Both the median and oblique flaps can be transferred without a delay procedure.

The median forehead is a good donor site for an island flap. This technique gives a one-stage repair without distortion of the eyebrows (Fig. 14-9). The island is tunneled to the defect, or the donor and recipient sites are joined by an incision for better exposure. The subcutaneous pedicle need not contain

a large vessel to support the graft. The donor site is closed primarily in the same manner as with the median rotation flap. In my experience the island flap frequently becomes edematous and may retain some of the extra bulk. I prefer a banner flap from the glabellar area for a one-stage repair of smaller defects on the upper portion of the nose, because the scars are better and edema is not seen (Fig. 14-10). This flap can be helpful, however, only if the glabellar

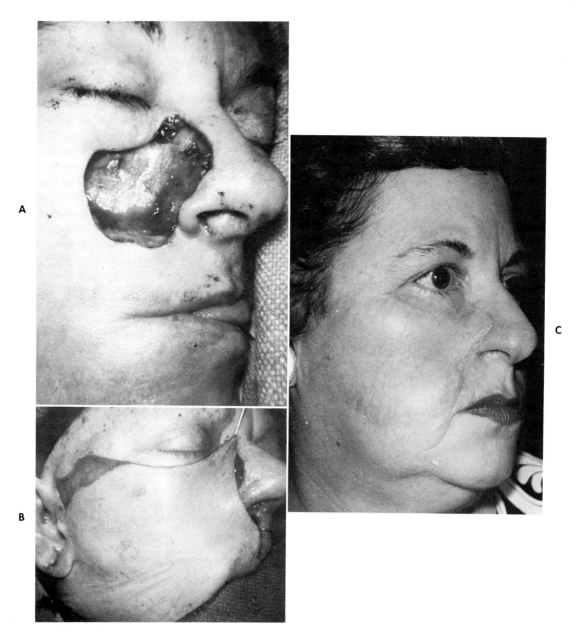

Fig. 14-11. Rotation-advancement cheek flap. **A,** Defect of the nose and cheek with exposed bone. **B,** Flap design and transfer after wide undermining. **C,** Result 1 year later.

region is free of brow hairs. The island flap from a higher region of the forehead avoids this area between the brows; thus it becomes the flap of choice in selected patients.

In general, I have been pleased with the results obtained with forehead flaps. Restoration is rapid and effective. The residual deformity on the forehead has always seemed to be a reasonable price to pay for a good-quality nasal repair.

Cheek flaps

A variety of flaps useful for the repair of lateral nasal defects may be obtained from the cheek. These flaps include rotation advancement flaps, banner flaps, and island flaps.

A large rotation advancement flap is created by a transverse incision across the lower eyelid and temple region and is supplemented by a vertical preauricular incision as needed (Fig. 14-11). The incision in the temple region extends above the level of the outer canthus to avoid ectropion of the lower eyelid because rotation of this inferiorly based flap is accompanied by some downward displacement of the flap. The donor site is closed by a radial placement of sutures. An excision of excess tissue is required along the nasolabial fold, and a wedge excision of excess tissue along the superior border is occasionally helpful in the temple area. The tissue delivered to the nose is from the thin lower eyelid, a disadvantage for the repair of some defects.

Perhaps the most commonly used cheek flap is the banner design, which follows the nasolabial fold (Fig. 14-12). In patients with lax tissue rather sizable superiorly based flaps may be obtained without appreciable deformity in the donor site. Long flaps are available, but in the male patient care must be taken to avoid transfer of beard tissue to the nose. Whenever possible, the flap is delivered above the paranasal groove to obviate a second procedure to reconstruct this groove. For the repair of small cover defects on the ala, the selection of a banner flap of nasal tissue prevents this troublesome deformity. In selected cases the tip of a nasolabial flap may be thinned and folded upon itself for alar lining, but this does add bulk; lining the flap with a split graft is an alternative. For the repair of a larger through-and-through defect, a turnover banner flap or island flap from the nasolabial fold can be used for lining

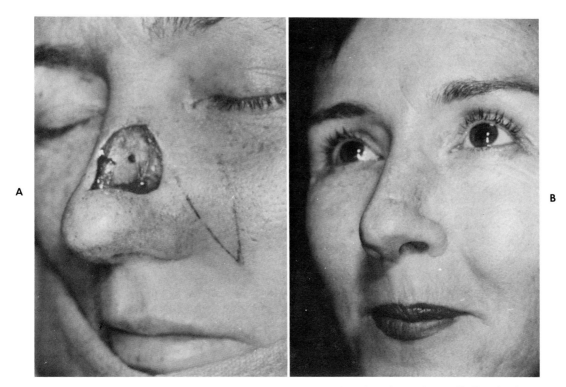

Fig. 14-12. Cheek banner flap. **A,** Defect (with exposed bone) and flap design. **B,** Result 18 months after the procedure.

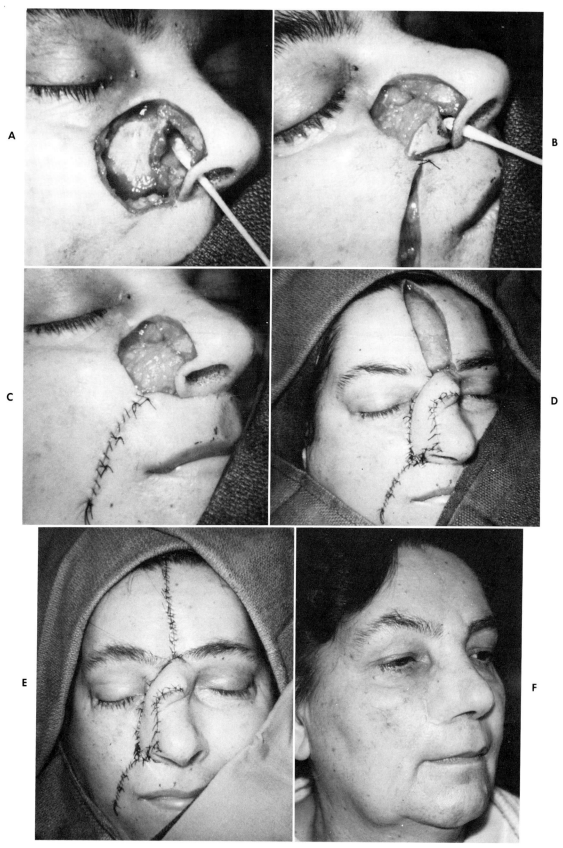

Fig. 14-13. Turnover island cheek flap and median forehead flap. **A,** Through-and-through defect with faint outline of nasolabial fold island flap. **B,** Mobilized nasolabial fold island flap being inset for lining. **C,** Completion of lining closure. **D,** Median forehead flap; donor defect is open. **E,** Completion of forehead closure. **F,** Result 11 months after the procedure.

and a forehead flap transferred for the cover (Fig. 14-13).

Other flaps

In older patients a banner flap from a redundant upper eyelid may be used to repair small, deep losses on the side of the nose near the inner canthus. The need for primary closure of the donor site without creation of a significant secondary deformity limits the amount of available tissue.

FLAPS FROM A DISTANT SITE

Flaps of skin and fat from distant donor sites on the neck, arm, chest, and abdomen are selected only

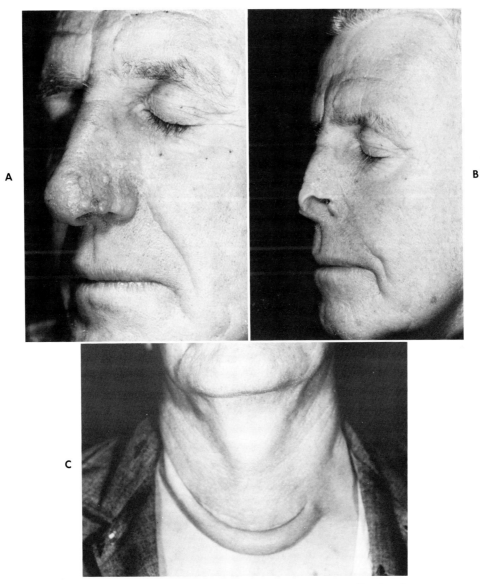

Continued.

Fig. 14-14. Neck tube pedicle. **A,** Basal cell cancer involving most of the nasal cover bilaterally. **B,** Six months after excision of the cover and both alae; temporary split-thickness skin graft has been used. **C,** Neck tube pedicle. **D,** Intermediate transfer of the right end of the pedicle to the left preauricular cheek. Left cervical tissue was later transferred to the nasal cover and the split-thickness graft was reflected bilaterally for alar lining. **E and F,** Result 1 year after the procedure.

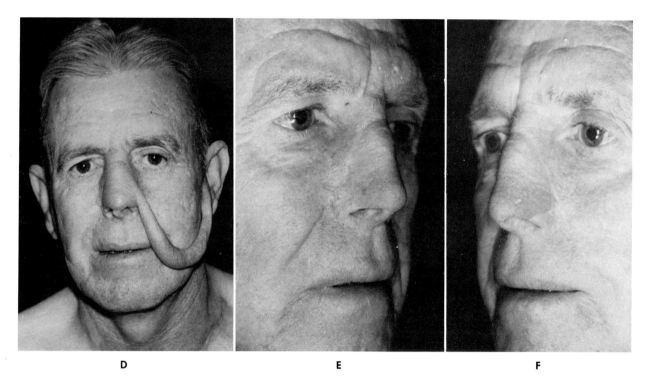

D   E   F

Fig. 14-14, cont'd. For legend see p. 93.

when regional flaps cannot deliver the quantity or quality of tissue required for the repair. These flaps require multiple stages and tend to be flabby. Only cervical tissue gives a reasonable match of color and texture.

Neck tube pedicles

Tissue from the lateral neck below the beard can be delivered to the nose by means of a low cervical tube pedicle (Fig. 14-14). The color match is usually excellent. These grafts are relatively soft and flabby; but in selected cases where most of the supporting structures are intact, they afford a good repair. If a skin graft is used on the neck, enough tissue can be obtained to resurface the entire nose. Primary closure of the pedicle donor site is routine, and the low cervical scar is relatively easy to conceal. Long tube pedicles will require a temporary bridge in the central portion. The graft is usually prepared with two additional delay procedures. Intermediate transfer of the pedicle to the cheek may prevent tension on the pedicle during the final placement. The multiple stages required for neck tube pedicle reconstruction is an obvious disadvantages, but this may be the best available tissue for the repair.

Arm tube pedicles

Grafts from the arm have the single advantage of preventing additional scars on the head and neck. The tissue obtained from the anteromedial aspect of the arm is too pale and flabby for an ideal repair, and multiple stages are required for the preparation and transfer of the graft. Awkward positioning of the arm for the transfer adds a significant disadvantage, which may introduce problems of joint rehabilitation in the aged. Use of arm tissue should be reserved for the patient who lacks integrity of the more usual donor sites (Fig. 14-15).

Other flaps

Flaps from the chest or abdomen require many operations, supply too much bulk, and afford a poor color match. Indications for their selection are rare.

SUMMARY

The nasal deformities created by cancer and its treatment are diverse. After adequate local excision of malignancy arising in the skin, reconstruction is seldom delayed, because the prognosis for cure is excellent. The plan for reconstruction must be individualized. Defects limited to the nasal cover are

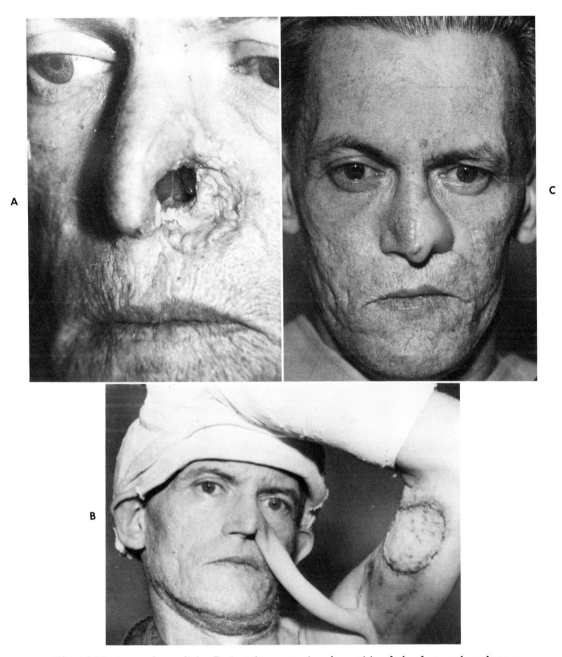

Fig. 14-15. Arm tube pedicle. Patient has extensive dermatitis of the face and neck as a result of irradiation. **A,** Surgical defect after excision of the malignant tumor. Temporary skin graft on the cheek. **B,** Transfer of the arm pedicle; skin graft was reflected for nasal lining. **C,** Flap 9 months later. Note poor match of color and texture.

repaired by primary closure, free grafts, or local flaps. Extensive defects commonly require the use of regional flaps from appropriate donor sites. Selected cases will require flaps from a distance. Prosthetic replacement must be considered occasionally.

REFERENCES

1. Brown, J. C., and McDowell, F.: Plastic surgery of the nose, St. Louis, 1951, The C. V. Mosby Co., p. 299.
2. Converse, J. M., and Casson, P. R.: Reconstructive

surgery; an integral part of treatment of cancer of the nose. In Gaisford, J. C., editor: Symposium on cancer of the head and neck, vol. 2, St. Louis, 1969, The C. V. Mosby Co.

3. Davenport, G., and Bernard, F. D.: Improving the take of composite grafts, Plast. Reconstr. Surg. **24:** 175, 1959.

4. Dupertuis, S. M.: Free ear lobe grafts of skin and fat, Plast. Reconstr. Surg. **1:**135, 1946.

5. Elliott, R. A.: Rotation flaps of the nose, Plast. Reconstr. Surg. **44:**147, 1969.

6. Figi, F. A., and Moorman, W. L.: The median forehead flap—indications and limitations, Plast. Reconstr. Surg. **24:**163, 1959.

7. Kraissl, C. J.: The selection of appropriate lines for elective surgical incisions, Plast. Reconstr. Surg. **8:**10, 1951.

8. MacFee, W. F.: The surgical treatment of cancer of the nose with emphasis on methods of repair, Ann. Surg. **140:**475, 1954.

9. New, G. B.: Sickle flap for nasal reconstruction, Surg. Gynecol. Obstet. **80:**498, 1945.

10. O'Connor, G. B., and McGregor, M. W.: Reconstruction of subtotal nasal defects, Am. J. Surg. **92:** 60, 1956.

11. Willis, R. A.: Pathology of tumors, St. Louis, 1948, The C. V. Mosby Co., pp. 355-356.

Chapter 15

Eyelid tumors and their treatment

Frederick J. McCoy, M.D.

Virtually all lesions found on the skin of the face can also be found on the eyelids. In addition, there are a few rare ones that originate from the meibomian glands and other structures peculiar to the lid components. Listed in the approximate order of frequency, these lesions are as follows: cutaneous papilloma and verrucua, hyperkeratosis, nevus, xanthoma, epithelioma (basal cell, squamous cell), melanoma, keratoacanthoma, trichoepithelioma, neurofibroma, syringoma, dermoid cyst, and sarcoma. Chalazion and a myriad of inflammatory and dermatologic conditions also occur but are not generally of concern to the reconstructive surgeon.

The following are the various modalities of treatment for these lesions: surgical extirpation, radiotherapy, electrocautery, cryotherapy, and fluorouracil.

In dealing with benign lesions, the physician may at various times find any one of these modalities to be useful. Pedunculated papillomas are simply clipped with Iris scissors and the bases cauterized. Verrucae and hyperkeratoses are cauterized with low-potential desiccation. Cysts are excised with the sac intact, in the same manner as in any other part of the face. Rarely, if ever, do these lesions create a tissue defect of significance unless it is produced iatrogenically by an injudicious choice or application of a method of treatment. The removal of malignant lesions, however, may entail the sacrifice of significant portions of the eyelids. Their immediate restoration to protect the globe is a matter of urgent necessity, and the treating physician must be prepared to meet the challenge.

I would like to acknowledge my appreciation to Dr. Jorge Lopez y Garcia for his assistance with the illustrations.

Although a skilled radiologist can achieve satisfactory results in many eyelid lesions, untoward reactions to dosage or method may result in an ineffectual response with recurrence or excessive scarring, tissue atrophy, late malignant degeneration, or loss of vision caused by cataract formation. At the worst, all of these conditions may exist simultaneously. Moreover, the healing problems encountered in irradiated tissues are always difficult and sometimes insurmountable.

Cryotherapy, in the form of Dry Ice or liquid nitrogen, has been proposed by various authors. Recently, Zacarian[16] has demonstrated good results with the latter material, using a special applicator. The acceptability of cryotherapy as a treatment of choice, however, has not been established.

Fluorouracil is effective in the treatment of keratotic lesions; but its use in the treatment of neoplastic disease must be regarded as uncertain, and its application about the eyelids is potentially hazardous.

The standard by which any treatment must be measured is whether it *reliably* separates the patient from his disease and restores normal function and appearance. Ideally, it should permit qualitative (biopsy for cell type) as well as quantitative (microscopic evidence of adequacy of removal) analysis. If a competent reconstructive surgeon is available, most neoplastic lesions of the eyelids are best managed surgically.

RECONSTRUCTION

A review of the literature reveals a bewildering array of ingenious procedures to reconstruct the eyelid, but basically these procedures involve four fundamental maneuvers:

1. Simple edge-to-edge approximation
2. Free skin grafts
3. Z-plasty
4. Flap transposition

These are used alone or in combination for all lid reconstructions.

CLASSIFICATION OF DEFECTS

Since the choice of a method of reconstruction depends primarily on one's analysis of the defect, it may be useful to categorize these defects in two broad groups.

CLASSIFICATION OF DEFECTS

I. Defects of skin only
   A. Simple approximation
   B. Z-plasty
   C. Local flaps from the following alternative donor sites:
     1. Another eyelid
     2. Cheek
     3. Forehead
II. Full-thickness or compound defects
   A. Class I—30% or less; adequate local tissue for
     1. Simple closure

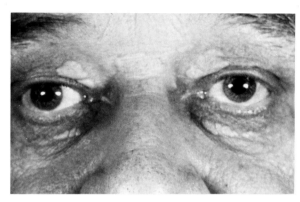

Fig. 15-1. Moderately extensive xanthelasma involving all four eyelids, which can be excised and sutured without grafts or flaps. Extending the incision across the concavities at the medial and lateral canthal areas would produce contractures and must be avoided.

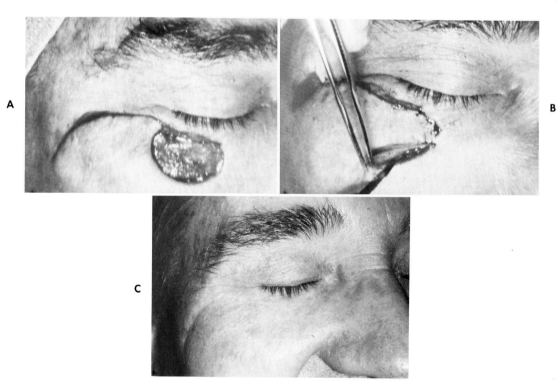

Fig. 15-2. A, Defect in lower lid, requiring rotational flap, is in the transitional area where thin lid skin is thickening to facial skin; adjacent cheek is an ideal donor area. Incision can be made in lines of tension. **B,** Flap mobilized and anchored; "dogear" is trimmed. **C,** Result 1 year later: scar is minimal; no distortion of lid.

2. Closure with canthotomy
3. Closure with Z-plasty
B. Class II—30% to 65%
  1. Switch flap (Esser)
  2. Alternatives:
     a. Imre
     b. Mustarde
     c. Lid-sharing procedure—Dupuy-Dutemps, Hughes
C. Class III—over 65%; lid-sharing procedure
  1. Dupuy-Dutemps with Fricke flap
  2. Hughes
  3. Köllner

Defects limited to the skin

Most lesions of the eyelids fall in the category of defects limited to the skin. In adults there is enough redundancy of skin that up to 25 to 30 mm.² in the upper eyelid and half of this amount in the lower lid can be removed, and the defect can still be repaired by simple wound closure without distortion of the palpebral margins (Fig. 15-1). Scars should parallel lid creases as nearly as possible to prevent contractures. When the defect exceeds the limit of simple closure, flap rotation can be utilized to add tissue and to convert a vertical pull to a transverse one, avoiding distortion of the lid margin (Fig. 15-

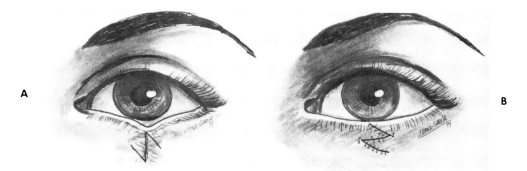

Fig. 15-3. Z-plasty gains length at the expense of width. Entire depth of the scar must be included rather than just the skin.

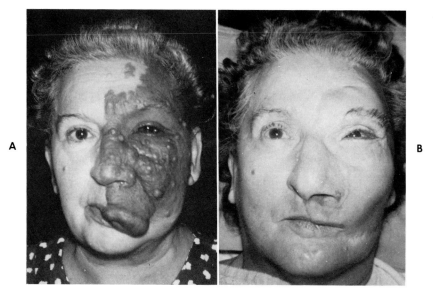

Fig. 15-4. A, Extensive hemangioma of the face and eyelids. **B,** Donor sites chosen for the grafts shown here were: contralateral upper eyelid for upper lid coverage; postauricular sulcus for the lower lid; supraclavicular fossa for the nose; tubed abdominal skin for the forehead and cheek; lower lip (Abbe-Estlander flap) for left upper lip replacement.

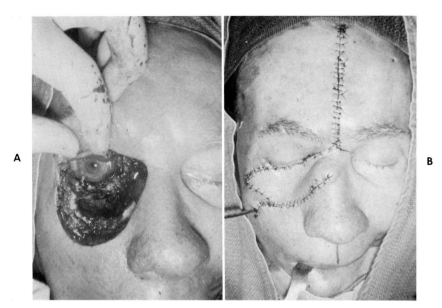

Fig. 15-5. **A,** Recurrent basal cell carcinoma and radionecrosis necessitated excision of the lower lid, cheek, and a portion of the underlying maxilla. The exposed antrum can be seen. **B,** Midline forehead flap provides reliable soft tissue cover; later bone grafting and lid reconstruction is anticipated. The eye is virtually sightless from radiation effect and exposure.

2). The Z-plasty is frequently adaptable, and the principle is the same as that for correcting a perpendicular scar contracture (Fig. 15-3). The repair of defects beyond this range requires tissue transplantation as a free graft or pedicled flap. The indications for these two types of repair are less precise and vary with different surgeons. In general, the deeper defects are repaired with flaps, but those that are larger and more superficial require free grafts.

Free grafts. In order of preference, the donor sites to be considered for full-thickness free grafts are the following:

1. The ipsilateral or contralateral upper eyelids
2. Postauricular skin
3. Supraclavicular skin (Fig. 15-4)

Thick split-thickness grafts from a hairless portion of the trunk or extremities are a fourth choice. In general, split grafts have poor color and texture match and a much greater tendency to contract.

Pedicled flaps. Where deep structures such as tarsus, palpebral ligaments, lacrimal apparatus, or bone are exposed, better cosmetic as well as functional results will be obtained with pedicled flaps from adjacent areas on the same or opposite lid, the cheek, or the forehead (Fig. 15-5).

Whole-thickness or compound defects

Class I defects. (See outline above.[10]) A lesion involving the lid margin, as well as one extending to the muscular or tarsoconjunctival layers, requires full lid–thickness excision. When this defect does not exceed 20% of the length of the eyelid, it can usually be closed by simple approximation in layers.[12] It is neither necessary nor desirable to offset the margins (as in the Wheeler "halving operation"[15]), which involves needless sacrifice of scarce tissue. A horizontal mattress suture at the lid margin everts the edge and prevents notching, provided that a competent, two-layer closure of the entire length of the defect is obtained (Fig. 15-6).

If the loss is 20% to 30% of the lid margin, it may be necessary to do a lateral canthotomy (Fig. 15-7). A simple test to determine if this procedure is necessary is to push gently upward (or downward if in the upper lid) on the sutured lid margin with a cotton-tipped applicator. If it does not slide easily up over the convexity of the globe, a relaxing canthotomy should be done (Fig. 15-8).[10,12]

If the perpendicular line of closure extends more than 4 mm. from the lid margin, the line of excision should be turned (Fig. 15-8, *A*), or a Z-plasty should be done to avoid contracture where the scar crosses the lid crease.

Class II defects. (See outline on p. 99.[10]) In defects that involve 30% to 65% of the lid margin, closure is not possible, and neighboring tissues must be called on to replace the various components. For reconstructive considerations, these components can

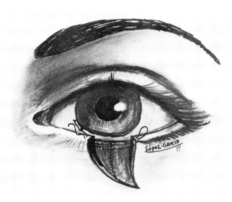

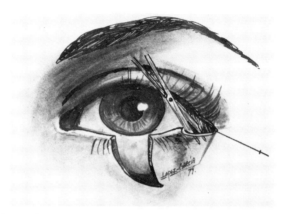

Fig. 15-6. Class I defects can be closed in two layers. Continuous sutures of 6-0 chromic catgut with knots buried is used to close the tarsoconjunctival layers. A horizontal mattress suture at the margin assures eversion and prevents notching. The musculocutaneous layer is closed with 5-0 silk or nylon. The point of the excised wedge is turned to avoid crossing creases.

Fig. 15-7. Relaxation when needed in either Class I or Class II defects may be obtained by doing a classical lateral canthotomy.

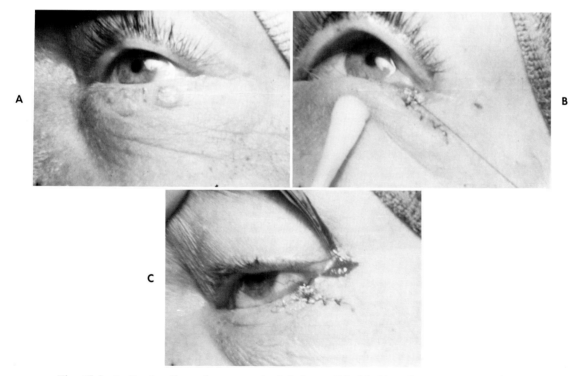

Fig. 15-8. A, Basal cell carcinoma on the left lower lid. Marking shows the point of the wedge turning off laterally to avoid a perpendicular crease crossing the scar. **B,** Testing for tension: bowstringing prevents the margin from sliding easily over the globe convexity, necessitating a lateral, relaxing canthotomy, **C.**

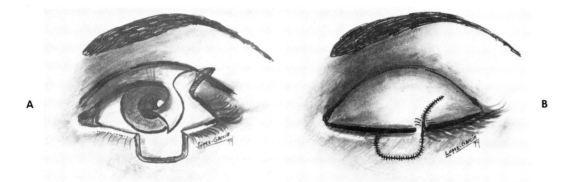

Fig. 15-9. A, Wound edges are prepared so that they are perpendicular to the lid margin for 2 or 3 mm. for accurate approximation. The flap is outlined and cut on the opposing lid (either upper or lower) so that the 3-mm. pedicle lies directly opposite a point midway between the center and either border of the defect, depending on whether the pedicle is directed medially or laterally. The width of the flap should be half that of the tissue lost in order to reduce both lids by the same amount. B, Donor area is closed as shown in Fig. 15-6. The flap is then set into the defect. A lateral canthotomy may also be required for adequate relaxation.

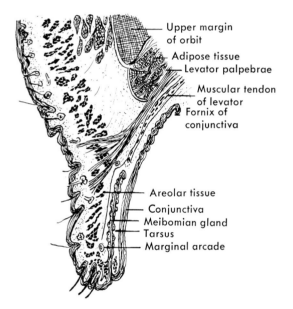

Fig. 15-10. Anatomic cross section of the upper eyelid shows the location of the marginal vascular arcade. (From McCoy, F., and Crow, M.: Plast. Reconstr. Surg. 35(6): 633-639. © 1965, The Williams & Wilkins Co., Baltimore.)

be divided into the following:
1. The tarsoconjunctival layer
2. The musculocutaneous layer
3. A well-aligned row of lashes

Ideally, the reparative process should replace all three components if the surgeon's dual responsibility of cosmetic and functional restoration is to be met. An equally important consideration in selecting any method of repair is repetitive reliability.

Without question, the switch flap, as originally described by Stein, Estlander, and Abbe[1,10] for lip reconstruction and by Esser and Hueston[4,6] for eyelid reconstruction, most closely satisfies these criteria, and when properly done, it produces the fewest complications. It also has the advantage of not introducing additional scarring on the cheek and elsewhere, as in the case of lateral advancement flaps, such as those of Von Imre,[14] Esser,[4] Mustarde,[12] and others.[9,13] The thickness of these skin flaps (and their lining composite grafts) makes them imperfect substitutes for a normal lid. In addition, such flaps fail to provide lashes. Transplantation attempts at lash replacement notoriously fall short of critical acceptability.[5]

Technique. The switch flap replaces lid tissue with lid tissue and can be used for either upper or lower eyelid reconstruction. It has produced uniformly superior results. The wound edges of the defect must be carefully prepared to receive the flap. It is of utmost importance that the wound margins be exactly perpendicular to the palpebral border for a distance of at least 2 mm. to avoid irregularity in healing. The flap is then outlined on the opposite lid so that the 3-mm. pedicle (containing the vascular supply) lies directly opposite a point midway between the center and one or the other of the borders of the recipient defects, depending on

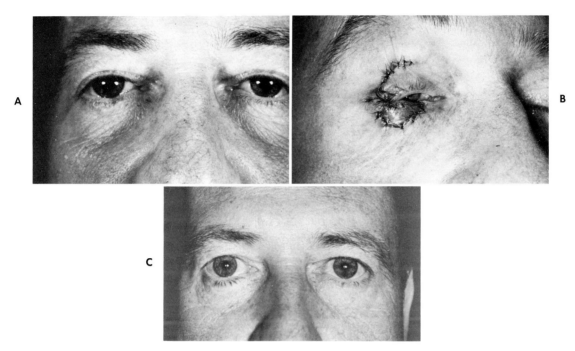

Fig. 15-11. **A,** A basal cell epithelioma involving 55% of the horizontal dimension (full thickness) of the right lower eyelid. **B,** Immediate postoperative appearance after re-section of 65% of the lid and utilization of a switch flap based medially; a canthotomy was also done. **C,** Three months later. Note the normal-looking lid margin, palpebral aperture and lash line. No scarring is visible to the average observer. (From McCoy, F., and Crow, M.: Plast. Reconstr. Surg. **35**(6):633-639. © 1965, The Williams & Wilkins Co., Baltimore.)

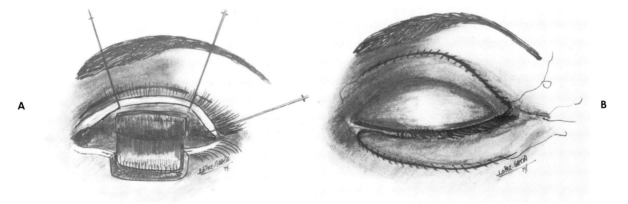

Fig. 15-12. **A,** Class III defect of the lower lid with tarsoconjunctival flap pulled down from the upper lid and sutured to the stump of the conjunctiva in the inferior fornix (6-0 chromic catgut). Incision in the upper lid is never less than 4 mm. from the lid margin. **B,** Skin coverage utilizing a skin flap from the upper lid.

whether the flap is based medially or laterally (Fig. 15-9).

The width of the flap along the palpebral margin should be one half that of the defect and should rarely exceed 11 mm. The incision should follow a line perpendicular to the lid margin for 2 mm. The musculocutaneous layer incision is tapered off horizontally to avoid a vertical scar crossing the normal lid crease with resultant contracture. The incision in the tarsoconjunctival component is continued per-

pendicularly to the attached border of the tarsus, then joined in triangular fashion at the conjunctival fornix. The flap is then rotated 180 degrees into position. If the 3-mm. pedicle appears too rigid, the *tarsus* (only) may be cut further, using the point of a No. 11 blade. Care must be taken not to disrupt the blood supply, which is carried primarily in the marginal arcade between the tarsus and the muscular layer (Fig. 15-10).

After it has been trimmed according to an accu-

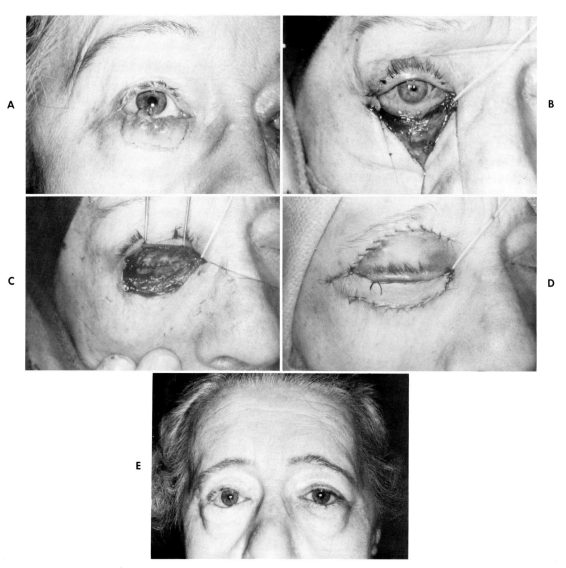

Fig. 15-13. **A,** Extensive basal cell epithelioma; line of resection is outlined in methylene blue. **B,** Defect after resection with frozen section control. Lower pointer indicates the stump of the lower canaliculus; upper pointer is retracting the upper lid for photographic purposes. **C,** Tarsoconjunctival flap is sutured to the cut edge of the lower lid conjunctiva. **D,** Skin coverage is obtained by rotating the flap from the upper lid. Note flap viability despite the 1:6 width-to-length ratio. **E,** Eleven year follow-up: good function; no recurrence.

rate pattern, the tarsoconjunctival layer is approximated precisely and sutured with continuous sutures of 6-0 chromic catgut with knots buried to prevent corneal or conjunctival irritation. The musculocutaneous layer is then sutured with interrupted sutures of 5-0 nylon (Fig. 15-11). A horizontal mattress suture of fine silk at the lid margin will ensure eversion of the edges and prevent "notching," which is always conspicuous in any free border. A gentle pressure dressing is applied for 48 hours, and then a simple eye pad is used. The skin sutures are removed in 5 days. After 14 days the pedicle is divided, and the 2 margins are trimmed and accurately sutured.

Class III defects. (See outline on p. 99.[10]) For complete or nearly complete lid reconstruction, some form of *lid-sharing* procedure is used. Variations of this method have been described by Dupuy-Dutemps,[12] Hughes,[7,8] Köllner,[13] and others (Fig. 15-12).

Technique. After the lid is removed, the stump of the conjunctiva (including the cut end of the levator aponeurosis in the case of upper lid) is identified. With the opposite or donor lid everted, an incision is made through the tarsoconjunctival layer no less than 4 mm. from and exactly parallel to the palpebral margin. The length should be equal to that of the defect. The tissues are mobilized by being undermined between the tarsal plate and the orbicularis muscles, which allows the cut tarsoconjunctival edge to be approximated to the conjunctival stump on the resected side and sutured with continuous sutures of 6-0 chromic catgut with knots buried.

A raw surface is thereby exposed between the intact donor lid margin and the resected margin, representing the musculocutaneous deficit. This raw surface is covered by a modified Fricke flap from the upper eyelid, based laterally. Width-to-length ratios for these flaps of 1 to 6 or more are perfectly safe, allowing for accurate tailoring (Fig. 15-13).

After 2 weeks the lids are separated and the margins trimmed and closed with continuous 6-0 silk sutures.

SUMMARY

An attempt has been made to simplify the approach to the treatment of tumors of the eyelids rather than to present a compendium of the many techniques found in the literature. To this end the surgical defects have been divided into those defects that involve skin only and those defects that include the whole thickness of the lid. The latter have been subdivided into three classes according to the extent of lid loss, and the different methods required for the correction of each have been outlined. The procedures suggested have been selected over 25-years of experience, on the basis of reliability and uniformity of excellence in the results. Complications, if the surgeon is competent, should be minimal.

REFERENCES

1. Brown, J. B.: Switching of vermillion bordered lip flaps, Surg. Gynecol. Obstet. **46:**701, 1928.
2. Callahan, A.: The free composite lid graft, Arch. Ophthalmol. **45:**539, 1951.
3. Esser, J. F S.: Ueber Eine Gestielte Uberpflanzung Eines Senkrecht, Angelegten Keils aus dem Oberen Augenlid in des Gleichseitige Unterlid oder Umgekehrt, Klin. Monatsbl. Augenheilkd. **63:**379-381, 1919.
4. Esser, J. F. S.: Eyelid flaps, Rev. Chir. Plastique **1:**295-297, January 1934.
5. Fox, S. A.: Ophthalmic plastic surgery, ed. 3, New York, 1963, Grune & Stratton, Inc.
6. Hueston, G. T.: Abbe flap technique in upper eyelid repair, Br. J. Plast. Surg. **13:**347, 1960-1961.
7. Hughes, W. L: A new method of rebuilding a lower lid, Arch. Ophthalmol. **17:**1008, 1937.
8. Hughes, W. L.: Reconstructive surgery of the eyelids, St. Louis, 1943, The C. V. Mosby Co.
9. Kirschner, M.: Operationslehr, vol. 3, Berlin, 1935, J. Springer, p. 1.
10. McCoy, F., and Crow, M.: Adaptation of the "switch flap" to eyelid reconstruction, Plast. Reconstr. Surg. **35**(6):633-639, 1965.
11. Smith, B.: Eyelid surgery, Surg. Clin. North Am. **39:**367, 1959.
12. Smith, B., and Cherubini, T. D.: Ocuplastic surgery, St. Louis, 1970, The C. V. Mosby Co.
13. Smith, F.: Manual of standard practice of plastic and maxillofacial surgery, Philadelphia, 1942, W. B. Saunders Co.
14. Von Imre, J.: Lidplastik, Budapest, 1928, Budapest "Studium", Verlag.
15. Wheeler, J. M.: Halving wounds in facial plastic surgery, Proc. Second Congress, Pan-Pacific Surg. Assoc., 1936.
16. Zacarian, S. A.: Cryogenic approach to treatment of lid tumors, Ann. Ophthalmol. **2:**706-713, October 1970.

Chapter 16

Cancer of the tongue: results of surgical treatment

Charles C. Harrold, Jr., M.D.

Progress has never been immediately evident in the treatment of cancer, because of the nature of the disease, the available modes of treatment, and the time needed to evaluate end results. It is therefore difficult for anyone, however brilliant, to speak or write on the subject every few months and contribute something that is new, different, and significant.

CANCER INCIDENCE

One fact, however, cannot be overemphasized: cancer of the tongue killed an estimated 1,750 people in 1972[9] and retained its title as the cancer responsible for the greatest number of deaths in the head and neck area. A large percentage of these deaths must have occurred among patients controlled by many of you readers, and with each death you must have asked yourselves the inescapable question, "What else could I or should I have done for that patient?" You are concerned now because you have other patients with tongue cancer, and you were involved in the care of an estimated 2,800 new patients during 1973.[9] This subject is therefore of continuing importance, and this presentation concentrates on survival rates and some of the salient points, whether old or new, in surgical treatment. It concludes with some remarks on the more general problems presented by cancer of the tongue.

SURVIVAL RATES

The latest survival rates of patients with cancer of the tongue reported from the head and neck service at Memorial Cancer Center[8] show little change from the figures based on patients seen from 1952 through 1961 and reported at this symposium in 1968. Statistics given by Strong in 1971[8] (Table 16-1) were based on patients seen from 1957 through 1963 and added 2 years of more recent experience but did not include the 6 years of older experience previously reported. The overall survival rates quoted in the 1968 and 1971 reports are 40%[5] and 40.5%,[8] respectively. In 1968 48% of the clinical material taken from patients was composed of metastatic nodes on admission; in 1971 46% was composed of metastatic cancerous nodes. Survival rates of patients who had cancer of the base of the tongue and who were surgically treated were 25% in 1968 and 29% in 1971. An exact detailed comparison is not valid, but there seems to be little evidence to substantiate a claim for any dramatic change in quantitative end results.

One observation worthy of note is the unexplained increasing incidence of the disease in women; the male to female ratio is now 2.8:1.[8]

Table 16-1. 582 cancers of the tongue

	1957-1963	
Indeterminate		100
Determinate		482
Failures		287
"Cures"		195
Absolute	195/582 =	33.5%
Determinate	195/482 =	40.5%

From Strong, E. W., and Spiro, R. H.: Rev. Med. **31**:1913-1920, 1971.

106

CURRENT METHODS OF SURGICAL TREATMENT

The trend toward a greater use of surgery continues with surgery now accounting for 82.3% of all patients treated (Table 16-2); if one includes in this category those patients treated by preoperative irradiation and surgery, the figure rises to almost 90%.[8]

Treatment of cancer of the anterior two thirds of the tongue

Cancers that are localized to the anterior two thirds of the tongue should not present problems in treatment. For the great majority of these patients, transoral access provides adequate exposure for excision. For acceptable function to be obtained, the tongue must remain mobile. When the floor of the mouth is intact, the preservation of one hypoglossal nerve and enough musculature to allow a remaining portion of the tongue to approximate the hard palate or a palatal substitute ensures a short convalescence, a minimum of morbidity, and good function in speech and deglutition.

Partial glossectomy. Spiro[7] has reported on the efficiency of treatment by isolated partial glossectomy. For lesions under 4.0 cm. the operation gave local control in 81% of patients; but when the primary site was larger than 4.0 cm., there was a local recurrence rate of 50% and an incidence of cervical node metastasis in 77%, some of whom had local recurrence in the primary site (Table 16-3). For most of the patients with lesions larger than 4.0 cm. a more extensive procedure had been advocated but for a variety of reasons had not been carried out.

Elective neck dissection and the combined operation. Spiro's[7] operation provides greater specificity for a policy regarding the indications for elective radical neck dissection—a policy that now may be described as follows: In the anterior two thirds of the tongue, a cancer larger than 4.0 cm. but still confined to the tongue requires a wider excision than can be gained by the transoral route. This necessi-tates a cervical approach, which in turn makes neck dissection preferable at the same sitting. Under these particular circumstances, a partial glossectomy accomplished by means of a median mandibulotomy combined with radical neck dissection can be a rational solution.

When the cancer extends beyond the anterior two thirds of the tongue, a host of potential problems arise. The indications then become more positive for a composite or combined operation, the old standby for treatment of advanced oral cancer. The most commonly used operation is the classic partial glossectomy with neck dissection and partial segmental mandibulectomy; the latter procedure allows tongue mobility but causes varying degrees of facial deformity. Use of the marginal mandibulectomy improves the cosmetic appearance, but a resulting loss of tongue mobility may cause some function to be sacrificed.

These well-known combined operations are mentioned only to emphasize again that another alternative exists in the family of combined operations and ensures both a good cosmetic and functional result without compromising the excision. Involving the use of the cervical skin flap in conjunction with a deltopectoral flap, it allows preservation of a normal mandible and is suitable for adaptation in all patients except those with hairy necks. The procedure has been so well publicized[2] that it no longer requires further elaboration. For the repair of more massive defects, some surgeons may prefer a forehead flap. All of these repairs will be reviewed in detail by other authors.

Treatment of cancer of the base of the tongue

The treatment of cancer of the base of the tongue deserves greater attention, even at the risk of repetition.

Patients having locally advanced cancers with both unilateral and bilateral cervical metastatic cancerous nodes on admission are more common.[4] Therefore, treatment must be aggressive in the exci-

Table 16-2. Initial treatment at Memorial Center

	Cases	Percent
Surgery	479	82.3
Preoperative irradiation and surgery	44	7.5
Irradiation	38	6.5
Chemotherapy	2	0.3
None	19	3.4

From Strong, E. W., and Spiro, R. H.: Rev. Med. **31:**1913-1920, 1971.

Table 16-3. Control by partial glossectomy

Stage	I	II	III	Total
Determinate cases	74	61	10	145
Local recurrence	6	11	3	20
"Cured" by subsequent treatment	0	1	0	1
Dead of disease (no other information)	5	4	2	11
Percent controlled	85.1	77.0	50.0	79.3

Adapted from Spiro, R. H., and Strong, E. W.: Am. J. Surg. **122:**707-710, 1971.

sion as well as knowledgeable and imaginative in the reconstruction if a satisfactory result is to be obtained.

Role of the larynx. In rehabilitation of the patient after excision of the base of the tongue, the larynx plays an important role. If it has been preserved the larynx must be competent to allow deglutition without aspiration of saliva and food into the tracheobronchial tree.

In our work over 40% of these excisions were combined with laryngectomies, and over 40% of the laryngectomies required multistaged procedures for closure of either elective pharyngostomies or persistent salivary fistulas.[4] The most commonly employed operation continues to be excision of the primary cancer combined with partial segmental mandibulectomy and neck dissection, but some surgeons are reconstructing the oral defect by using cervical and deltopectoral flaps through a median mandibulotomy approach. Others, when performing a laryngectomy, prefer a neck dissection route through an anterior and lateral pharyngotomy, avoiding a mandibular approach. In patients with large pharyngostomies, repair by bilateral deltopectoral and forehead flaps have become commonplace.

OPERATIVE RISKS

As more experience is gained, a better appraisal can be made of the risk to reward ratio in the surgical treatment of advanced tongue cancer.

In this respect the overall operative mortality for patients treated surgically is 3.3%; this percentage rises with the increasing extent of the surgery.[6] For example, for all patients with oral cancer treated by combined operations, the operative mortality was 8%. For those patients treated by combined operations for advanced cancer (clinically and histologically positive metastatic cancerous nodes plus locally advanced primary tumors) the rate increased to 10%. For 28 patients treated by bilateral radical neck dissections performed simultaneously with excisions of the base of the tongue (and total laryngectomy in 26 of these) the rate rose to 14%.[4] For those patients treated by combined operations for cancer that was not advanced, the rate was 6%.

Quality of survivals

Successes. If these are the risks, what are the rewards? The surgical treatment of cancer of the base of the tongue may serve as an example. In some circles, the diagnosis of bilateral metastatic nodes at the time of the patient's admission is regarded as a death sentence. However, in our hands,

of 52 patients with this extent of disease on admission, 5 patients, or 10%, were well at 5 years.[4]

Seventy-two percent of those successfully treated for cancer of the base of the tongue were sufficiently rehabilitated to return to full-time employment and 18%, to part-time work.[4]

Disability that does result from this type of surgery is sometimes caused by aspiration of food and saliva into a larynx whose value in communication is completely negated by the associated danger of recurrent pneumonia. Because of neuromuscular and sensory deficits, total laryngectomy may become a life-saving measure for these patients.

In another study Donaldson[1] has reported on his experience with 14 patients who had total glossectomy. Two died of pneumonia, another had a laryngectomy at the time of total glossectomy, and still another had a later laryngectomy because of recurrent pneumonia. Six had to be permanently fed by tubes. There were 5 survivors, 3 of whom had had metastatic cervical nodes. His experience was similar to ours. It is true that in some instances of total or nearly total glossectomy the larynx can be preserved when it has not been invaded by cancer, and the patient may have an impaired but intelligible laryngeal speech but at a price of a more prolonged morbidity, a higher incidence of permanent tube feeding, and a greater risk of respiratory problems.

Failures. What happens with the failures is yet another story. With cumulative experience in this phase of the problem, one becomes impressed with the need to have a flexible philosophy about surgical treatment. For example, ideally speaking, the surgeon should choose the operation that would give the best chance for cure, and he should give secondary consideration to those surgical modifications that can ensure acceptable function and cosmesis. However, when the surgeon is confronted with a patient whose chances of survival are small, he should temper this philosophy with a decision to avoid, if treatment fails, a postsurgical status that would be worse than the preoperative one or a status involving plans for staged reconstruction that most likely would never be completed. Situations such as these should be avoided if at all possible, for they keep the patient in a hospital when he could be with his friends; and in the final analysis these situations are incompatible with good palliation.

When treatment fails in the patient who has had advanced tongue cancer, it characteristically fails early; in over 80% of the patients, death occurs within the first 24 months. There has been no change in this observation, which dates back to 1951, when we first started reviewing the results of our combined operations.[3] Disease-free intervals in these failures are usually not greater than 6 months; intervals shorter than this usually indicates a death occurring early in the 24-month period.

When cancer recurs in the oral cavity, hypopharynx, or neck, palliation is better and more prolonged in the patient who has had a laryngectomy. This is a fact that should not be overlooked in the treatment of cancer of the base of the tongue; it should be carefully weighed by the surgeon when he is faced with deciding whether to sacrifice or preserve a larynx.

Local recurrence remains the chief cause of treatment failure. Preoperative irradiation has decreased local recurrence and possibly has improved the quality of survival in those patients who will later die of distant metastases, other primary or metastatic tumors in the opposite side of the neck, or various combinations of these. In our experience, treatment of these local recurrences by surgery, irradiation, and chemotherapy has produced few cures in the past 20 years. Some of these patients who have recurrences in both the mouth and neck are often transported to treatment centers at great expense and made to wait for irradiation delivered by massive and impressive machines, but the end result is ultimately the same. It is my personal opinion that it is more practical to manage these patients as long as possible by any type of ambulatory chemoimmunotherapy that is available. Under these circumstances treatment with the latest chemical agents in varying combinations and dosages should be regarded by the patient and his physician as a possible chance for survival; for in the past the use of either irradiation or surgery alone or in combination has yielded no long-term survivors.

CONCLUSION

Cancer of the tongue has an unexplained increasing incidence in women and remains the leading cause of death among patients with cancer of the head and neck.

A better utilization of the surgical options available in treatment is being reflected in a lower operative mortality and an improvement in the quality of survival, whether that survival is palliative or curative.

For the patient with either advanced regional or disseminated tongue cancer, there has been no reported appreciable change in quantitative survival since the symposium sponsored by this foundation 5 years ago. Significant improvements in this group await the discovery of new chemotherapeutic and immunotherapeutic agents that will either supplement surgery or replace it.

REFERENCES

1. Bakamjian, V., and Littlewood, M.: Cervical skin flap for intraoral pharyngeal repair following cancer surgery, Br. J. Plast. Surg. 17:191-210, 1964.
2. Donaldson, R. C., Skelly, M., and Paletta, F. X.: Total glossectomy for cancer, Am. J. Surg. 116:585-590, 1968.
3. Harrold, C. C.: Present-day methods of surgical treatment of intraoral cancer, proceedings of the Second National Cancer Conference, vol. 1, New York, 1952, American Cancer Society, Inc., pp. 444-455.
4. Harrold, C. C.: Surgical treatment of cancer of the base of the tongue, Am. J. Surg. 114:493-497, 1967.
5. Harrold, C. C.: Cancer of the tongue; some comments on surgical treatment. In Gaisford, J. C., editor: Symposium on cancer of the head and neck, St. Louis, 1968, The C. V. Mosby Co., pp. 185-190.
6. Spiro, R. H., and Frazell, E. L.: Evaluation of radical surgical treatment of advanced cancer of the mouth, Am. J. Surg. 116:571-577, 1968.
7. Spiro, R. H., and Strong, E. W.: Epidermoid carcinoma of the mobile tongue; treatment by partial glossectomy alone, Am. J. Surg. 122:707-710, 1971.
8. Strong, E. W., and Spiro, R. H.: Notre experience du cancer de la langue au Memorial Hospital, Rev. Med. 31:1913-1920, 1971.
9. Silverberg, E., and Hollet, A.: Cancer statistics 1973, CA 23(1):16-17.

Chapter 17

Cancer of the floor of the mouth

Dwight C. Hanna, M.D.

Improvement in the management of cancer of the floor of the mouth continues to be the goal of all therapists, at least until the day arrives when the causative factors are better understood and prevented. In 1974 it is estimated that 7,900 deaths occurred from oral cancer; 525 of these deaths were attributed to lesions originating in the floor of the mouth.[2] Thus oral cancer remains responsible for over 2% of the total cancer mortality. Whereas the vast majority of lesions formerly occurred in men (ratios were as high as 16:1), many investigators are now reporting a much higher incidence in women; ratios such as 7:1 and 4:1 have been reported recently.[3,4] The reason for this change and its relationship to any of the suspected causative factors has not been established.

The highest goal sought by therapists is the eradication of the tumor with minimal disturbance of the function or appearance of the patient. However, when one considers the anatomical location of the area defined as the floor of the mouth, which is a narrow U shaped band of mucosa surrounded medially by the mobile tongue, laterally by the gingiva, inferiorly by the sublingual and submandibular glands, the lingual nerve, and the geniohyoid and mylohyoid muscles, and posteriorly by the palatine folds, one can readily understand why tumors of the area can so easily disturb the function or appearance of the area. It has been estimated that the lesion will have involved 75% of one or more of these adjacent structures by the time of diagnosis and initiation of treatment.[4]

ETIOLOGY AND INCIDENCE

Cancer of the floor of the mouth is a disease primarily affecting older patients, the median age being about 60 years for men and slightly younger for women. Most of the patients are between 50 and 70 years of age. Most lesions are believed to start from ulcerative, traumatic, inflammatory, luetic, and keratotic lesions of the mouth that either go untreated or fail to respond to good local care during a period of 2 weeks.[5]

Leukoplakia, the most common dyskeratotic lesion of the mouth, consistently indicates a premalignant lesion. Clinically, leukoplakia appears as a whitish or gray patch adherent to the mucosa and most commonly results from heavy smoking (1 to 2 packs of cigarettes daily). This keratotic reaction is believed to be a defense mechanism against local irritants, such as tobacco. When thickening or ulcerations appear, a biopsy is definitely indicated because a malignant change may have already occurred, in which case removal of the irritation will produce little improvement.

Lichen planus is a similar lesion and sometimes can be differentiated from leukoplakia only by a biopsy. When conservative management of leukoplakia fails to produce an immediate improvement or disappearance of the lesion, excision is indicated, particularly if the lesion can be excised and primarily closed. Failure to eliminate the irritant (such as tobacco), however, will result in a recurrence of the leukoplakia. If there is a recurrence, reexcision is definitely indicated, and the mucosa should be replaced by skin grafting, if necessary.

Systemic chemotherapy such as with methotrexate, has been used in the past, but this treatment has proven quite disappointing over a long period of time.

Squamous cell carcinoma of the floor of the mouth is the most common intraoral lesion; nearly

Table 17-1. Definition of the TNM categories of malignant tumors about the oral cavity*

T (Primary tumor)		*N* (Regional lymph nodes)		*M* (Distant metastasis)	
TIS	Carcinoma in situ	N0	No clinically palpable cervical lymph node(s); or palpable node(s) but metastasis not suspected	M0	No distant metastasis
T1	Tumor 2 cm. or less in greatest diameter			M1	Clinical or radiographic evidence, or both, of metastasis other than to cervical lymph nodes
T2	Tumor greater than 2 cm. but not greater than 4 cm. in greatest diameter	N1	Clinically palpable homolateral cervical lymph node(s) that are not fixed; metastasis suspected		
T3	Tumor greater than 4 cm. in greatest diameter	N2	Clinically palpable contralateral or bilateral cervical lymph node(s) that are not fixed; metastasis suspected		
		N3	Clinically palpable lymph node(s) that are fixed; metastasis suspected		

Stage I:	T1	N0	M0	Stage IV:	T1	N2	M0	T1 N3 M0
Stage II:	T2	N0	M0		T2	N2	M0	T2 N3 M0
Stage III:	T3	N0	M0		T3	N2	M0	T2 N3 M0
	T1	N1	M0		Or, any T or N category with M1			
	T2	N1	M0					
	T3	N1	M0					

*Data from Cancer statistics, 1974, New York, 1974, American Cancer Society, Inc.

40% of all oral carcinomas seen are of this type. It is often multifocal in origin, and any patient who develops one carcinoma has a significantly greater chance of developing a second primary lesion.

STAGING OF THE TUMOR

Clinical staging of the tumors of the oral cavity is desirable, and the staging system of the American Cancer Society shown in Table 17-1 is the system used by most surgical services.

Other variations have appeared in the literature, particularly in reports by radiologists, and these variations sometimes lead to confusion when a comparison of results is attempted.[3] Nevertheless, the TNM system of staging does offer a satisfactory means for comparison when used by all reports. Because better survival rates have been reported in the treatment of earlier and smaller lesions, much publicity has been directed toward bringing patients under treatment at an earlier date. In a recent report from Memorial Hospital in New York, Harrold cited little increase in the number of TI patients seen in their clinic over the past 29 years.[4] Reports from radiotherapy centers appear to indicate a larger number of TI, T2 lesions than most reports from surgical centers, which can be interpreted to mean that more of the early lesions are being treated by irradiation than by surgery.[3]

HISTORY

Various methods of treatment of oral cancers have been popular over the years. Prior to 1940 most oral cancers were treated by radiation therapy; both the primary lesion and neck involvement were irradiated, and surgery was not performed. During the 1940's Memorial Hospital, under the leadership of Hayes Martin, Director of the Head and Neck Service, began to utilize a more radical surgical approach to lesions of the floor of the mouth; by 1944, an equal number of patients were treated by surgery as were treated by irradiation.[4] The trend continued until 1950, when over 90% of patients were treated by surgery, not only at Memorial Hospital, but throughout the country. As the concept of the radical neck dissection became popular and wide resections of the primary lesion were accepted, better 5- and 10-year survival figures were observed. However, this treatment also lead to a greater incidence of deformities of appearance and function. Such deformities proved unacceptable to many patients and referring physicians, as well as to the surgeons themselves, and stimulated a search for not only better means of treatment, but better methods of reconstruction. Thus during the 1950's and 1960's more imagination was displayed in the development of methods of restoring function and appearance, first as a secondary procedure and then as part of the primary management of intraoral cancers. Coincident with this trend was the appearance of high-energy radiation therapy, which allows a greater concentration of radiation to the tumor area with a less damaging effect on the surrounding normal tissue. In many sophisticated radiation therapy centers, tumor-free 5- and 10-year survival figures that were as high as those from surgical centers were being reported, and frequently these patients had less obvious cosmetic deformities. However, even this form of treatment is not without its morbidity and permanent impairment of function and appearance. The need for improved methods of management still exists, and neither irradiation nor surgery holds any great edge in results. Often the final decision on the method of treatment of cancer of the floor of the mouth is based on the availability of the most competent people in any given area of the country.

TREATMENT

Because we have had good departments of radiation therapy available at the institutions where we have concentrated our work, programs of management involving either surgery or radiation therapy have been possible. We have concentrated our interests in trying to develop a system of proper selection of patients for each modality of treatment rather than in developing a combined program for treatment, believing that by this approach we can offer the patient the best chance of survival with the least possible deformity. This plan of management has been further supported by the observation that neither surgery nor radiation therapy have much to offer the patient if the first major form of treatment has failed to control the tumor.

Therefore, the following plan of management, with only brief variations at any given time, has evolved over the past 20 years. Almost all T1 and T2, N0 lesions involving the anterior floor of the mouth, as well as selected T1, N0 lesions anterior to the posterior border of the mylohyoid muscle have been referred to radiation therapy. These patients have been followed very closely for possible recurrence or lymph node involvement, and either a radical neck dissection or a composite resection has been carried out as soon as a recurrence or metastasis has been proved. The most difficult differential diagnosis has been between obstruction of Wharton's duct accompanied by an enlargement of the submandibular gland after treatment of anterior lesions and possible metastatic cancerous lymph nodes found in the submaxillary triangle. Careful palpation and experience allows one to make this differentiation with good accuracy and thus save the patient from treatment that is too aggressive. If any doubt exists, however, we prefer to err with treatment that is too aggressive rather than too late. Success with this plan of treatment requires a meticulous follow-up program, which in our clinic

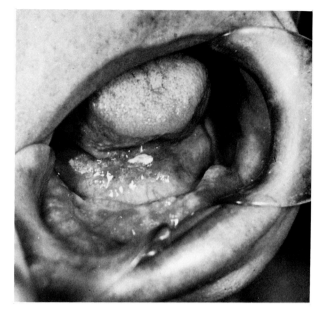

Fig. 17-1. T2 N0 squamous cell carcinoma of the right floor of the mouth.

means monthly checks for the first 3 months, checks every 2 months for the next 6 months, and checks every 6 to 12 months indefinitely. Our experience has shown that most recurrences or metastases are observed in the first 2 years after the initial treatment and that subsequent treatment can be successful only if detected early.

All Stage III lesions and selected Stage II and Stage IV lesions where lymph nodes have not been fixed have been operated on. When the size of the primary lesion necessitates removal of enough tissue that replacement of soft tissue is necessary to maintain freedom of the tongue and a satisfactory sulcus in the floor of the mouth, pedicle coverage becomes the procedure of choice (Fig. 17-1). Frequently the gingiva and the inner table of the mandible will be removed with the specimen, leaving raw bone, which requires pedicle coverage. At least 1 cm. of tumor-free soft tissue is taken with the specimen, and frequent frozen section biopsies are utilized to check the remaining borders for submucosal extension of the tumor. Elective neck dissections are carried out, even if lymph node involvement is not detected, to obtain pedicle coverage intraorally.

Surgical procedure

Incisions on the neck are determined by the cervical pedicle used intraorally (Fig. 17-2). This pedicle is based on the mastoid process and the infra-

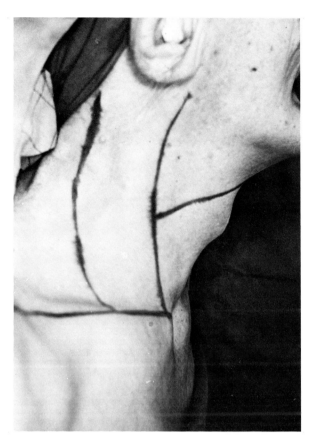

Fig. 17-2. Outline of neck incisions.

auricular area; the anterior border of the pedicle runs parallel to the anterior border of the sternocleido-mastoid muscle. The pedicle is kept just posterior to the beard on the male. The incision is carried down to the upper border of the clavicle and then posteriorly. The pedicle is designed to obtain as near a 3:1 length to width ratio as possible, not exceeding a 4:1 ratio. The anterior part of the neck is exposed by an incision extending from the middle anterior border of the cervical pedicle to the underside of the chin on the opposite side. The posterior triangle of the neck is exposed by an extension of the lower incision of the cervical pedicle toward the shoulder, which then becomes the upper border of a shoulder deltopectoral pedicle based on the sternum. This pedicle is used to resurface the neck at the conclusion of the operation.

A routine neck dissection is carried out; care is taken to protect the postauricular artery, which is vital to the survival of the cervical pedicle. When the neck specimen is dissected to the underside of the mandible, the mouth is entered and a buccal incision is made to remove the inner table of the jaw if the tumor is adjacent to the jaw. If the tumor has grown into the bone, demonstrated either clinically or by x-ray examination, a full-thickness section of the jaw is removed with the specimen. After complete removal of the specimen, hemostasis is completed; the wound is then carefully flushed out with copious amounts of saline solution. A complete change of gowns and gloves is made, and closure is begun.

The cervical pedicle is advanced into the mouth, and the bony prominence of the angles of the mandible is removed if it appears to impinge on the base of the pedicle (Fig. 17-3, *A*). The pedicle is trimmed to fit and will resurface the entire side of the mandible and tongue, as well as the entire anterior floor of the mouth if it is necessary (Fig. 17-3, *B*). This procedure leaves an oral cutaneous fistula, which is closed surgically 3 to 6 weeks after the initial surgery. The neck incisions are closed by means of a deltopectoral pedicle based on the sternum (Fig. 17-3, *C*). A split-thickness skin graft is obtained from the abdomen and used to resurface the shoulder (Fig. 17-3, *D*); it is held in place by a tie-over gauze dressing. Once all incisions are closed, a tracheostomy is done; the nasal endotracheal tube is then removed. A Hemovac drain is inserted for 48 hours for suction drainage. Normally, 2 to 4 units of blood are used during the procedure. Antibiotic drugs are given preoperatively and for 5 days postoperatively. Closure of the oral cutaneous fistula is accomplished during the same admission if the patient is still confined to the hospital 3 weeks after surgery. Normally, however, the patient is discharged about 2 weeks after the operation and readmitted 4 weeks later for closure of the fistula.

Complications

Bone necrosis of the mandible remains the most consistent complication of radiotherapy;[1] it is apparently caused by dental caries. A very strict routine of dental extraction of decayed teeth is carried out in the area of treatment before irradiation is begun; a routine of dental prophylaxis is aimed at eliminating decay and death of teeth after irradiation. A program of brushing, oral lavage, and fluoride applications is encouraged. If dental caries develop after irradiation, they are repaired before decay is advanced, so that the need for extraction may hopefully be avoided. Where radionecrosis has occurred, removal of small spicules of bone has allowed spontaneous healing to occur. However, when conservative management has failed, wide resection of the involved bone has become necessary to control pain and recurrent infections.

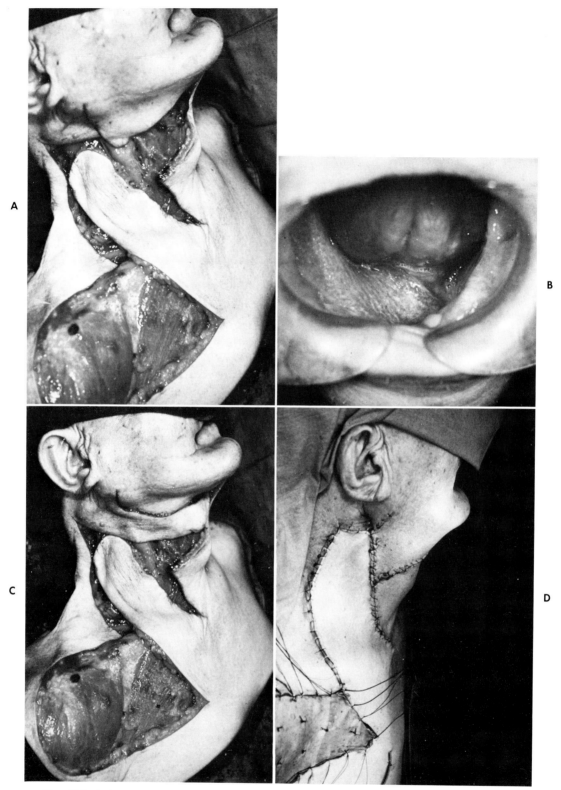

Fig. 17-3. A, Neck flaps elevated with the cervical flap inserted into the mouth. **B,** Cervical flap in right floor of the mouth. **C,** Deltopectoral flap inserted on the neck. **D,** Skin graft on shoulder donor site.

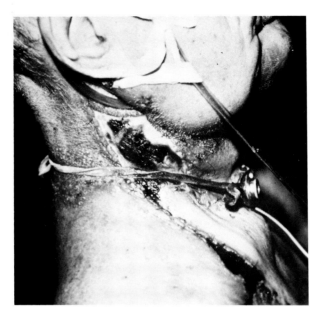

Fig. 17-4. Necrosis deltopectoral flap from tracheostomy strap.

Complication rates of 6% to 38% have been reported. We have seen a 10% rate of complications in our clinic.

The most frequently seen complication of the surgical management of these tumors has been the complete or partial loss of the cervical pedicle. This loss has occurred in 20% of the cases and has been caused primarily by the interruption of the postauricular artery. The length to width ratio is increased beyond 4:1, and angulation of the pedicle is produced where the angle of the jaw places too much tension on the base of the pedicle. No permanent fistulas have resulted from this complication that could not be closed when the intentional fistula was closed. Nevertheless, the mobility of the tongue or an adequate sulcus has been lost when a large portion of the pedicle has been lost. Three deltopectoral pedicles were partially lost when the straps from the tracheostomy tubes strangled the tips of the pedicles (Fig. 17-4). No losses of this pedicle have occurred since the tubes have been sutured in, and the three cases mentioned above were easily managed by split-thickness skin grafts; there was no rupture of the carotid artery in any instance. All cervical and deltopectoral pedicles have been raised and transferred without delays.

Surgical resections performed after radiation has failed to control the primary lesion have forced a more posteriorly placed cervical pedicle to be elevated. If this elevation was impossible, a forehead pedicle or deltopectoral pedicle has been used for lining inside the mouth. Both pedicles have obvious limitations; the forehead pedicle leaves an obvious deformity of the forehead, and the deltopectoral pedicle has its origin so far from its insertion that many stages of grafting are necessary. These pedicles have been necessary primarily in Stage III lesions or radiation failures.

No bilateral 1-stage neck dissections have been done for the past 15 years, because of the high morbidity and mortality and low cure rates. Most of these patients were declared incurable and were treated symptomatically from the beginning. Although no deaths have occurred from radiation therapy, our operative mortality of 3% to 4% still exists, primarily because of aspiration in the immediate postoperative period. These deaths have all been of inpatients with Stage III lesions involving the anterior floor of the mouth where the anterior jaw has been removed. In each of these patients, a K wire has been used for support; but removal of the mylohyoid, geniohyoid, and genioglossus muscles have produced a significant impairment of function, causing serious aspiration and swallowing difficulties in a large number of patients.

These significant complications have primarily occurred in patients with Stage III and Stage IV lesions who have had other debilitating disease, such as diabetes, cirrhosis, and malnutrition, or previous irradiation. The majority of the complications seen in our clinic have been wound infections, delayed wound healing, and partial losses of skin grafts and pedicles with fistulas.

Results

Many different methods of reporting results have appeared in the literature; therefore, it is very difficult to compare results from different centers. However, it is quite clear that Stage I lesions have the best prognosis. (Our radiation department reports a 5-year survival rate of 60.8% of patients with T1 and T2, N0 lesions.) Stage II lesions offer a less favorable result. Five-year survival rates of 50% to 60% are reported; slightly higher rates are reported by radiation therapy than by surgery. The best results from radiotherapy are reported of patients with T1, T2, and occasionally T3 lesions where no lymph node involvement is determined at the time treatment begins. Surgery offers a much better prognosis for T2 and T3 lesions with N1 or N2 lymph node involvement; patients with Stage III lesions treated by surgery have a 24% 5-year survival rate as compared with the 12% survival rate of those treated by radiotherapy.

Our experience has been that a few patients with Stage I and Stage II lesions who were initially treated by radiation therapy have been saved by surgery when recurrences were detected early but that there have been no survivals after surgical failure. Radiotherapy in these patients has given only temporary palliation. Furthermore, patients treated initially for T1 and T2, N0 lesions, who subsequently develop lymph node involvement can be helped by a radical neck dissection; and the prognosis is good, provided that there is no subsequent recurrence of the primary lesion.

SUMMARY

During the past 25 years there has been a fourfold increase in the incidence of cancer of the floor of the mouth in women. Patients with T1 and T2, N0 lesions can be treated by radiotherapy and have 5-year survival rates as good as the survival rates of those treated by surgery (70+% for patients with T1 lesions and 50+% for patients with T2 lesions). All primary lesions with lymph node involvement are best treated by surgery. Most surgical excisions of T2 and T4 lesions will require soft tissue replacement to prevent significant impairment of function or change in appearance. Such techniques are now available and should be utilized at the time of initial surgery. A system of selecting patients for radiation therapy or surgery has been suggested in an attempt to fit the treatment to the patient rather than the patient to the treatment. Most radiotherapists tend to minimize the complaints patients have after radiation therapy, and surgeons tend to minimize complaints patients have after surgery. Both modalities offer good and bad results, and we are attempting to capitalize on the best that each service has to offer.

REFERENCES

1. Campos, J. L., Lampe, I., and Fayos, J. V.: Radiotherapy of carcinoma of the floor of the mouth, Radiology **99**:677, 1971.
2. Cancer statistics, 1974, New York, 1974, American Cancer Society, Inc., p. 10.
3. Fayos, J. V.: Management of squamous cell carcinoma of the floor of the mouth, Am. J. Surg. **123**:706, 1972.
4. Harrold, C. C.: Management of cancer of the floor of the mouth, Am. J. Surg. **122**:487, 1971.
5. Landa, S. J. F., and Zarem, H. A.: Cancer of the floor of the mouth and the gingiva, Surg. Clin. North Am. **53**:135, 1973.

Chapter 18

Cancer of the paranasal sinuses and nasopharynx

Robert G. Chambers, M.D.

Carcinoma of the paranasal sinus fortunately is not common; it accounts for only 0.3% of all cancers occurring in the human body.[10] Prognosis of these neoplasms is very poor, principally because of their insidious onset, inaccessibility, and advanced stage when diagnosed. Since 1946 a total of 241 malignant tumors of this type have been followed through to death or to a 5-year survival without disease. These tumors are discussed according to their primary sites.

Nasopharynx

The dome-shaped vault of the nasopharynx joins the oropharynx and nasal cavities, except for the soft palate floor and is a rigid structure; it does not lend itself to any type of extirpative surgery.[16] Malignancies of the nasopharynx seem to be best handled by irradiation. At best, the survival rate does not exceed 25%.[13] Contiguous vital structures at the base of the skull are rapidly involved, and most patients succumb to their disease within 2 years. Between 1946 and 1965 27 patients were seen with carcinoma of the nasopharynx; only 7 of these patients lived 5 years. Since 1965 hydroxyurea therapy has been given concomitantly with cobalt 60 therapy, and 23 of 40 patients (58%) lived 5 years without disease. Patients who have neck metastases without distant spread and who show excellent rapid control of the primary nasopharyngeal carcinoma should be considered candidates for appropriate neck dissections. Twenty of 67 patients received a neck dissection; 6 of these patients have survived 5 years.

Frontal sinus

In this study, 5 cases of primary frontal sinus carcinoma were noted. The commonest early complaint of these patients was constant unilateral frontal headache. Swelling and proptosis of one eye, displacement of bony walls, broadening of the base of the nose, and purulent nasal discharge are late findings.[13] After diagnosis of carcinoma is established, radium can be applied directly in the frontal sinus, followed by x-ray therapy.[16] None of these patients with primary frontal sinus carcinoma survived beyond 3 years.

Sphenoid sinus

Primary carcinoma of the sphenoid sinus is rare; 4 of the 241 patients fell in this category. Except for surgical opening of the sinus for biopsy, the treatment of sphenoid cancer is radiologic.[16] All 4 patients succumbed to their disease.

Ethmoid sinus

Primary carcinoma of the ethmoid labyrinth is the second most frequently occurring sinus cancer.[16] In this group of 20 cases, the mean age was 49 years. In order of frequency the symptoms are nasal obstruction, nasal bleeding, pain, swelling of one eye, and anosmia.[16] Most often these patients have a purulent discharge and a bleeding growth in one side of the nose. Other findings, such as local cellulitis, proptosis, papilledema, turbinate enlargement, and nasopharyngeal and palatine masses, may be present. X-ray findings include ethmoid and adjacent sinus clouding, orbital wall destruction, destruction of the base of the skull, destruction of the posterior antral wall, and obliteration of the foramen.[11]

The treatment of cancer of the ethmoid sinus is often a combination of surgery and irradiation. The extent of the tumor is determined by a lateral rhinotomy and an appropriate antrostomy.[16] Postoperative roentgen therapy is given through anterior ports.[13] The external irradiation is supplemented with intranasal therapy in the form of intracavitary radium.[16] If possible the radiation dose should reach 6,000 to 8,000 R. Fifteen of the 20 patients were treated in this manner, and 5 of these survived. The remaining 5 patients were given a course of preoperative irradiation after appropriate surgical diagnosis; 6 weeks later a combined cranial transfacial resection was done. Three of these patients survived 5 years.

An uncommon tumor often showing symptoms similar to ethmoid cancer is the esthesioneuroblastoma of the cribriform plate.[12,14] During the past 23 years I have accumulated a total of 14 patients who have had this tumor. Age range has been 8 to 80 years, and male patients have outnumbered female patients 2 to 1. Clinical symptoms in order of frequency are long-standing nasal obstruction on one side, frequent epistaxis, history of recurrent nasal polyps, excessive lacrimation, rhinorrhea, and occasionally anosmia. Late symptoms are exophthalmos, bony and ocular distortion, headaches and pain.[1-9]

Esthesioneuroblastomas appear with fairly constant physical findings. In its early stage it is seen as a small tumor high on the septal side. The tumor is soft, friable, and bleeds easily. Larger tumors will fill the nasal vault and involve the adjacent sinuses with a nonulcerating, pinkish gray tumor covered by smooth mucosa.[12,14]

A radiological examination will not show any bone destruction until late in the course of the disease.

The treatment of these tumors is in doubt. In my experience, the most successful treatment has been concomitant chemotheraphy and preoperative irradiation followed by as limited a surgical procedure as possible. Usually a combined craniotomy and rhinotomy approach is the least surgical procedure that can be done. For the more extensive lesion a craniomaxillary facial resection must be carried out. I have had no success with a simple maxillary rhinotomy.

Five of the 14 patients in this series are free of disease after 4 years or more. Six patients are dead.

The cause of death was intracranical extension and metastases.

Carcinoma of the antrum

The maxillary sinus is the largest paranasal sinus and the one most frequently involved with cancer.[11,16] The symptoms and signs of antral cancer can also be highly suggestive of sinusitis. Careful x-ray studies, particularly tomography, adds vital information as to the presence and degree of bone involvement. At least 70% of antral carcinomas will have evidence of destruction of some portion of the bony vault.[13,16] In the absence of definite evidence of cancer it is justified to employ a very brief trial of antibiotics, allergic management, and drainage. However, in the absence of a definite response to this regimen an exploratory sinusotomy should be done.[13]

Once the diagnosis of cancer is made, the antrum and adjacent structures are carefully mapped out for serial biopsies to determine the extent of involvement. The status of all the bony walls is evaluated by selective biopsy and finger palpation through the sinusotomy opening. The orbit can be spared only when there is no tumor involvement of the roof of the antrum. When the orbit is preserved, a calculated risk is assumed.

Antral cancer is treated by surgery, surgery and postoperative irradiation, and preoperative irradiation followed by surgery; each modality has its proponents.[13] It is generally agreed, however, that the following conditions are contraindications to curative treatment[13]: (1) destruction of the pterygoid plate, (2) destruction of the base of the skull, (3) nasopharyngeal extension, (4) tumor in the temporal fossa, (5) inoperable regional metastases, (6) extensive involvement of the dermal lymphatics of the overlying skin, and (7) generalized metastases.

I prefer to treat cancer of the maxillary sinus with a planned full dose of preoperative irradiation followed by appropriate radical surgery about 6 weeks later. The extent of the resection is determined by the original diagnostic studies. After the specimen has been removed, the wound cavities are covered with a split-thickness skin graft. I am opposed to the immediate obliteration of the palatine defect by the use of nasal septum or migrated skin flaps. Whenever possible, a preoperatively manufactured dental prosthesis is inserted immediately. If a prosthesis cannot be manufactured preoperatively, one should be fitted within 3 to 4 weeks. In selective cases additional irradiation in the form of intracavitary radium is of benefit postoperatively. Electrosurgery or cryosurgery, or both, are adjuncts that can be used for persistent local disease or recurrences.

During the past 23 years 150 consecutive cases of antral cancer have been examined, treated, and personally followed. All have been treated in the manner outlined; the absolute survival rate has been 50%.

SUMMARY

A group of 241 cases of paranasal sinus carcinoma and nasopharyngeal carcinoma have been discussed. Although the results leave much to be desired, principally because of the late stage of the disease at the onset of treatment, some gratifying results can be obtained by the judicious and meticulous selection of appropriate therapy.

REFERENCES

1. Becher, M. H., and Jacox, H. W.: Olfactory esthesioneuroepithelioma; experiences in the management of a rare malignant neoplasm, Radiology **82:** 77-83, 1964.
2. Bidstrup, R. J., and Wilkins, S. A., Jr.: Olfactory esthesioneuroma, South. Med. J. **63:**1426-1430, 1970.
3. Castro, L., De la Pava, S., and Webster, J. H.: Esthesioneuroblastoma; are part of 7 cases, Am. J. Roentgenol. Radium Ther. Nucl. Med. **105:**7-13, 1969.
4. Doyle, P. J.: Approach to tumors of the nose, nasopharynx, and paranasal sinuses, Laryngoscope **78:** 1756-1762, 1968.
5. Doyle, P. J., and Paxton H. D.: Combined surgical approach to esthesioneuroepithelioma, Trans. Am. Acad. Ophthalmol. Otolaryngol. **75:**526-531, 1971.
6. Farr, H. W.: Soft part sarcoma of the head and neck, Am. J. Surg. **122:**714-718, 1971.
7. Fitz-Hugh, G. S., Allen, M. S., Rucker, T. N., and Sprinkle, P. M.: Olfactory neuroblastoma (esthesioneuroepithelioma), Arch. Otolaryngol. **81:**161-168, 1965.
8. Gerard-Marchant, R., and Micheau, C.: Microscopical diagnosis of olfactory esthesioneuromas; general review and report of five cases, J. Natl. Cancer Inst. **35:**75-82, 1965.
9. Harpman, J. A.: Malignant neoplasm around the cribriform plate, Arch. Otolaryngol. **84:**189-192, 1966.
10. Harrison, D. F. N.: The management of malignant tumors of the nasal sinusus, Otolaryngol. Clin. North Am. **4**(1):159, 1971.
11. Helger, J. A.: Maxilloethmoidal carcinoma, Otolaryngol. Clin. North Am. **4**(1): 159, 1971.
12. Hutter, R. V., and others: Esthesioneuroblastoma; a clinical and pathological study, Am. J. Surg. **106:**748-753, 1963.
13. Maccomb, W. S., and Fletcher, G. H.: Cancer of the head and neck., Baltimore, 1967, The Williams & Wilkins Co.
14. Schenck, N. L., and Ogura, J. H.: Esthesioneuroblastoma, Arch. Otolaryngol. **96:**322, October, 1972.
15. Tabb, H. C., and Barroneo, S. J.: Cancer of the maxillary sinus, Laryngoscope **60:**119, 1950.
16. Ward, G. E., and Hendrick, J. W.: Tumors of the head and neck, Baltimore, 1950, The Williams & Wilkins Co.

Chapter 19

Carcinoma of the hypopharynx and cervical esophagus

John M. Loré, Jr., M.D.

The incidence of squamous cell cancer of the hypopharynx and cervical esophagus is low in comparison with other carcinomas of the head and neck. For carcinoma of the hypopharynx the age-adjusted death rates (based on 100,000 deaths) in the United States for the years 1950 to 1967 were as follows[2]:

Men	Percent	Women	Percent
White	0.304	White	0.046
Nonwhite	0.282	Nonwhite	0.045

Carcinoma of the cervical esophagus was responsible for approximately 0.6% of the deaths from all types of cancer of 100,000 men in the United States.[11]

The etiology of these squamous cell carcinomas is the same as for other cancers of the upper respiratory and digestive tracts: tobacco and alcohol. Deficiency diseases, such as the Plummer-Vinson syndrome associated with vitamin deficiency and iron deficiency anemias (especially in elderly women), and lye burns of the esophagus also appear to be causative factors. One patient sustained a severe caustic burn as a child and later, in the third decade of life, developed a cervical esophageal cancer (Fig. 19-1).

ANATOMY
Hypopharynx

The hypopharynx is that portion of the pharynx that extends from a horizontal line superiorly at the level of the tip of the epiglottis or the superior border of the hyoid bone and inferiorly to the lower border of the cricoid cartilage (Fig. 19-2). Laterally, the pharyngoepiglottic (glossoepiglottic) folds form the boundaries between the hypopharynx and the oropharynx. The exact boundaries superiorly are somewhat arbitrary and vary according to author.[5,9] On the posterior wall the superior extent of the hypopharynx is somewhat higher than the anterolateral portion. The anatomic description from the American Joint Committee for Cancer Staging and End Results is as follows.[1]

Pyriform sinus. The pyriform sinus is bound superiorly by the pharyngoepiglottic fold, anterolaterally between the inner surface of the arytenoid and cricoid cartilages. Inferiorly it extends to the upper edge of the esophagus.

Postcricoid area. The postcricoid site is the posterior surface of the larynx. It extends from the posterior surface of the arytenoid cartilages and their connecting folds to the inferior surface of the cricoid. The lateral margin is the anterior part of the pyriform sinus.

Posterior pharyngeal wall. The posterior pharyngeal wall extends from the level of the tip of the epiglottis, superiorly, down to the posterior margins of the pyriform sinus.

Thus tumors of the lateral wall are classified as tumors of the pyriform sinus. However, there is laterally a segment of the hypopharynx that does not appear to be a part of the pyriform sinus. The hypopharynx thus consists of a posterior wall, two lateral walls, an anterior wall that is for all practical purposes a portion of the larynx (the laryngeal surface of the epiglottis), the mucosa covering the posterior aspect of the cricoid cartilage, aryepiglottic folds, and pharyngoepiglottic folds (Fig. 19-2, *A*). The truly pharyngeal anterior boundaries are the anterior portion of the pyriform sinus and the mucosa covering the posterior aspect of the cricoid cartilage.

Although some authors[1] describe three distinct parts of the hypopharynx (the pyriform sinus, the post-

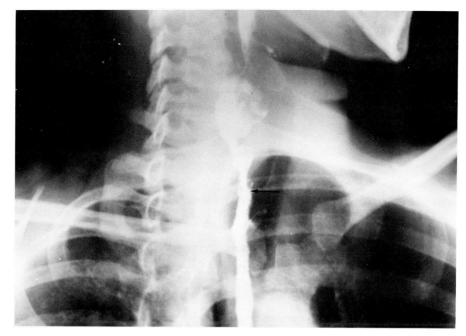

Fig. 19-1. Arrow points to a cervical esophageal carcinoma extending into the thorax. Etiology related to caustic burn the patient suffered as a child.

Fig. 19-2. A, Anterior view of the anatomy of the hypopharynx. **B,** Lateral view of the anatomy of the hypopharynx.

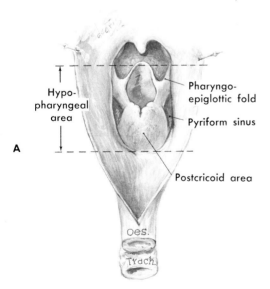

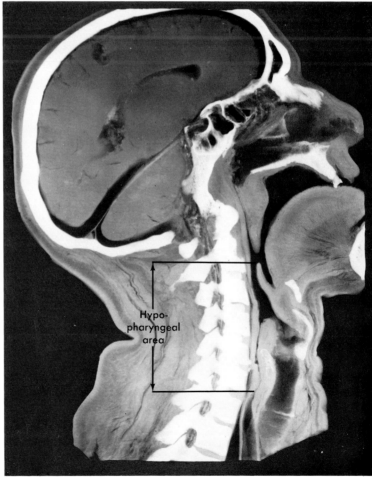

Table 19-1. Carcinoma of the hypopharynx and cervical esophagus*

Region and site	Total number of patients	Stage I		Stage II		Stage III		Stage IV	
		Number†	Percent‡	Number	Percent	Number	Percent	Number	Percent
Pyriform sinus	325	19	71	82	46	142	32	82	4
Postcricoid area	58	1	100	19	31	20	22	18	6
Posterior pharyngeal wall	81	15	38	18	33	29	20	19	0

*Data from American Joint Committee on Clinical Staging and End Results; clinical staging system for carcinoma of the pharynx, Chicago, 1965, the Committee.
†Number of patients in each group.
‡Survival rate at 60 months.

cricoid area, and the posterior pharyngeal wall), another part, the lateral walls, appears quite distinctly above the level of the pyriform sinus.

Cervical esophagus

The cervical esophagus superiorly is continuous with the hypopharynx at the inferior border of the cricoid cartilage. It extends inferiorly slightly to the left to a purely arbitrary level at the edge of the manubrium sterni, measuring in length from 4.7 to 7.5 cm. in men and 4 to 7 cm. in women.[6]

PATHOLOGIC ANATOMY

Squamous cell cancer of the hypopharynx and especially of the cervical esophagus appears to have a propensity for spreading submucosally (Fig. 19-3). These cancers may still become exfoliated, however; hypopharynx cancer that has become tremendous in size has been seen. (One patient had a lesion measuring 6 × 4 cm., which makes one wonder how the patient was able to swallow at all and why a fatal bout of aspiration did not occur (Fig. 19-4). In other instances the primary lesion of the hypopharyngeal cancer can be minute but have massive metastasis (Fig. 19-5). Spread can also occur by direct extension to contiguous structures. For example, a lesion can extend anteriorly to the larynx and superiorly to the oropharynx to involve the base of the tongue and the palatine tonsil; it can then extend into the nasopharynx, as well as spread from the hypopharynx to the cervical esophagus and vice versa. A lesion of the medial wall of the pyriform sinus or the postcricoid area can directly extend to involve and fix the arytenoid cartilages. Nodal metastasis can occur via the parapharyngeal and retropharyngeal lymph channels superiorly to the base of the skull and inferiorly via the tracheoesophageal lymph channels into the mediastinum. Spread to the internal jugular chain of lymph nodes also occurs. Carcinoma of the cervical esophagus may appear with initial enlargement of the supraclavicular lymph nodes and fullness in Burns' space.

On two occasions, carcinoma that originated in a pharyngoesophageal diverticulum has been seen.

Submucosal spread of hypopharyngeal cancer may result in what appears to be multiple separate primary lesions as the tumor involves isolated areas of mucosa. Multiple primary lesions can occur, however.

Goodner, in his review of cancer of the cervical esophagus,[4] reported that of 178 patients, 173

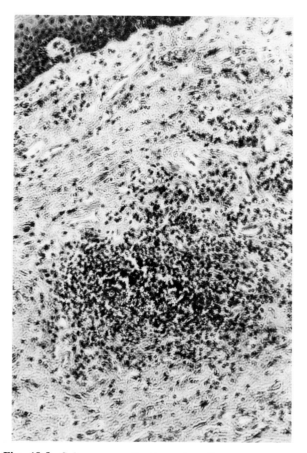

Fig. 19-3. Submucosa collection of malignant squamous cells in cervical esophageal carcinoma.

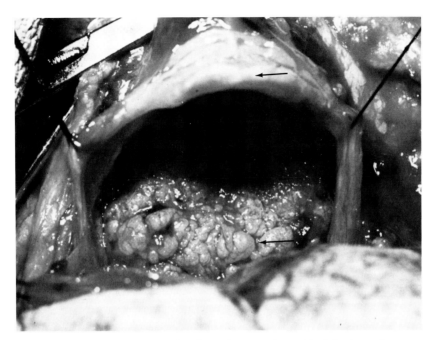

Fig. 19-4. Massive carcinoma originating from the posterior wall of the hypopharynx as seen through a transhyoid pharyngotomy during surgery. Upper arrow indicates the epiglottis; lower arrow indicates a tumor on the posterior hypopharyngeal wall.

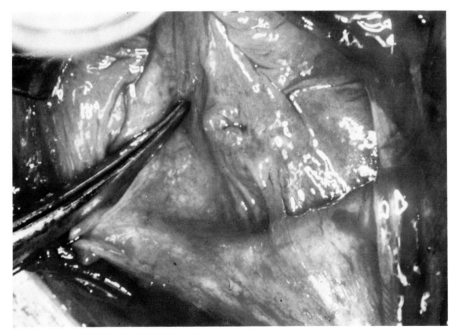

Fig. 19-5. Small primary carcinoma of the medial wall of the pyriform sinus opposite the tip of the instrument.

had confirmed squamous or epidermoid carcinomas by histologic examination. There were 3 patients who had adenocarcinomas, 1 who had fibrosarcoma, and 1 who had mucoepidermoid carcinoma.

SURVIVAL

The pathologic anatomy and natural history of these cancers indicate a poor prognosis. The usual history of late diagnosis and the fact that the pyriform sinus is one of the so-called unknown primary sites in head and neck cancer add to this poor prognosis. The carcinoma depicted in Fig. 19-5 is an example of how such cancer eludes diagnosis. A small primary lesion that was not seen by mirror laryngoscopy appeared by direct laryngoscopy as a small cyst with intact overlying mucosa, but on biopsy it proved to be squamous cell carcinoma (Fig. 19-5).

Table 19-1 shows the 5-year survival rates of patients with hypopharyngeal squamous cell carcinoma according to the American Joint Committee on Clinical Staging and End Results.[1] The Committee has stated that a poorer prognosis seems to be associated with the less-differentiated types of squamous cell carcinoma. It is interesting to note that pyriform sinus carcinoma has a somewhat better prognosis than carcinoma of the other sites despite the fact that the pyriform sinus is one of the hidden primary regions. The survival rate of patients who have carcinoma of the cervical esophagus, according to Goodner,[4] is 15.3% when surgery is used alone and 19.2% when surgery is combined with radiation therapy.

SIGNS AND SYMPTOMS
Hypopharyngeal carcinoma

Patients who have symptoms associated with carcinoma of the hypopharynx can be divided into two main groups: those patients who have a significantly sized primary lesion and those who have a cervical mass associated with an extremely small primary lesion.

The symptoms of patients in the first group include a persistent sore throat, sometimes described as a burning sensation. It is usually associated with dysphagia of varying degree and expectorations that are excessive but seldom with blood. Pain may be present on the side of the neck where the bulk of the tumor lies and may occasionally radiate to the homolateral ear. Hoarseness is not common and when present usually indicates paralysis of a vocal cord, caused by fixation of an arytenoid cartilage by direct extension to the larynx. This condition contraindicates an operation that would preserve the larynx.

Sore throat, dysphagia, and voice changes are absent in the group with extremely small primary lesions (2 to 3 mm. in size). The only complaint may be a mass in the neck that initially may be of unknown origin.

Cervical esophageal carcinoma

The primary symptom of cervical esophageal carcinoma is dysphagia of variable degrees. As the degree of esophageal obstruction increases, aspiration can occur with hoarseness caused by irritation of the vocal cords. Cord paralysis is possible, and the lesion may extend to involve the laryngeal nerves. Early diagnosis of a small esophageal cancer is quite rare.

Medical histories of patients who had carcinoma of the hypopharynx and cervical esophagus (especially the former) indicate that there was an unacceptable delay in diagnosis from the time of the onset of the first symptom. The delay ranged from 4 months to more than 12 months. The fault appears to have been, all too frequently, that of the physician who was first consulted. From situations where no adequate examination was made and the patient was advised to gargle with a mouthwash to situations where an apparently competent examination was made, the diagnosis was missed. The complaint of a sore throat is simply too common for most physicians to conduct or recommend an adequate examination, yet a sore throat persisting for more than 2 to 3 weeks indicates the necessity of further meticulous examination.

PHYSICAL FINDINGS AND DIAGNOSIS

The significant physical findings revealed by initial office examination of the head and neck are based on four maneuvers:

1. Palpation for cervical lymphadenopathy
2. Direct inspection (with a tongue depressor) of the superior portion of the posterior and lateral hypopharyngeal walls
3. Mirror laryngoscopy with careful and complete visualization of all parts of the hypopharynx (posterior wall, lateral walls, pyriform sinus and postcricoid area) as well as the larynx and base of the tongue for spread of disease
4. Palpation of the superior portion of the posterior and lateral hypopharyngeal walls as well as the base of the tongue and the palatine tonsils for spread of disease

Cervical lymphadenopathy ranges from small nodes to nodes as large as 6.5 × 8.5 cm. in diameter. In hypopharynx cancer the more commonly palpable lymph nodes are the middle internal jugular and

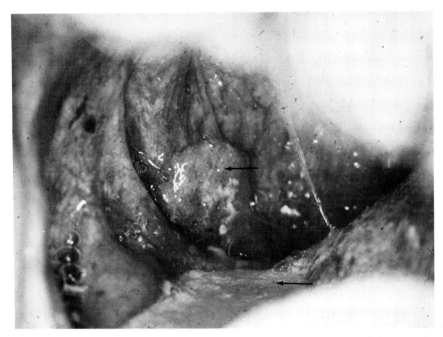

Fig. 19-6. Carcinoma of the superior portion of the posterior lateral wall of the hypopharynx as visualized by depressing the tongue. Upper arrow indicates tumor; lower arrow indicates the base of the tongue.

subdigastric group; in cervical esophageal cancer low internal jugular and supraclavicular nodes may be detected. The parapharyngeal, retropharyngeal, tracheoesophageal, and superior mediastinal node enlargements are not usually palpable.

Direct inspection utilizing a tongue depressor can detect some lesions of the superior portion of the hypopharynx (Fig. 19-6). The use of topical anesthesia with 10% cocaine or 2% tetracaine (Pontocaine) hydrochloride will reduce the gag reflex and aid in this inspection. Valium can be utilized to further relax the patient. Mirror laryngoscopy is the main office procedure for all lesions below the most superior portion of the hypopharynx. A problem of mirror laryngoscopy is that most examiners, because of the name of the procedure and habit, concentrate only on the larynx. The importance of visualization of the walls of the pyriform sinus is recognized during phonation, which tends to open these recesses. However, visualization of the midportion of the posterior and lateral walls of the hypopharynx is apt to be overlooked. This oversight may in part be caused by the angulation of the mirror, which must be directed downward and more posteriorly to visualize these often-missed regions.

The apex or inferior tip of the pyriform sinus

must be carefully scrutinized. Adequate visualization with the laryngeal mirror may not be feasible, and direct laryngoscopy and direct pharyngoscopy are always necessary when cervical lymphadenopathy of unknown origin exists or unexplained symptoms persist. Only the superior aspect of the postericoid area can be visualized by mirror examination. However, inflammation, edema, or an accumulation of saliva at the base of the arytenoid cartilages posteriorly will indicate that something is wrong.

Filling of the pyriform sinus with saliva (positive Jackson's sign) is almost prima facie evidence of some type of esophageal obstruction and requires further evaluation with esophagram and esophagoscopy. However, depending on the extent of obstruction, this sign may be absent in esophageal cancer.

Histologic diagnosis is made from a biopsy by means of either a laryngoscope or a pharyngoscope for the hypopharynx and an esophagoscope for the esophagus. At the time of direct examination it is imperative that indirect mirror examination be repeated with the patient under topical anesthesia (8 to 10 ml. of 10% cocaine). The patient is premedicated, and under these circumstances indirect examination may be very rewarding. Indirect examination affords an excellent overall view of the larynx and hypopharynx and a functional evaluation of the larynx as to whether there is a paralyzed or sluggish vocal cord. The direct examination then follows. If the lesion is obvious, topical anesthesia suffices; otherwise, general anesthesia via a small endotracheal tube is the choice. When a lesion originates high on the posterior or lateral walls of the hypopharynx, direct biopsy through the oral cavity is sometimes feasible. It is most important that repeated biopsies be obtained when a diagnosis of carcinoma is suspected and the initial biopsy report is negative.

As an initial procedure open surgical excisional biopsy of a mass in the neck is condemned. If there is a question regarding the etiology of a cervical mass and a complete examination has failed to reveal a primary lesion, a needle aspiration may be performed. When all else (a complete head and neck examination including direct laryngoscopy, bronchoscopy, esophagoscopy, nasopharyngoscopy, radiologic examination, needle aspiration, and complete physical examination) fails, then an open surgical, frozen section biopsy of a mass in the neck is justified.

The physician should not attempt to pass the esophagoscope beyond the tumor, because it could perforate the esophagus. Deep biopsy should also be avoided for the same reason. Often a physician can make a diagnosis by utilizing a small fragment of Gelfoam ($20 \times 60 \times 7$ mm.) grasped in a foreign body "peanut type" forceps.[8] The Gelfoam is gently rubbed on the ulcerative tumor and picks up cells that are then smeared on a slide for a Papanicolaou stain.

RADIOGRAPHIC EXAMINATION

Radiographic examination must be performed before any direct examination with a laryngoscope or pharyngoscope and biopsies are made; otherwise, false findings of the size and extent of the tumor may result from edema.

Soft tissue examination of the lateral wall of the neck

Soft tissue examination of the lateral wall of the neck is the simplest type of radiographic examination and is mainly used to confirm the larger lesions revealed by mirror examination. Fig. 19-7 shows a large, bulky lesion of the posterior wall overhanging the supraglottic region. Fig. 19-8 shows the shadow of a large lateral hypopharyngeal wall tumor that involves the pyriform sinus and epiglottis and extends superiorly to the palatine tonsil. In addition to

conventional radiograms, xerograms render improved soft tissue detail.

Coronal planogram

Coronal planograms are also based on the soft tissue shadow of the tumor best seen in the larger lesions. These examinations give some evidence of the extent of the tumor and may at times detect a

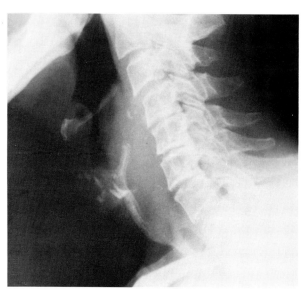

Fig. 19-7. Soft tissue x-ray film of a large bulky lesion of the posterior wall overhanging the supraglottic region.

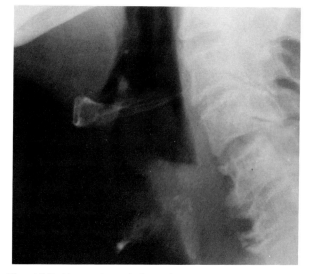

Fig. 19-8. Large lateral hypopharyngeal carcinoma that extends superiorly to the palatine tonsil and inferiorly into the pyriform sinus.

smaller tumor, especially one involving the intrinsic part of the larynx. Obliteration or encroachment of any of the usual air-filled areas, such as the pyriform sinus, the ventricle, margins of the arytenoids, aryepiglottic folds, the epiglottis, and true and false cords, are usually seen. Subglottic fullness is of great aid in these radiographic examinations to delineate spread of disease. Fig. 19-9 shows a large lesion of the right lateral hypopharyngeal wall, involving the epiglottis, the arytenoid area, and the ventricle. Another film showed that the pyriform sinus was also invaded. It must be emphasized that differentiation between edema and tumor is hardly possible. Fig. 19-10 depicts a large ulcerative carcinoma of the right pyriform sinus, which is virtually totally obliterated; the carcinoma extends superiorly along the lateral hypopharyngeal wall. There is evidence of involvement of the right false cord and encroachment into the right ventricle.

Barium swallow procedure

The use of barium as a contrast material will aid in the confirmation of lesions that obliterate a pyri-

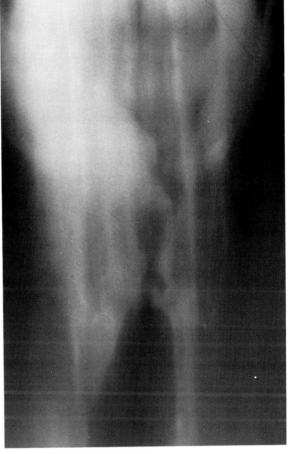

Fig. 19-9. Coronal planogram depicting a posterior hypopharyngeal carcinoma with involvement of the arytenoid area and obliteration of the ventricle.

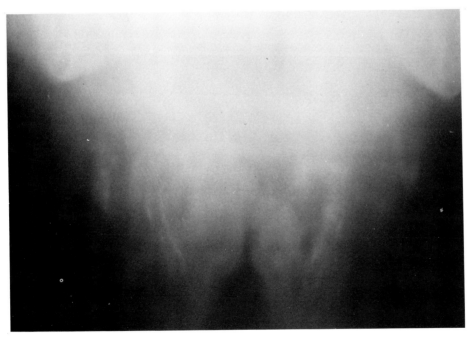

Fig. 19-10. Coronal planogram depicting a hypopharyngeal tumor involving the right pyriform sinus.

form sinus or will reveal a defect caused by a larger tumor involving the posterior or lateral walls of the hypopharynx. This modality is the primary diagnostic x-ray procedure for tumors of the esophagus. The barium visibly passing through the glottis is obvious evidence of aspiration associated with an obstructing lesion. Fig. 19-11, *A*, depicts, in an anteroposterior view, a large hypopharyngeal tumor of the posterior wall of the hypopharynx; there is encroachment on the left lateral wall and the pyriform sinus. Fig. 19-11, *B*, a lateral view after deglutition, shows a thin layer of barium adherent to a tumor of the lateral hypopharyngeal wall; the tumor involves the epiglottis and the pyriform sinus.

Laryngogram

The laryngogram has been recognized by some[14] as one of the most helpful radiologic examinations to detect very small lesions of the hypopharynx and larynx as well as to delineate the extent of the tumor.

This modality requires painstaking effort on the part of the radiologist, both to take the films and to interpret them. We have not been as successful as others in this technique and have not pursued it as vigorously as we might have.

Cinefluorogram

The cinefluorogram is of special interest to the surgeon since he can review the finding of fluoroscopy with a barium swallow of both the hypopharynx and the cervical esophagus, aiding to delineate the extent of the disease.

TREATMENT

In general, the treatment of hypopharyngeal and cervical esophageal carcinoma is surgery or radiation, or both. I prefer to utilize surgery alone for smaller lesions and a combination of surgery followed by radiation therapy when the primary or metastatic lesion is excessively large or when it is questionable that

Fig. 19-11. (Same patient as depicted in Fig. 19-9.) **A,** Barium swallow procedure indicating a large posterior hypopharyngeal carcinoma extending to the left lateral wall and the pyriform sinus. **B,** Barium swallow procedure depicting a lateral view after deglutition; barium is adherent to the tumor of the hypopharynx. The epiglottis and pyriform sinus are involved.

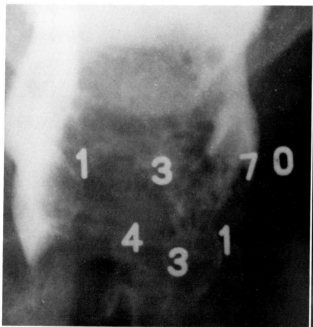

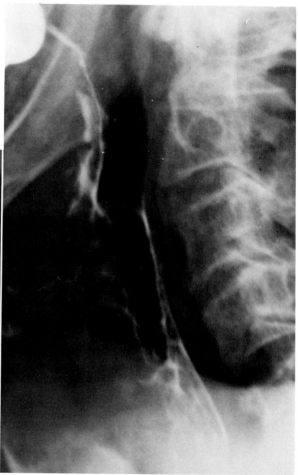

the surgical margins are clear of disease. A discussion of the merits of preoperative[7] or postoperative radiotherapy is beyond the scope of this presentation, but because of the tendency of the disease to spread submucosally, radiation therapy plays an important role in the treatment of these lesions. By the same token, the surgeon must take this spread into account and make free use of frozen sections, using the cryostat, to attempt to resect this sometimes hidden extension of hypopharyngeal cancer to the base of the tongue, oropharynx, and nasopharynx superiorly and to the larynx and esophagus inferiorly. In a similar manner, using the cryostat and frozen sections, an extension of esophageal cancer is resected to the mediastinal lymph nodes inferiorly and to the larynx and hypopharyx superiorly.

The fields of radiation therapy should usually include the base of the skull for hypopharyngeal cancer and the mediastinum for esophageal cancer. The failures in both surgery and radiation therapy may well be related to the limited areas encompassed by both modalities. The surgeon may unfortunately limit his field of resection because of the complexity of reconstruction of the digestive tract and the fact that the disease at the time of therapy has spread beyond the area of resection. Radical neck dissection is always performed with clinically palpable nodes at the time of resection of the primary lesion and is advisable in the absence of clinically palpable nodes.[12] Although most physicians relegate chemotherapy and forms of immunotherapy to surgical and radiation failures, one wonders whether these modalities should not be utilized earlier in the treatment of those tumors that have the poorer prognoses.

Probably nowhere else in head and neck surgery is reconstruction so taxing to the surgeon and the patient as is reconstruction of the digestive tract when large areas require resection. The simpler the reconstructive procedure the better, but this idea leads to a paradox when one must encompass large

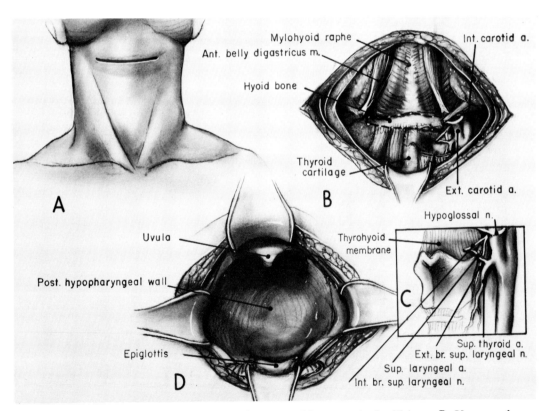

Fig. 19-12. Transhyoid pharyngotomy. **A,** Skin incision over the hyoid bone. **B,** Upper and lower skin flaps retracted, showing the portion of the hyoid bone to be removed. **C,** Anatomy of the superior laryngeal and hypoglossal nerves, which should not be injured. **D,** Surgical exposure of the posterior and lateral walls of the hypopharynx. (From Loré, J. M., Jr.: An atlas of head and neck surgery, ed. 2, Philadelphia, 1973, W. B. Saunders Co.)

areas of the hypopharynx and the esophagus. The multiplicity of the methods of reconstruction emphasizes the problem. A digestive cripple or a many-staged procedure requiring that the patient spend his last months mostly in the hospital can hardly be considered successful management.

SURGICAL TECHNIQUES ACCORDING TO ANATOMIC LOCATION
Hypopharynx

Posterior or lateral wall. Resection of primary lesions of the posterior or lateral wall of the hypopharynx are done by means of the following procedures: (1) transhyoid or suprahyoid pharyngotomy, (2) median labiomandibular glossotomy, and (3) lateral pharyngotomy—especially when combined with radical neck dissection.

The transhyoid or suprahyoid approach is mainly utilized for small primary lesions of the posterior wall in the absence of metastatic disease. This approach may serve as a modality for precise visualization of the tumor to evaluate its size and extent. If the lesion is small, it can then be resected with the prevertebral fascia, and the defect in the posterior wall can be covered with either a split-thickness or dermal graft, or it can be simply allowed to granulate without any covering. If the lesion is larger or extends into the lateral wall, the operative technique of a lateral pharyngeal approach and neck dissection can be utilized. Fig. 19-12 demonstrates the surgical technique of the transhyoid pharyngotomy.

The median labiomandibular glossotomy does not adapt itself well when combined with a radical neck dissection because of the possible interruption of the blood supply to the homolateral portion of the tongue. Fig. 19-13 demonstrates the technique of the median labiomandibular glossotomy.

Fig. 19-14 demonstrates the technique of the lateral pharyngotomy approach for a resection of carcinoma of the posterior or lateral wall of the hypopharynx. A radical neck dissection is being performed concomitantly.

A serious problem associated with a significant number of resections of the hypopharynx that preserve the larynx is postoperative dysphagia and aspiration. At times a cricopharyngeal myotomy may be of some aid if, in fact, this portion of the hypopharynx has not been resected. It then becomes a matter of judgment as to whether a total laryngectomy should be performed; the physician must take into account the size of the resected area, the age of the patient, and the presence or absence of

pulmonary disease. The preservation of the larynx in some instances has later required total laryngectomy; in these instances it would have been better to have performed a total laryngopharyngectomy at the onset.

Pyriform sinus. Both total and partial laryngopharyngectomies are usually combined with radical neck dissection, whether or not there are clinically palpable nodes, because of the high incidence of nodal metastasis. Because carcinoma originating in the pyriform sinus may go undetected by the unexperienced examiner, these lesions may then, by direct extension, involve a significant portion of the larynx, thus necessitating a total laryngectomy and pharyngectomy, as well as resection of several centimeters of the superior portion of the cervical esophagus. On the other hand, small lesions (1 to 2 mm.) have been detected arising in the walls of the pyriform sinus and associated with large cervical metastasis. In recent years as conservation surgery of the larynx has developed, partial laryngectomy and partial pharyngectomy have been utilized for these small primary lesions.[13]

The technique of a total laryngopharyngectomy is essentially that of a total laryngectomy, extending the resection to include either part or all of the hypopharynx. Since carcinoma of the larynx is to be covered in another chapter, the technique of total or partial laryngectomy is given here only in very brief detail. In a small lesion of the pyriform sinus the entire pyriform sinus is resected with or without a portion of the arytenoid cartilage, the aryepiglottic fold, and the posterior cricoarytenoid muscle. A cricopharyngeal myotomy is done. The approach is via a lateral pharyngotomy, and extreme care is taken not to cut near or into the tumor. A transhyoid pharyngotomy for inspection purposes can be performed, but it has not been of help in visualization of a small lesion of the medial wall of the pyriform sinus.

A radical neck dissection is virtually always performed regardless of whether or not there is clinically palpable cervical disease. When a total laryngopharyngectomy is performed, the neck dissection is in continuity; when a partial laryngectomy is done, the neck dissection may be best performed in discontinuity.

Postcricoid area. The surgical management of carcinoma of the postcricoid area always involves total laryngectomy since the lesion is located on the anterior wall of this region of the hypopharynx, which in turn is part of the posterior portion of the larynx. Depending on the extent of the lesion, a portion of the posterior and lateral walls and the pyri-

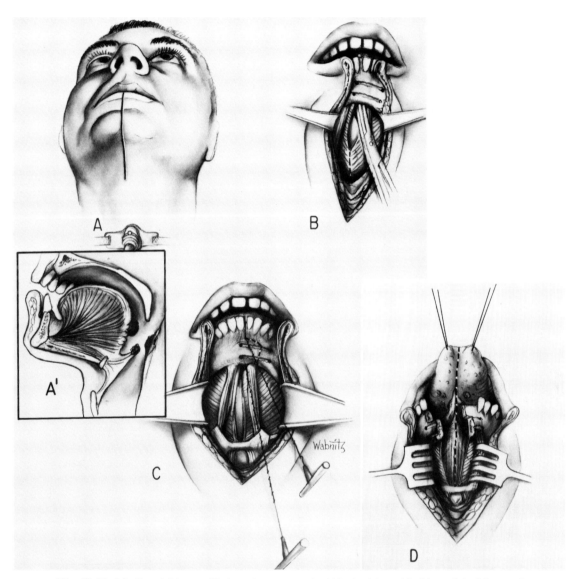

Fig. 19-13. Median labiomandibular glossotomy. **A,** Skin incision. **A¹,** Line of incision and location of three types of lesions amenable to this surgical approach; posterior pharyngeal wall, base of the tongue, and tip of the epiglottis. **B,** After drill holes and kerfs (used for closure with tie wires) are made in the mandible, a curved clamp is inserted under the symphysis for introduction of a Gigli saw. **C,** Exposure and transection of the mandible in step fashion. **D,** The tongue and floor of the mouth are incised in the midline. This incision affords an excellent exposure of the posterior and lateral walls of the hypopharynx and oropharynx. (From Loré, J. M., Jr.: An atlas of head and neck surgery, ed. 2, Philadelphia, 1973, W. B. Saunders Co.)

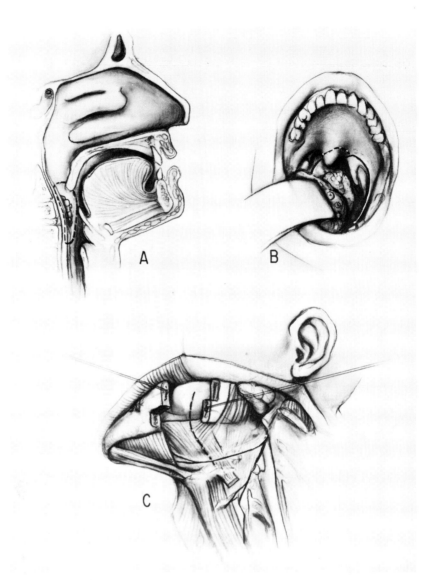

Fig. 19-14. Lateral pharyngotomy. **A,** Cross-sectional anatomy, which depicts a posterior wall carcinoma of the hypopharynx and oropharynx. **B,** Intraoral view of a lesion extending to the left lateral wall and the edge of the posterior tonsillar pillar. The solid and dotted lines outline the area of resection. When the lesion is restricted to the hypopharynx, the resections may not be carried quite so high. **C,** A left radical neck dissection has been performed. The contents of the neck dissection have been removed for clarity, yet it may be impractical and unnecessary to maintain continuity. The dotted line indicates the incision for the pharyngotomy. It is most important that this incision is well away from the tumor. A transhyoid pharyngotomy may be necessary to ascertain the exact extent of the disease. **D,** Initial exposure of a portion of the tumor. The lingual nerve can be transected. **E,** Additional exposure with the line of resection, which may include the underlying prevertebral fascia. A hot knife is used to outline the mucosal incision. The parapharyngeal and lateral pharyngeal lymph nodes are resected, as well as the palatine tonsil and posterior pillar. Care must be taken not to injure the internal carotid artery in the lateral extent of the resection. **F,** The free edges of the mucosa are sutured to any remaining underlying fascia. The defect is covered with a free dermal graft or a deltopectoral flap if more of the lateral wall of the pharynx is resected. The carotid artery may be protected with a dermal graft or levator scapulae muscle flap. (From Loré, J. M., Jr.: An atlas of head and neck surgery, ed. 2, Philadelphia, 1973, W. B. Saunders Co.)

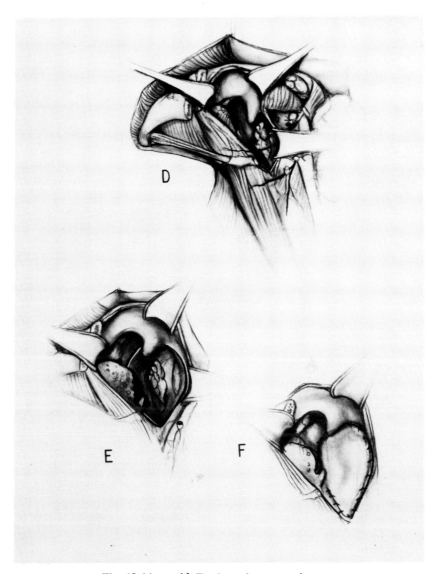

Fig. 19-14, cont'd. For legend see opposite page.

form sinuses are resected with at least 2-cm. margins. Free use of frozen sections, especially of a circumferential portion of the esophagus, is necessary to evaluate submucosal spread. Even though an esophagoscopy has been performed, very careful evaluation of the downward extent of disease at the time of transection of the esophagus is mandatory to avoid cutting into the tumor.

Cervical esophagus

When the tumor of the cervical esophagus is located superiorly, a total laryngectomy is necessary because of the proximity anteriorly of the cricoid cartilage of the larynx. Dysphagia and aspiration, associated with any type of reconstruction of this portion of the cervical esophagus with preservation of the larynx, are also problems. Substitution of the anterior portion of the larynx and trachea for the resected portion of the esophagus has not proved feasible. Free use of frozen sections on a circumferential rim of the remaining distal esophagus is mandatory.

When the tumor is located in the midregion of the cervical esophagus, preservation of the larynx may be feasible, depending on the size of the local tumor and its metastasis to the tracheoesophageal lymph nodes. If this spread involves the recurrent nerves,

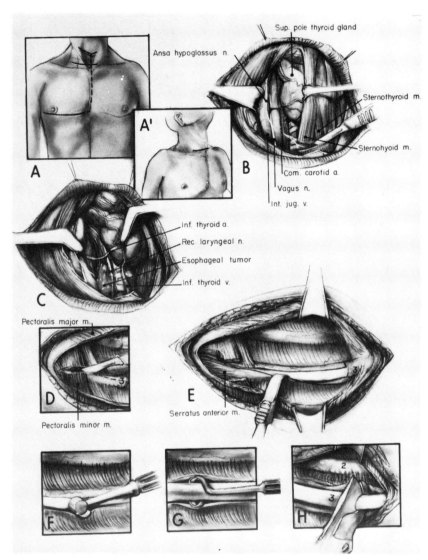

Fig. 19-15. Resection of a carcinoma involving the cervical portion and extending to the thoracic inlet. **A¹,** Initial incision to evaluate the extent of the cervical portion of the tumor and its resectability after an esophagoscopy, laryngoscopy, bronchoscopy, and possibly mediastinoscopy. **A,** A right thoracotomy through an **inframammary** incision is then made to evaluate the thoracic extent of disease. The dotted lines depict a sternal splitting incision if necessary. **B** and **C,** Exposure of the anatomy and tumor in the cervical region. **D-I,** Technique for the right thoracotomy is depicted. **J,** Extension of the thoracotomy superiorly transecting the second rib. **K,** The mediastinal pleura is incised, exposing the trachea, esophagus, and the right bronchus down to the azygos vein. **L** and **M,** If necessary the sternum is split for additional exposure. **N,** Complete cervical and thoracic exposure of the surgical field.

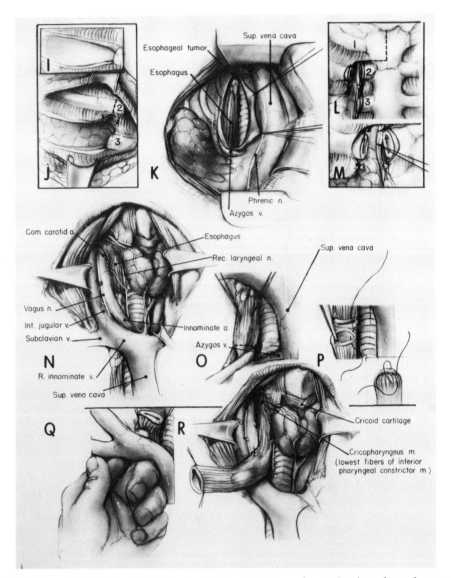

Fig. 19-15, cont'd. O, The dotted line depicts the distal line of resection just above the azygos vein. **P,** The distal esophageal lumen is closed and allowed to drop back into the mediastinum as a permanent blind end. **Q** and **R,** Mobilization of the proximal esophagus from behind the right innominate vein and innominate artery. If there are adequate margins superiorly, the segment of the esophagus is then resected. Reconstruction is with a section of colon via substernal tunnel. When the tumor approaches the cricoid cartilage level a total laryngectomy is performed. Reconstruction is with the colon; a pharyngocolectomy is performed. This type of reconstruction may be staged, depending on the general condition of the patient.[4] When an excessive length of trachea is resected with the laryngectomy, turned in cervical flaps are used to reach the deeply located end of the trachea to form the tracheostoma. (From Loré, J. M., Jr.: An atlas of head and neck surgery, ed. 2, Philadelphia, 1973, W. B. Saunders Co.)

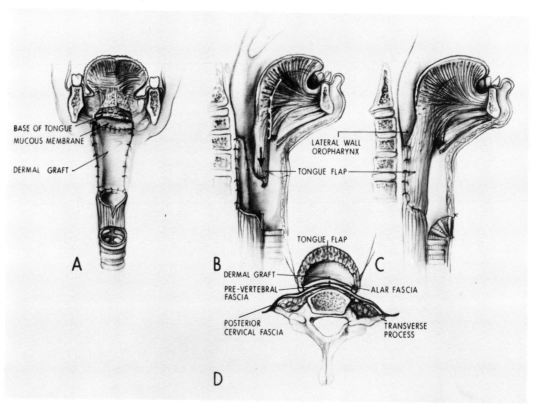

Fig. 19-16. Tongue flap and dermal graft for reconstruction of the entire hypopharynx, a portion of the oropharynx, and a portion of the cervical esophagus. **A,** A laryngopharyngectomy has been performed. The oropharynx and esophagus have been mobilized, and their free edges have been sutured to the prevertebral fascia. This procedure fixes these structures and minimizes tension on the mucosa to dermal graft sutures. The dermal graft is sutured laterally to the prevertebral fascia, and the upper and lower ends are sutured to the mucosa of the oropharynx and esophagus. The anterior wall of the esophagus is split vertically in the middle for a distance of 1 or 2 cm. to enlarge its lumen. The horizontal dotted line across the base of the tongue indicates the incision to form the tongue flap. **B,** Lateral view of mobilization of the tongue flap. **C,** The tongue flap has been tubed about 270 degrees to form the anterior and lateral walls of the newly constructed gullet. The dermal graft forms the posterior wall. The tongue flap is sutured not only to the dermal graft but also to the prevertebral fascia. Distally it is sutured to the esophagus with through-and-through sutures of either interrupted or continuous Connell sutures. If continuous sutures are used, they should be in two sections, right and left, to avoid a purse effect and narrowing the lumen. The distal tip of the tongue flap is pulled into the vertical esophageal incision to widen the lumen. A second layer of three interrupted sutures through esophageal and tongue musculature may be used for reinforcement, although the initial mucosa-to-mucosa sutures are more important. A small section of free dermal graft may also be used as an overlay on this suture line. **D,** Cross section through the new gullet. The tongue flap forms the anterior and lateral walls, and the dermal graft forms the posterior wall. The so-called prevertebral fascia is actually the posterior cervical fascia and is made up of two layers: the alar fascia and the true prevertebral fascia, which are separated by loose connective tissue.[5] Each layer is attached to the ends of the transverse processes of the vertebrae. When portions of the prevertebral fascia are resected with the tumor, the dermal graft is then sutured to the anterior longitudinal ligament. (From Loré, J. M., Jr.: An atlas of head and neck surgery, ed. 2, Philadelphia, 1973, W. B. Saunders Co.)

such a finding would tend to support laryngectomy. If the larynx is preserved in the presence of bilateral abductor vocal cord paralysis, an arytenoidopexy or similar procedure is performed to establish a glottic airway. Aspiration, however, may be serious.

When the tumor is located in that portion of the cervical esophagus at the thoracic inlet, the larynx may be preserved. The distal limit of resection depends on the gross size of the tumor within the lumen and on the submucosal spread. If the latter feature is extensive, subtotal esophagectomy or even total esophagectomy must be considered.[15] Radiation therapy alone may then be the treatment of choice because of the general condition of the patient and the magnitude of the surgery necessary. On the other hand, if the disease is sufficiently confined, the level of transection is in the region of the azygos vein.

If the tumor is deemed nonresectable and radiation therapy is not feasible or is a failure, palliation to reestablish the continuity of the digestive tract, using the terminal ileum and the right colon, has been suggested. This procedure can be applied to lesions of the lower cervical and thoracic esophagus.

Fig. 19-15 demonstrates the surgical technique of resection of a tumor at the level of the thoracic inlet.

RECONSTRUCTION

Although this chapter is not concerned with the various types of reconstruction of the hypopharynx and esophagus, the following is a listing of these procedures:

1. Primary end-to-end closure with flexion of the neck and head
2. Local rotated pharyngeal flaps (This procedure is combined with the first one.)[10]
3. Lateral cervical (Wookey type) skin flaps[16] and deltopectoral skin flaps
4. Thoracic cervical skin tube
5. Free skin graft—split-thickness or dermal graft over tantalum mesh
6. Tongue flap combined with dermal graft; especially suited to laryngopharyngectomy (Fig. 19-16)
7. Colon transplant
8. Stomach
9. Free jejunal after the technique of Nakayama
10. Various types of plastic tubes, such as Negus and Montgomery

REFERENCES

1. American Joint Committee for Cancer Staging and End Results: Clinical staging system for carcinoma of the pharynx, Chicago, 1965, the Committee, pp. 10 and 16.
2. Burbank, F.: Patterns in cancer mortality in the United States: 1950-1967, monograph 33, Bethesda, Md., U.S. Department of Health, Education, and Welfare, Public Health Service, National Institutes of Health.
3. Burdette, W. J.: Palliative operation for carcinoma of cervical and thoracic esophagus, Ann. Surg. **173**(5): 714-732, 1971.
4. Goodner, J. T.: Treatment and survival in cancer of the cervical esophagus, Am. J. Surg. **118**(5):673-675, 1969.
5. Hollinshead, W. H.: Anatomy for surgeons. the head and neck, ed. 2, vol. 1, New York, 1968, Harper & Row, Publishers, p. 44.
6. Lerche, W.: The esophagus and pharynx in action, Springfield, Ill., 1960, Charles C Thomas, Publisher.
7. Levitt, S. H., Beachley, M. C., Zimberg, Y., Pastore, P. N., DeGiorgi, L. S., and King, E. R.: Combination of preoperative irradiation and surgery in the treatment of cancer of the oropharynx, hypopharynx, and larynx, Cancer **27**(4):759-767, 1971.
8. Loré, J. M., Jr.: Atlas of head and neck surgery, ed. 1, Philadelphia, 1962, W. B. Saunders Co., p. 22.
8a. Loré, J. M., Jr.: Total reconstructon of the hypopharynx with tongue flap and dermal graft, Ann. Otol. Rhinol. Laryngol. **83**(4):476-480.
9. MacCoomb, W. S., and Fletcher, G. H.: Cancer of the head and neck, Baltimore, Md., 1967, The Williams & Wilkins Co., p. 217.
10. Marchetta, F. C., Sako, K., and Creedon, P. J.: Rotation of esophageal and pharyngeal flaps for reconstruction of the cervical esophagus, Am. J. Surg. **102** (6):854-858, 1961.
11. Moore, W. T., Arnold, G. E., and Day, L. H.: Surgical treatment of carcinoma of the cervical esophagus, South. Med. J., **60**(11):1159-1163, 1967.
12. Ogura, J. H., Biller, H. F., and Wette, R.: Elective neck dissection for pharyngeal and laryngeal cancers; an evaluation, Ann. Otolaryngol. **80**:646, October, 1971.
13. Ogura, J. H., Salzstein, S. L. and Spjut, H. J.: Experiences with conservation surgery in laryngeal and pharyngeal cancer, Laryngoscope **71**:258-276, 1961.
14. Powers, W. E., Holtz, S., and Ogura, J.: Contrast examination of the larynx and pharynx; inspiratory phonation, Am. J. Roentgenol. Radium Ther. Nucl. Med. **92**(1):40-42, 1964.
15. Scanlon, E. F., Morton, D. R., Walker, J. M., and Watson, W. L.: The case against segmental resection for esophageal carcinoma, Surg. Gynecol. Obstet. **101**: 99-103, 1958.
16. Wookey, H.: Surgical treatment of carcinoma of the hypopharynx and esophagus Br. J. Surg. **35**:249, 1948.

Chapter 20

Cancer of the larynx and hypopharynx

Joseph H. Ogura, M.D.
Donald G. Sessions, M.D.

Major problems in discussing long-term results in the treatment of cancer of the larynx and hypopharynx include the difficulties of arriving at a universally acceptable staging and classification system and of obtaining a uniform method for end results reporting. In an effort to find the most desirable method of staging and classifying carcinomas of this area, we have begun a retrospective and prospective study of our own material to ascertain if the classification that we have been using is correct in terms of disease, treatment, and results. This chapter is a preliminary report of our effort to date.

STAGING AND CLASSIFICATION

Recent proposals before the Internatonal Union Against Cancer (UICC)[2] in May 1971 and revisions by the American Joint Committee for Cancer Staging and End Results Reporting (AJC)[1] in November 1971 concerning staging and classification of carcinomas of the larynx have made the methods of these two organizations almost identical. Despite the fact that these two groups have come to an apparent initial agreement on staging and classification for the larynx, our extensive experience with these lesions has led us to disagree with the classification on several points. One of the major problems in this field has been inadequate definition of the various anatomic boundaries of the larynx and particularly of the hypopharynx. The TNM system of staging the

We wish to acknowledge Ms. Caroline Bradley, Secretary, Head and Neck Cancer Registry, Department of Otolaryngology, Washington University School of Medicine, for her assistance.

disease and categorizing the lesions and the extent of involvement requires precise description of the tumor in its relation to specific anatomic landmarks, its regional nodal involvement, and its distant metastasis.

Larynx anatomy and staging problems

Supraglottis. The UICC proposal (May 1971) divides the larynx into three regions and subdivides the regions into sites. The supraglottis is subdivided into the epilarynx (the posterior surface of the suprahyoid epiglottis and the aryepiglottic fold—the marginal zone and the arytenoid area) and the remaining supraglottis; the epilarynx (the infrahyoid epiglottis, ventricular bands, and ventricular cavities) is excluded.

The AJC proposal similarly subdivides the larynx according to regions and sites. Proposed UICC and AJC staging for primary tumors of the supraglottis is summarized in the following list:

TIS Preinvasive carcinomas (carcinoma in situ)
T1   Tumor limited to region; normal mobility
    T1a Tumor confined to laryngeal surface of epiglottis, an aryepiglottic fold, a ventricular cavity, or a ventricular band
    T1b Tumor involving epiglottis and extending to ventricular cavities or bands
T2   Tumor of epiglottis and/or ventricles or ventricular bands and extending to vocal cords; no fixation
T3   Tumor limited to larynx; fixation and/or destruction or other evidence of deep invasion
T4   Tumor with direct extension beyond larynx (to pyriform sinus, postcricoid region, vallecula, or base of tongue)

We disagree with the UICC and AJC proposal that lesions of the anterior or lingual surface of the epiglottis are supraglottic. We place these lesions in an anatomic region called the superior hypopharynx because they carry a much poorer prognosis.

We agree with the UICC that supraglottic lesions that extend onto the true vocal cords without loss of mobility should be classified as supraglottic T2 lesions. These rare tumors are amenable to a three-quarter laryngectomy with fold-over reconstruction.

Marginal lesions. The UICC describes tumors of the aryepiglottic fold with greater than 5 mm. extension into the pyriform fossa as supraglottic T4 tumors. Because of the bad biologic behavior of these marginal lesions, we prefer to call them lesions of the inferior hypopharynx or the pyriform fossa. We agree with describing tumors of the arytenoid area as being in the marginal region.

Glottis. The UICC proposal subdivides the glottis into the vocal cords, the anterior commissure, and the posterior commissure. The AJC proposal does not mention the posterior commissure as part of the glottis. The following list summarizes UICC and AJC proposed classification for tumors of the glottis:

TIS Preinvasive carcinoma (carcinoma in situ)
T1   Tumor limited to region; normal mobility
     T1a Tumor confined to one cord
     T1b Tumor involving both cords
T2   Tumor extending to either subglottis or supraglottic regions (to ventricular bands or ventricles); normal or impaired mobility
T3   Tumor limited to larynx; fixation of one or both cords
T4   Tumor extending beyond larynx (into cartilage, pyriform sinus, postcricoid region, or skin)

We can see no clinically useful reason to create an entirely new classification region called T1b. In our experience, tumors not limited to one vocal cord (a glottic tumor involving more than one site) carry a poorer prognosis and should thus be classified as glottis T2. We would prefer to delete the T1b category.

We agree that some endolaryngeal tumors extending beyond the region of origin without fixation (some small transglottic tumors) can be changed to T2. We agree that tumors of the vocal process of the arytenoid area should be classified with tumors of the glottic region.

Subglottis. The UICC and the AJC proposes that the subglottis is the subglottic region exclusive of the undersurface of the true cords. UICC and AJC staging for tumors of the subglottis is indicated in the following list:

TIS Preinvasive carcinoma (carcinoma in situ)
T1   T1a Tumor limited to one side of subglottic region and not involving undersurface of cord
     T1b Tumor extending to both sides of subglottic region and not involving undersurface cords
T2   Tumor involving subglottic region and extending to one or both cords
T3   Tumor limited to larynx; fixation of one or both cords
T4   Tumor extending beyond larynx (to postcricoid region, trachea, or skin)

We feel that the subglottic area is the cylindrical area whose caudal border is the lower edge of the cricoid cartilage and whose cephalic border is an imaginary circle 5 mm. below the free border of the vocal folds in men and 4 mm. below the free border in women. Tumors that originate more than 5 mm. below the free margin of the vocal fold are described as subglottic in origin. Tumors originating at the glottic level that involve the mucosa greater than 5 mm. below the free margin of the vocal fold are described as glottic tumors with subglottic involvement.

Hypopharynx anatomy and staging problems

The hypopharynx is divided into four regions: the superior hypopharynx, the inferior hypopharynx, the posterior pharyngeal wall, and the postcricoid area.

Superior hypopharynx. The superior hypopharynx is bounded posteriorly by the lingual surface of the epiglottis, inferiorly by the vallecula, laterally by the glossoepiglottic folds, and anteriorly by an imaginary line projected from the tip of the epiglottis anterior to the base of the tongue about 1 cm. posterior to the circumvallate line. The proposed classification of tumors of the region is as follows:

T1   One site only (vallecula, lingual epiglottis, *or* base of tongue)
T2   Two sites involved
T3   Three sites involved
T4   Extending beyond superior hypopharynx into base of tongue, inferior hypopharynx, or larynx

Inferior hypopharynx. The inferior hypopharynx is an inverted three-sided pyramid bounded superiorly by the glossoepiglottic folds (including the pyriform fossa from the aryepiglottic folds medially and laterally to the lateral pharyngeal wall) and inferiorly by the apex of the pyriform fossa. The proposed classification of tumors of this region is as follows:

T1   One site only (aryepiglottic fold, medial wall, pyriform, *or* lateral wall pyriform only)

T2   Two sites involved (aryepiglottic fold and medial wall, *or* medial wall *and* anterior wall)

T3   Three sites involved (aryepiglottic fold, medial wall, *and* a third area such as apex)

T4   Tumor outside inferior hypopharynx (postcricoid region or into larynx or base of tongue)

Posterior pharyngeal wall. The posterior pharyngeal wall of the hypopharynx is bounded laterally by the lateral pharyngeal wall, inferiorly by the cricopharyngeal wall, and superiorly by an imaginary line projected posteriorly from the tip of the epiglottis. Above this region is the posterior pharyngeal wall of the oropharynx. The following list shows the proposed classification of tumors of this region:

T1   Lesions up to 2 cm. in size
T2   Lesions over 2 cm.
T3   Invasion beyond region
T4   Invasion of bone

Postcricoid area. The postcricoid area includes the mucosa covering the posterior surface of the cricoid cartilage anteriorly and the inferior border and circumference of the cricopharyngeal wall. The proposed classification of tumors of the postcricoid area is shown in the following list:

T1   Lesion smaller than 2 cm. not extending below cricoid area
T2   Lesion over 2 cm. not extending beyond cricoid area
T3   Lesion extending into pyriform sinus or upper esophagus
T4   Lesion causing fixation

Regional lymph nodes

The list below shows the proposed classification for regional cervical lymph nodes. It should be noted that multiple suspected metastatic cancerous nodes and suspected ipsilateral lymph nodes greater than 4 cm. have been classified as N2, which is an addition to the UICC and AJC classification.

N0   No palpable nodes; metastasis not suspected
N1   Metastasis suspected; palpable cervical node—mobile, ipsilateral, single
N2   Metastasis suspected; palpable cervical node—mobile, contralateral, midline or bilateral, ipsilateral cervical node—4 cm. or multiple
N3   Metastasis suspected; papable cervical node(s)—fixed

Distant metastasis

Proposed classification of distant metastasis is shown in the list below and does not differ from UICC and AJC classification.

M0   No distinct metastasis
M1   Clinical and/or radiographic evidence of metastasis other than to cervical nodes

Cancer of the larynx and hypopharynx

Staging. Staging for carcinoma of the larynx and hypopharynx is shown in the list below and is in agreement with UICC and AJC suggestions.

Stage I   T1 N0, N1 or N2 M0
Stage II   T2 N0, N1 or N2 M0
Stage III   T3 N0, N1 or N2 M0
            T4 N0, N1 or N2 M0
            T1 T2 T3 or T4 N1b or N2b M0
Stage IV   T1 T2 T3 or T4 N3 M0
            or
            T1 T2 T3 or T4 N0 N1
            N2 N3 M1

Treatment. The following outline indicates the treatment currently employed for patients with carcinoma of the larynx and hypopharynx. We have discussed the technical aspects of these various operations elsewhere.[3,4]

TREATMENT FOR CANCER OF THE LARYNX AND HYPOPHARYNX

I. Cancer of the larynx
  A. Supraglottic cancer
    1. T1 and T2: subtotal supraglottic laryngectomy (SSL) or ND, or both
    2. T3: extended SSL or ND, or both; total laryngectomy (TL) and ND
    3. T4: TL and ND
  B. Glottic cancer
    1. T0: vocal cord stripping
    2. T1: hemilaryngectomy (hemi); radiation
    3. T2: hemi
    4. T3 and T4: TL
  C. Subglottic cancer—T1 to T4: TL and ND
II. Cancer of the hypopharynx
  A. Superior hypopharynx cancer
    1. T1 to T3: extended SSL and ND
    2. T4: extended SSL and ND; TL and ND; total laryngopharyngectomy (TLP) and ND
  B. Inferior hypopharynx (pyriform fossa) cancer
    1. T1 and T2: partial laryngopharyngectomy (PLP) and ND
    2. T3: PLP and ND; TLP and ND
    3. T4: TLP and ND
  C. Posterior pharyngeal wall cancer
    1. T1 to T3: partial pharyngectomy (PP) and ND
    2. T4: total pharyngectomy (TP) and ND

D. Postcricoid cancer
  1. T1: TL with laryngotracheal autograft (LTA)
  2. T2: TLP with LTA and ND
  3. T3: TLP and ND with pharyngoesophageal reconstruction (PER)
  4. T4: TLP with ND with PER

Table 20-1. Head and Neck Cancer Registry, August 1973

	Number of cases
Computer registered	713
Follow-up in progress	671
1971 to 1972	368
Affiliated hospitals (City–Starkloff Memorial, Veterans Administration, St. Louis County)	500
Missing records	205
Total	*2,457*

Table 20-2. First-degree surgical procedure—therapy

	Number of cases
VC stripping	7
TL	155
SSL	127
PLP	65
Hemi	163
Total	*517*

STUDY OF RESULTS

To obtain the most informative material in terms of staging, classification, treatment, and long-term results of treatment of cancer of the larynx and hypopharynx, a Head and Neck Cancer Registry was created in the Department of Otolaryngology of the Washington University Medical School in the fall of 1972. Initially, a retrospective study was established so that pertinent information could be acquired from the patient's past office and hospital records. All patients from 1955 to the present who have been diagnosed histopathologically as having carcinoma of the larynx and hypopharynx have been included in the study.

The primary data package includes a primary data sheet, a drawing of the primary lesion as it is described or diagramed in the office or hospital record, and a copy of the surgical pathology biopsy and specimen records. The information from the records has been remarkably adequate. After the primary data package was assembled, all lesions were classified by senior members of the Department of Otolaryngology, and all pertinent data reviewed. Follow-up was a physician examination or a telephone call by a full-time Cancer Registry secretary.

Information from the primary data sheet is key-punched on computer cards. The Washington University Department of Computer Services, utilizing a standard computer program, analyzed the data.

Table 20-3. Long-term results of therapy

Procedure	Alive; no cancer	Alive; first-degree cancer	Alive; metastasis	Alive; second-degree cancer	Dead; no cancer	Dead; cancer	Total first-degree surgical procedures
VC stripping	6					1	7
TL	64	5	4		25	57	155
SSL	69	3	1	1	10	43	127
PLP	26	3	2		14	20	65
Hemi	111	6	5	5	18	17	163
						Total	*517*

Table 20-4. Long-term results of therapy; survival after treatment of tumor

Procedure	T0 Survival 3 yr.	T0 Survival 5 yr.	T1 Survival 3 yr.	T1 Survival 5 yr.	T2 Survival 3 yr.	T2 Survival 5 yr.	T3 Survival 3 yr.	T3 Survival 5 yr.	T4 Survival 3 yr.	T4 Survival 5 yr.	Total survival rate
VC stripping	2	2	2								6/7 86%
TL			4	7	8	10	5	30	1	5	100/155 65%
SSL			9	29	9	16	2	6	4	8	85/127 67%
PLP			4	3	1	6	2	6	4	11	37/65 56%
Hemi			40	68	11	15	1	1	1	1	141/163 86%

Table 20-5. Long-term results of therapy; survival after treatment of cancerous nodes

Procedure	N0 Survival		N1 Survival		N2 Survival		N3 Survival		Total survival rate	
	3 yr.	5 yr.	3 yr.	5 yr.	3 yr.	5 yr.	3 yr.	5 yr.		
VC stripping	4	2							6/7	86%
TL	21	49	8	12	2	4	2		98/155	63%
SSL	22	42	4	12	3	1	1	1	86/127	68%
PLP	8	14	7	6	1		1	3	30/65	46%
Hemi	63	78		1		1		1	144/163	88%

Table 20-6. Site of recurrence after treatment

Procedure	Local	Neck	Stomal	Distant	Local and neck	Local and distant	Local, neck, and distant	Total
VC stripping	1							1
TL	16	18	6	8	4		2	54
SSL	9	20		2	2			34
PLP	5	3		1	3		1	13
Hemi	13	8						21

Table 20-7. Cause of death

Procedure	Primary cancer uncontrolled	Neck metastasis uncontrolled	Distant metastasis	Complications of treatment	Intercurrent disease	Second-degree cancer	Other
VC stripping					2		
TL	12	20	21	1	13	7	10
SSL	3	14	11	4	13	4	5
PLP	3	3	11	7	6	1	6
Hemi	1	2	7	1	14	4	12

RESULTS

The present status of the study is shown in Table 20-1. The information is complete on 713 cases, and they have been entered into the study. Information is available but incomplete because of inadequate follow-up on 671 cases. Three hundred and sixty-eight cases managed and treated in the past 3 years are ready for computer registration. In the next year we plan to add about 500 cases to the study from our resident-affiliated outside hospitals.

The types and numbers of surgical procedures employed are shown in Table 20-2. Long-term results of therapy are shown in Tables 20-3 through 20-5. These patients have all been followed for a minimum of 3 years after initial therapy. In viewing the excellent results of the partial laryngopharyngectomy (for inferior hypopharyngeal lesions), one must remember that we use very strict preoperative criteria in this surgery. Similarly, it is clear that nodal metastasis (Table 20-5) plays an important part in the survival of patients requiring surgery (PLP) for inferior hypopharyngeal cancers. Tables 20-6 and 20-7 summarize the sites of recurrence of these tumors after specific operations and the causes of death.

SUMMARY

Staging and classification of carcinoma of the larynx and hypopharynx have been discussed. Several areas of disagreement between our classification and that of the UICC and the AJC have been presented, and some constructive recommendations have been made.

The current treatment regimen presently utilized for cancer of the larynx and hypopharynx has been outlined.

The organization of our Head and Neck Cancer Registry, particularly as it pertains to cancer of the larynx and hypopharynx, has been presented and some preliminary results of the study of these tumors have been given.

REFERENCES

1. American Joint Committee for Cancer Staging and End Results Reporting: Clinical Staging System for Carcinoma of the Larynx (revision), Chicago, 1972, the Committee.
2. International Union Against Cancer, American Joint Committee on Cancer Staging and End Results Reporting: TNM classification of malignant tumors of breast, larynx, stomach, cervix uteri, corpus uteri, Geneva, Switzerland, 1972, the Union pp. 13-17.
3. Ogura, J. H., and Biller, H. F.: Conservation surgery in cancer of the head and neck; Otolaryngol. Clin. North Am. 641-665, October, 1969.
4. Ogura, J. H., and Sessions, D. G.: Conservation surgery of the larynx and pharynx. In Proceedings of the Tenth World Congress of Otorhinolaryngology, Venice, 1973, Amsterdam, Excerpta Medica Foundation, in press.

Chapter 21

Cancer of the salivary glands

John C. Gaisford, M.D.

Numerous articles on salivary gland tumors have been published over the years, and excellent books on the subject exist. One can find a variety of classifications of these tumors, usually in publications by pathologists, dentists, and various surgical specialists (general surgeons, otolaryngologists, and plastic surgeons). Individual authors have used their favorite terminologies for these publications and some have reported on no more than one case of a parotid tumor.

The following classification of malignant tumors is one that my associates and I have included in previously published papers; it has changed very little over the years.

Malignant tumors of the salivary glands
Mucoepidermoid carcinoma
Squamous cell carcinoma
Malignant mixed tumor
Undifferentiated carcinoma
Hodgkin's disease
Acinic cell cancer
Cylindromatous carcinoma (adenocystic)
Lymphosarcoma
Rhabdomyosarcoma
Reticulum cell sarcoma
Fibrosarcoma
Melanoma
Adenocarcinoma

The classification of the benign tumors is subject to a greater variation and is not included here, with the exception of Table 21-1, in which the incidence of benign salivary gland tumors is compared with that of malignant ones.

DIAGNOSIS

Nearly all diagnoses of salivary gland tumors are made as a result of the patient finding a lump in the vicinity of a salivary gland. Most of these lumps are completely asymptomatic, especially in the early stages and before they involve contiguous structures. The clinical differentiation between a benign and a malignant tumor may be, and usually is, impossible. Several developments (especially facial nerve paralysis, rapid growth, and pain) may indicate malignancy. These findings are not absolutely indicative of malignancy; more than 12 of the histologically benign tumors in our series had nerve involvement, compared with 40 of the malignant parotid tumors. Rapid enlargement of a salivary gland is frequently a sign of malignancy, but it also occurs with benign cysts, Warthin's tumor, fatty infiltration, and infection. Pain is rarely a symptom, but when it does occur, particularly in the region of the parotid gland, one should seriously consider a cancer to be present deep within the gland, even when there is no definite tumor mass present. The patient should be carefully examined at frequent intervals (every 3 weeks), and if pain persists, removal of the gland should be considered. Three such cases have been found on our service over the years.

Biopsies of salivary gland tumors and sialograms are not employed. Biopsies are considered unsafe (the facial nerve could be cut, and the tumor may spread or not be found); and sialograms, although expensive and sometimes painful, are not routinely helpful (they are nonspecific and can really indicate only that a lump may be present).

PATHOLOGY

The vast majority of salivary gland cancers are of the mucoepidermoid variety (Table 21-2); and although it is true that many of these act in a relatively benign fashion clinically (for this reason some

Table 21-1. Incidence of benign and malignant tumors of salivary glands

Type	Benign	Malignant	Total
Parotid	467	153	620
Submaxillary	52	18	70
Minor	40	22	62
Total	*559*	*193*	*752*

Table 21-2. Malignant tumors of salivary glands

Type	Parotid	Submaxillary	Minor
Mucoepidermoid	52	3	6
Adenoid cystic	15	6	11
Miscellaneous	36	5	1
Total	*153*	*18*	*22*

surgeons and pathologists elect to talk about them as though they were completely benign), we have seen a sufficient number of them spread and kill so that we consider them malignant. The most dangerous variety of cancer is the adenoid cystic type, which spreads by insinuating tongues of tumor along fascial planes, nerve filaments, and into other soft tissue areas. The other malignant tumors are serious but do not make up large groups.

MANAGEMENT

Salivary gland malignant tumors must generally be considered surgical problems. Because we perform an extensive operation for any salivary gland problem, we frequently do not know the histologic type of tumor being treated until the pathologist has received the gland and enclosed tumor and has examined the tumor microscopically.

Because of oral anatomy, it may be impossible to plan a proper operation for an intraoral tumor without a biopsy. A preliminary biopsy is practical in this situation because extensive reconstructive surgery may have to be planned, and one would not wish to resect maxilla and possibly other important structures needlessly.

The submaxillary gland, with its tumor, is totally removed. If a clinically positive node exists in the neck, the node is removed at that time; if a frozen section biopsy reveals a metastatic tumor, a complete radical neck dissection is carried out immediately.

The parotid gland presents a completely different picture because of its configuration and adjacent anatomical structures (facial nerve, mandible, and so on). The least surgery that is performed is the removal of the parotid tissue superficial to the facial nerve (even for tumors thought to be benign). If the enclosed tumor is malignant and does not extend outside of the removed tissue, no further surgery is performed. If the frozen section biopsy reveals that the tumor is adenoid cystic, undifferentiated, or squamous cell carcinoma, the performance of a complete radical neck dissection is considered for the immediate or very near future. If any parotid cancer has a metastasis in the neck, a neck dissection should be done. The adenoid cystic, undifferentiated, and squamous cell cancers metastasize so frequently that neck dissection should at least be considered in the definitive treatment.

The facial nerve (the entire nerve or only a peripheral branch) is removed only when it is obviously involved by a malignant tumor or tumors adherent to the nerve. If enough nerve is resected to cause troublesome paralysis and the nerve cannot be primarily anastomosed, an immediate graft from the cervical area is performed and results are routinely good.

RESULTS OF TREATMENT

Because of the natural course of salivary gland tumor growth, it is rather difficult to express the significance of disease-free intervals by comparing the length of these intervals with that of many other types of malignant neoplasms. Whether or not it is significant that a patient who has been operated on for a cellular mucoepidermoid cancer of the parotid gland is free of disease 10 years later is highly questionable. However, our rather aggressive surgical approach to the salivary gland tumor problem has had acceptable results.

Of the patients followed for 5 years after surgery, 62% of those treated for malignant parotid gland tumors were free of disease, as were 55% of those treated for submaxillary gland tumors and 55% of those treated for minor salivary gland cancers. A considerable additional number of patients in each category were living but had recurrent disease.

CONCLUSION

Cancer of the salivary glands is a surgical problem that must be attacked initially in a radical fashion to obtain good results. The diagnosis of a salivary gland cancer may be impossible to make clinically, but any swelling of a gland must be considered a possible cancer (25% to 30% of parotid gland tumors are malignant, and the percentage is considerably higher in minor salivary, sublingual, and submaxillary gland tumors).

Chapter 22

Carotid body tumors

Robin Anderson, M.D.
Edwin G. Beven, M.D.

Tumors of the carotid body are uncommon; for example, only 37 patients who had this tumor were seen at Memorial Hospital in New York during a period of 30 years.[4] The tumor is not rare, however, and anyone who does much head and neck surgery is certain to encounter at least a few patients with this disease. In spite of considerable standardization of technique, removal of a carotid body tumor is difficult, bloody, and fraught with disaster.

The history of carotid body tumor surgery has been reviewed by many authors. The first report, by Riegner in 1880, was of an unsuccessful procedure.[8] The first successful removal was that carried out by Maydl in 1886.[2] In 1903 Scudder reported on a successful operation performed in the United States.[2]

There has not always been agreement as to whether or not patients who have this tumor should be operated on, primarily because the problems associated with hemiplegia often were far worse than those produced by the enlarging mass. For many years Hayes Martin advised conservative nonsurgical management.[6]

On the other hand, most surgeons doing this type of surgery have felt that the tumors, while not necessarily histologically malignant, produce signs and symptoms of significance if allowed to grow, and that they should be removed before they become inoperable. Furthermore, these surgeons have found that with increasing experience and skill, the operation can be carried out successfully in most instances without significant mortality or morbidity. In 1967 Farr[4] reviewed the treatment of the 37 patients at Memorial Hospital. In the early part of the series, serious complications were common; in the last 20 years of

the series, only 1 of the 22 patients who were operated on died. In 1968 Chambers and Mahoney[3] reviewed their treatment of 40 patients who had tumors; they reported no mortality or hemiparesis. Shamblin and colleagues reviewed the Mayo Clinic series in 1971.[7] Seventy patients were operated on, there was a total of 16 postoperative cerebral vascular accidents and 3 deaths. Five patients were left with permanent hemiplegia.

This chapter reports the continuing experience at the Cleveland Clinic since the review published in 1963.[1] At that time we had excised 13 tumors without mortality or significant morbidity. At this time we are adding 11 patients, all of whom had lesions that were removed surgically. The pathologic entity known as a carotid body tumor has been called many names: paraganglioma, chemodectoma, and chromaffinoma, among others. The degree of malignancy remains questionable, but there is no doubt that most of these tumors grow and that many are invasive. Their histology is generally that of the carotid body with a vascular stroma surrounding nests of "chief" or epithelioid cells. The pathologic picture and its variations are well reviewed by LeCompte.[5] Distant metastases of the tumor have been reported; the patient operated on in 1907 by George Crile, Sr., survived with distant metastases for 25 years.[1]

DIAGNOSIS

Most patients with carotid body tumors come to the surgeon's office with an asymptomatic mass in the neck. Pulsation or a bruit suggests the presence of a tumor but is not pathognomonic. The correct diagnosis will rarely be made preoperatively, however, unless the possibility is considered by the surgeon. Once his suspicions have been aroused, carotid angiography should be done. The radiographic picture showing a vascular tumor filling the crotch of the carotid bifurcation is characteristic (Fig. 22-1). We have one patient, however, whose angiogram was typical but whose surgically removed lesion was an oversized hypertrophic lymph node.

DATA

In our series reported in 1963, we had 15 patients, 13 of whom were operated on. In that series there were no vascular sequelae following 3 carotid ligations and 3 arterial replacements. We have had 11 additional cases in the past 10 years.

Our present technique is essentially the same as that reported previously. We feel even more strongly than we did at that time that the vascular surgeon should be a member of the treatment team from the

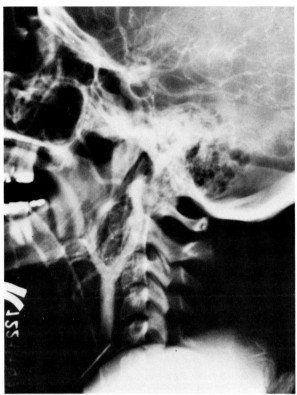

Fig. 22-1. Typical angiogram showing characteristic deformation of a carotid bifurcation by a vascular tumor.

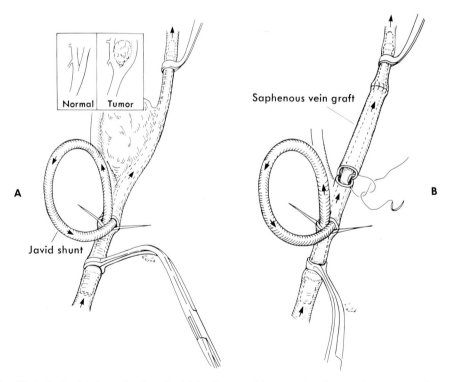

Fig. 22-2. A, Javid shunt is placed within the carotid artery in the usual manner to bypass the operative site. **B,** If a vein graft is necessary, it is threaded onto the shunt; and the two anastomoses are carried out.

time the diagnosis is seriously considered. He is responsible for the angiography and collaborates in the surgical planning. Since most of these tumors can be removed without endangering the carotid artery and without catastrophic hemorrhage, his presence is not always necessary in the operative field. On the other hand, if the dissection becomes critically difficult, he should be available to move into the field, bypass the lesion, resect the artery, and replace it with a vein autograft if necessary (Fig. 22-2). The vascular techniques employed are standard; the use of hypercarbia has not been indicated to date.

In this group of 11 patients, 2 patients have had bilateral tumors verified by angiography. In each instance, 1 side was treated. One patient may well require excision of the second side, but the tumor is small and asymptomatic at the present time. In the other patient the opposite lesion extends to the base of the skull and would unquestionably require carotid ligation. This hurdle will be met only if the lesion becomes symptomatic. The carotid artery was ligated in 3 instances without replacement because of extension of the tumor above the level at which a graft could be anastomosed. One carotid artery was grafted, and the graft has remained patent since the operation. There were 3 nerve X and 1 nerve XII paralyses without significant morbidity. One patient whose carotid artery was ligated developed a partial hemiplegia on the third postoperative day; it cleared within several days. The patient whose artery was replaced developed a hemiplegia immediately after surgery but returned to normal over a period of 3 months and made a complete recovery.

SUMMARY

Twenty-six patients who had carotid body tumors have been operated on at the Cleveland Clinic. In this series the carotid artery was ligated in 6 patients, and arterial replacement was necessary in 4 patients. Hemiplegia occurred in 2 patients. One patient's condition cleared in several days; the other required 3 months for a complete return to normalcy.

REFERENCES

1. Anderson, S., and Scarcella, J. V.: Carotid body tumors, Am. J. Surg. **106:**856, 1963.
2. Byrne, J. J.: Carotid body and allied tumors, Am. J. Surg. **95:**371, 1958.
3. Chambers, R. G., and Mahoney, W. D.: Carotid body tumors, Am. j. surg. **116:**554, 1968.
4. Farr, H. W.: Carotid body tumors—Am. J. of Surg. **114:**614, 1967.
5. LeCompte, P. M.: Tumors of the carotid body and related structures. In: Atlas of tumor pathology, sect. 4, fasc. 16, Washington, D.C., 1951, Armed Forces Institute of Pathology.
6. Martin, H.: Surgery of head and neck tumors, New York, 1957, Paul B. Hoeber, Inc.
7. Shamblin, W. R., Remine, W. H., Sheps, S. G., and Harrison E. G., Jr.: Carotid body tumors, Am. J. Surg. **122:**732, 1971.
8. Taylor, B. G.: The management of carotid body tumors, J. La. State Med. Soc. **114:**102, 1962.

Chapter 23

Malignant melanoma of the head and neck

John N. Simons, M.D.

A study in 1968[1] of 257 consecutive patients treated for melanoma of the head and neck revealed that the survival rate of patients treated by wide excision (with or without flap closure) and "elective" regional nodal dissection was highest. At that time this aggressive approach was proposed as the treatment of choice for patients with malignant melanoma of the head and neck, and this approach has continued to be the surgical choice for all such patients during the subsequent years. A follow-up study in 1972 confirmed that this aggressive approach was continuing to have a beneficial effect.[2] This chapter is an extension of the previous studies.

METHODS AND MATERIALS

The records of all patients with malignant melanoma of the head and neck who were seen at the Mayo Clinic from 1950 through 1970 were reviewed. As with the two previous series, patients were included only if definitive therapy was given and there was hope of a cure. Patients with superficial melanoma or Hutchinson's freckle (lentigo maligna) and patients who refused treatment or who had disseminated disease were excluded. Patients who had lesions of the conjunctiva were included only if the lesion involved the palpebral conjunctiva. The series consisted of 336 patients who met this criteria. Follow-up data were obtained on all but 6 patients.

FINDINGS AND COMMENT

Table 23-1 lists in decreasing order of frequency the sites of the melanoma. Five patients in whom the site of the primary lesion was unknown had regional metastasis at the time of first treatment. In this respect, I believe that the "disappearing mela-

Table 23-1. Locations of lesions in 336 patients with malignant melanoma of the head and neck

Location	Number
Neck	88
Cheek	86
Ear	36
Nasal cavity and antrum	35
Scalp	24
Temple	23
Forehead	15
Eyelid	8
Nose	6
Lip	3
Chin	3
Soft palate	2
Alveolar ridge	2
Unknown	5
Total	336

Table 23-2. Age and sex of patients with malignant melanoma of the head and neck

Age (years)	Male	Female	Total
0-9	0	1	1
10-19	9	2	11
20-29	18	7	25
30-39	36	17	53
40-49	27	21	48
50-59	48	25	73
60-69	40	26	66
70-79	32	16	48
80-89	4	5	9
90-99	1	1	2
Total	215	121	336

noma" is a distinct entity and that several of the lesions with unknown primary sites represented this rare occurrence.

Melanoma was found to be rare in the younger age group; only 12 of the 336 patients (4%) were under 20 years old (Table 23-2). The most common age group was the sixties; it included 73 patients (21%). Men predominated in a ratio of 1.8:1.

The patients were grouped into the following five main categories of initial treatment: (1) wide excision with or without skin grafting for closure of the primary wound; (2) wide excision with or without skin grafting, and dissection of regional clinically positive nodes; (3) dissection of regional clinically positive nodes without excision of the primary lesion (primary lesion under control or its site not known); (4) wide excision, with or without skin grafting, and prophylactic nodal dissection; and (5) wide excision, with or without skin grafting, and late nodal dissec-

tion after the development of clinically positive nodes. All patients in group 5 were also in group 1.

The lethality of malignant melanoma continues to be impressive; 162 of the 336 patients (48%) died of uncontrolled disease. Of these 162 patients, 27 (17%) died more than 3 years from the time of surgery, whereas 11 (7%) died 5 years or more from the time of operation. The mean interval from the time of surgery to the time of death was 2.2 years. Tables 22-3 and 22-4 summarize the data on 280 patients eligible for a 3-year follow-up and on 224 patients eligible for a 5-year follow-up.

The overall survival rates of all patients who were surgically treated for melanoma of the head and neck and who had a chance of being cured averaged 45% for the 3-year follow-up and 43% for the 5-year follow-up. Of 152 patients who were initially treated by excision alone without nodal dissection and who were eligible for the 3-year follow-up study,

Table 23-3. Three-year follow-up study of 280 patients with malignant melanoma of the head and neck

Procedure	Total number of patients	Dead; uncontrolled disease		Dead; other cause		Alive; disease		Alive; no disease	
		Number	Percent	Number	Percent	Number	Percent	Number	Percent
Excision without nodal dissection	152	47	31	10	7	20	13	75	49
Excision with nodal dissection for positive nodes	52	33	63	1	2	3	6	15	29
Regional nodal dissection—no treatment to primary lesion	31	23	74	0	0	3	10	5	16
Excision with prophylactic nodal dissection	45	10	22	2	4	1	2	32	71
Total	*280*	*113*	*40*	*13*	*5*	*27*	*10*	*127*	*45*
Excision with late dissection for positive nodes*	30	23	77	0	0	2	7	5	16

*Patients were in group that had undergone excision without nodal dissection.

Table 23-4. Five-year follow-up study of 233 patients with malignant melanoma of the head and neck

Procedure	Total number of patients	Dead; uncontrolled disease		Dead; other cause		Alive; disease		Alive; no disease	
		Number	Percent	Number	Percent	Number	Percent	Number	Percent
Excision without nodal dissection	134	54	40	13	10	6	4	61	46
Excision with nodal dissection for positive nodes	40	25	63	1	3	0	0	14	35
Regional nodal dissection—no treatment to primary lesion	29	23	79	0	0	2	7	4	12
Excision with prophylactic nodal dissection	30	6	20	2	7	0	0	22	73
Total	*233*	*108*	*46*	*16*	*7*	*8*	*3*	*101*	*43*
Excision with late dissection for positive nodes*	28	23	82	0	0	0	0	5	18

*Patients were in group that had undergone excision without nodal dissection.

75 (49%) survived free of disease. However, 47 of the 152 patients (31%) died of uncontrolled disease, and an additional 20 patients (13%) had an uncontrolled primary lesion or recurrent metastatic disease at the end of the 3-year study. The 5-year cure rate (46%) was not significantly lower than the 3-year rate of patients treated by excision alone. The increase in deaths from uncontrolled disease from the 3-year to the 5-year period (31% to 40%) primarily represents patients who were alive at the end of 3 years but who had active and uncontrolled disease and died of uncontrolled disease within the next 2 years. These findings are similar to those of the previous studies.[1,2]

In patients who had both a primary lesion and positive regional nodes or positive regional nodes and either a primary site that was unknown or a primary lesion that was under control, the survival rates decreased to levels of 29% and 16% for the 3-year follow-up and 35% and 12% for the 5-year follow-up, respectively. (For some unknown reason, in the present study 5-year cure rates of those patients who had a primary lesion and clinically positive nodes increased from the previous studies.) However, 7 of every 10 patients in the 5-year group who initially had positive nodes, with or without a positive primary lesion, died of uncontrolled disease. The overall survival rate of patients who had positive regional nodes decreased to 21%.

Forty-five patients in the fourth group—those initially treated by wide excision of the primary lesion and by prophylactic nodal dissection—were eligible for the 3-year follow-up, and 30 were eligible for the 5-year follow-up. Ten (22%) of those patients eligible for the 3-year follow-up died of uncontrolled disease, and only 1 additional patient who had active disease was alive at the time of the follow-up. Thirty-two of the 45 patients (71%) treated by this aggressive approach survived 3 years and were free of disease, and 22 of the 30 patients (73%) survived 5 years and were free of disease.

The survival rates in the "prophylactic" group do represent a significant improvement over the average survival rate for all four treatments; of particular significance is the improvement over the survival rate of patients treated by excision alone, the only other surgical treatment of the patient with clinically negative nodes that can be validly compared. The results of the present study indicate, however, that at least 20 additional patients out of each 100 patients who have melanoma of the head and neck will be cured if prophylactic nodal dissection is utilized in addition to the standard wide excision with or without skin grafting.

The experience with patients who were treated initially at the Mayo Clinic by simple excision and who were instructed to return only if regional nodes became positive were reviewed. In this group, there were 30 and 28 patients, respectively, at the 3-year and 5-year follow-up levels. The 3-year and 5-year survival rates decreased to below 20% of the patients treated in this sequence.

The most impressive results were obtained by prophylactic nodal dissections performed on 39 patients who were eligible for a 3-year follow-up study. Of the 5 patients in this group who had clinically negative but histologically positive regional nodes, 1 (20%) survived (Table 23-5). The survival rate, however, of patients with clinically and histologically negative nodes was 79%. Although only with the passage of time and more prophylactic nodal dissections will the meaning of these figures be evident, survival figures to date are most encouraging and strongly indicate the judicious role of prophylactic nodal dissection for malignant melanoma of the head and neck.

SUMMARY

Of 336 patients with malignant melanoma of the head and neck who were treated at the Mayo Clinic, 280 were eligible for a 3-year follow-up and 237 were eligible for a 5-year follow-up. Treatment consisted of three surgical approaches: (1) simple excision, (2) excision of clinically positive regional nodes, and (3) wide excision of the primary lesion combined

Table 23-5. Three-year follow-up study of 44 patients with malignant melanoma of the head and neck who underwent prophylactic nodal dissection

Status of nodes		Total number of patients	Dead; disease		Dead; other cause		Alive; disease		Alive; no disease	
Clinical	Histologic		Number	Percent	Number	Percent	Number	Percent	Number	Percent
Negative	Negative	39	6	15	2	5	0	0	31	79
Negative	Positive	5	4	80	0	0	0	0	1	20

with elective neck dissection. For both the 3-year and 5-year follow-up studies, the overall survival rates of the total group averaged nearly 45%. Once clinically positive nodes were detected, the survival rates decreased to less than half of this figure, whereas the survival rates of patients treated by prophylactic nodal dissection increased to 71% in the 3-year follow-up and 73% in the 5-year follow-up. Of those patients treated by prophylactic nodal dissection where histologically all nodes were found to be negative, the survival rate was 79%. Based on the continued finding of significantly increased survival rates obtained by prophylactic nodal dissection, this modality is the treatment of choice for the patient who has malignant melanoma of the head and neck.

REFERENCES

1. Simons, J. N.: Malignant melanoma of the head and neck, Am. J. Surg. **116:**494-498, 1968.
2. Simons, J. N.: Malignant melanoma of the head and neck, Am. J. Surg. **124:**485-488, 1972.

Chapter 24

Carcinomas of the thyroid

George Crile, Jr., M.D.
William A. Hawk, M.D.

It is difficult to reconcile the various points of view about the treatment of cancer of the thyroid unless surgeons stop talking about cancer of the thyroid as an entity and start to break it down into its component parts. The problem is that cancer of the thyroid is not like cancer of the stomach or cancer of the colon, in which most of the tumors follow the same patterns of metastases and are of approximately the same degree of malignancy. Cancer of the thyroid is more like cancer of the skin, in which there is a spectrum of tumors that includes such different entities as the highly malignant melanoma, the moderately malignant squamous-cell carcinoma, and the relatively benign basal-cell carcinoma.

No one would make a general statement as to how all types of cancer of the skin should be treated, or advise prophylactic dissection of lymph nodes in the treatment of a basal-cell cancer of the skin. Yet in the treatment of certain cancers of the thyroid, such as the encapsulated angioinvasive carcinoma, although metastasis to regional nodes is nearly as rare as it is in basal-cell cancer, some surgeons advocate prophylactic dissection of lymph nodes. The trouble is that they are thinking of thyroid cancer as an entity.

One of the chief difficulties lies in the nomenclature of thyroid carcinomas and in the lack of understanding between surgeons and pathologists. It is unfortunate that thyroid cancers are classified as papillary, follicular, or undifferentiated, in accordance with their morphologic characteristics rather than in accordance with their biological behavior. Pathologists who classify tumors morphologically may, in their final diagnoses, fail to discriminate between a well-differentiated nonencapsulated tumor (that is predominantly follicular with only a few papillary areas), and a well-differentiated, encapsulated follicular carcinoma; they tend to call both types follicular carcinoma. To be meaningful, a classification must take into account not only the morphologic characteristics but also the biological behavior of the neoplasm. The classification of carcinomas listed below includes such considerations.[1]

    I. Papillary carcinoma
        a. Usual papillary carcinoma, whether predominantly papillary or predominantly follicular or mixed
        b. Microcarcinoma
   II. Follicular carcinoma
        a. Encapsulated angioinvasive carcinoma
        b. Invasive carcinoma
 III. Medullary (solid) carcinoma
 IV. Anaplastic carcinoma
  V. Lymphomas

CARCINOMAS OF LOW MALIGNANCY
Papillary carcinomas

The commonest cancers of low malignancy are the papillary carcinomas, constituting 60 to 70 percent of all thyroid cancers. These tumors occur chiefly in young persons, often a few years after radiation therapy to the head, chest, or neck, given in childhood for some benign condition. Papillary carcinoma may be multicentric in the thyroid and tends to me-

Reprinted with permission from Cleveland Clinic Quarterly 38:97-104, July, 1971.

153

tastasize early to regional nodes. Distant metastasis is rare. Growth of the tumor tends to be readily suppressed by feeding of desiccated thyroid. In a patient between puberty and 45 years of age, papillary carcinoma, if treated by a proper operation and not cut into, implanted in the wound and thus disseminated, is associated with almost as good a 10- to 15-year life expectancy as the patient would have had if he had never had the cancer.[2]

In women the survival curves in regard to papillary carcinoma are superimposable, up to 15 years, on those of cancer-free women of the same age and race. In males or in patients of either sex who are very young (prepubertal) or beyond middle age, papillary carcinoma tends to be more invasive and to metastasize to lungs or bone. In females, between puberty and menopause, the disease tends to be almost benign in regard to distant metastasis. Fortunately, in both sexes the growth of tumors that occur in youth is generally suppressible by the feeding of desiccated thyroid.

The operations that one of us (G. C., Jr.) has recommended for the treatment of cervical metastases of papillary carcinoma of the thyroid are much more extensive than standard radical neck dissections, and entail removal (when involved) of the midline (Delphian) nodes, the superior mediastinal nodes, the paratracheal nodes, and the carotid and scalene nodes, as well as the nodes of the jugular chain that are routinely removed in conventional neck dissections. After making a high, wide, thyroidectomy incision, or in males, an incision parallel to the anterior border of the sternocleidomastoid muscle, the belly of the sternocleidomastoid muscle is freed from its attachments, and a band put around it. The muscle may then be elevated so that the nodes beneath it and posterior to it can be resected. In similar fashion the carotid artery and vagus nerve are mobilized and the jugular vein too, unless it is more convenient, on one side, to resect the vein. Often bilateral dissections are done through the same high transverse incision that is used for the thyroidectomy. The involved nodes are not removed individually but, insofar as possible, in groups within their envelopes of fatty and areolar tissue.

The lobe of the thyroid on the affected side is always removed completely together with the isthmus and part of the contralateral lobe. Only if there is gross bilateral involvement of thyroid or nodes is a true total thyroidectomy performed. It is often impossible to distinguish a parathyroid from an involved capsular node, and if all the thyroid is removed

without regard for the parathyroids the incidence of tetany is prohibitively high.

In a personal series of 307 consecutive patients with papillary cancer of the thyroid, all but three of whom have been followed for from 5 to 27 years after operation, there has been no death from local recurrence or from cervical metastases of papillary carcinoma. Two patients, each of whom had undergone four operations before consultation at the Cleveland Clinic, had had cancer implanted in their necks and there was advancing local recurrence at the time they died from systemic metastasis, but neither in these patients, nor in any patients in this series was local recurrence the cause of death.

Prophylactic neck dissection was not performed unless cervical nodes were grossly involved at the time of exploration. Tumor has appeared in the nodes of only 4 percent of the patients who did not at the time of operation have gross evidence of nodal involvement. In each case the cancer was permanently controlled and the patient has remained well for from 8 to 19 years after a small second operation for removal of the affected group of nodes.

Unless the recurrent laryngeal nerve was already paralyzed by invasion of cancer it was usually possible to preserve the nerve. Even when it was densely adherent to the primary tumor or to metastases in paratracheal nodes it was possible to tease the tumor off the nerve. There have been no local recurrences after this procedure. Although the trachea was never sacrificed there were no recurrences in the thyroid area.

Total thyroidectomy was performed in 9 percent of the patients, yet there was only one instance of recurrence of cancer in the residual thyroid (0.3 percent). It is now more than 20 years since the second operation and the patient appears to be free of cancer. Unilateral vocal cord paralysis (including that in patients who had incurred it preoperatively) occurred in 11 percent of the patients, and permanent tetany in 2 percent. In only 4 percent of the patients were the sternocleidomastoid muscles sacrificed, and in only 2 percent were the eleventh nerves resected. In only one operation was it necessary to perform a thoracotomy to gain access to mediastinal nodes. Thus, in the majority of patients the only morbidity of disfiguration was a thyroidectomy scar.

Life-table analysis of 140 consecutive patients operated on from 5 to 25 years before showed that in the 75 female patients upon whom the first definitive operation was performed by one of us (G. C., Jr.) the rate of survival up to 15 years was as high as would have been expected in a group of the same sex, race, and age who had not had papillary carcinoma. Beyond 15 years the number of patients is too small to be of statistical significance, but clinically only one patient (and she had been operated on several times elsewhere before being treated at Cleveland Clinic) died of thyroid cancer.

In the entire series of 307 patients with papillary cancer of the thyroid the 5-year survival rate was 94 percent. Seventy-six of the patients, however, had been admitted with recurrences after a thyroid operation elsewhere. Fourteen percent of these ultimately died of cancer as compared to only 5 of 231 (2 percent) of those upon whom one of us (G. C., Jr.) performed the first definitive operation on the thyroid. An additional 1 percent of the patients in this group are living with uncontrolled cancer.

Since 70 percent of the 307 patients had involvement of nodes, and 4 percent had preoperative pulmonary metastases, it is apparent that the patients in this series were not selected.

In recent years the results of treatment have been better than in the earlier period. Ninety patients with previously untreated papillary carcinoma were treated in the 5-year period 1960 through 1964. Operations were even less radical than in the earlier period, yet no patient has died of cancer and only one has progressing disease. Since in our entire experience we have never seen a patient who went for 5 years without recurrence and then had a fatal recurrence of the disease, it is safe to say that, short as the follow-up is, it indicates that the ultimate mortality rate from cancer will be less than the postoperative mortality that would be incurred by routinely performing total thyroidectomies and radical neck dissections.

Since the growth of many papillary carcinomas can be suppressed by feeding desiccated thyroid, it is important to prescribe full suppressive doses for the duration of the patients' lives. The incidence of recurrence after operations has been reduced by more than 50 percent since 3 gr of Armour's brand of desiccated thyroid or its equivalent has been given daily. In many patients with extensive metastasis the tumor has either regressed or stopped growing. After the growth of a tumor has been suppressed there has been little or no tendency for it to escape from control. Thirty-two patients, with distant metastases mainly to the lungs, have been treated by desiccated thyroid and have been followed for from 5 to 27 years. In 18 of them the metastases either have shrunk or remained unchanged. In 14 patients similarly treated the metastases did not respond. The best re-

sponses occurred in patients who gave a history of having had radiation in infancy or childhood for benign disease of the head and neck, and in the younger patients, especially if they were female.

Microcarcinomas

A group of the microcarcinomas of the thyroid have been called "nonencapsulated sclerosing tumors."[3,4] These tumors are from 1 to 10 mm in diameter and are present in about 3 percent of all thyroids examined at routine autopsy.[5] The tumors appear to be similar to the microcarcinomas of the prostate that are present so frequently in men more than 50 years of age. When a microcarcinoma is removed in the course of a thyroidectomy done for another reason, it should be considered as an incidental finding that requires no additional surgical treatment. We have not seen metastases from such tumors. On the other hand, as occult microfocus of true papillary carcinoma may give rise to extensive metastases in cervical nodes.[6] In the latter case the malignant potential is expressed in metastases long before the tumor is clinically evident; whereas in the former case, if no metastases are seen at the time of operation it is unlikely that they subsequently will develop.

Encapsulated angioinvasive carcinomas

Encapsulated angioinvasive carcinomas are almost never multicentric and seldom metastasize to regional nodes.[7] All that is required to give the patient with an encapsulated follicular carcinoma the best possible prospect of cure is to remove completely the affected lobe. Attempts to perform total thyroidectomy or node dissection are useless and merely increase morbidity. It is important, however, to remove the tumor with the capsule intact, preferably by lobectomy, so that tumor tissue does not become implanted in the wound and recur. When removal is complete the prognosis in these patients is almost as good as that in those of similar age and sex with papillary cancer.

The growth of encapsulated follicular cancers is rarely controlled by desiccated-thyroid feeding as is that of the papillary variety, but ^{131}I may be effective. The prognosis becomes more grave when the patients are elderly men. The average age of patients who were well 5 or more years after operations for encapsulated angioinvasive cancers was 44 years, whereas the average age of those who died of the cancers was 62 years. No patients less than 54 years of age died of this type of cancer. The prognosis was worse in men than in women: 33 percent of the men died of cancer, and 8 percent of the women.

CARCINOMAS OF INTERMEDIATE MALIGNANCY
Invasive follicular carcinoma

Although the invasive follicular carcinoma is so uniformly fatal that it hardly can be called a tumor of moderate malignancy, it grows so slowly that more than half of our patients who died of it had survived for more than 5 years after operation. Whether the encapsulated angioinvasive carcinoma is a chronologically early phase of the invasive follicular adenocarcinoma is difficult to say, but we doubt that it is. Analysis of age, sex, and duration of history suggests that each of the follicular types of thyroid tumors is an entity, and does not originate in another type. Invasive follicular carcinomas are tumors of high malignancy invading blood vessels and surrounding tissues, but their rate of growth may be relatively slow.

Between the years 1946 and 1958 at the Cleveland Clinic, diagnosis of atypical adenoma was made 15 times, that of encapsulated follicular carcinoma 38 times, and that of invasive follicular carcinoma 15 times. The characteristics of the tumor of each group are summarized in Table 24-1.

There is little about the duration of the goiters before operation, the age and sex of the patients, the relative size of the tumors in the different groups or their tendencies to metastasize to nodes or systemically to suggest that with the passing of time the tumors progress from one type to another. Although the invasive follicular carcinoma may grow slowly and patients may live with metastases for many years, our experience has shown it to be ultimately fatal, usually as a result of systemic metastasis. Angioinvasion is a prominent histologic feature of these tumors, and they seem to metastasize through the bloodstream before the diagnosis is made. Operations are mainly palliative. If lymph nodes are involved they should be removed along with the primary tumor as simply as possible so as not to add the morbidity of a radical operation to the burdens of a patient already having distant metastases.

Medullary (solid) carcinoma

The term medullary carcinoma is a misnomer because the tumor is not soft but stony hard.[8] *Solid carcinoma* would be a better name, or *amyloid-forming cancer*, because amyloid is almost always present. This tumor is undifferentiated in structure but its cells are regular and not anaplastic. It produces an amyloid stroma that can be shown by special stains. Medullary carcinoma metastasizes to lymph nodes and through the bloodstream, is locally invasive, and should be treated by radical removal of the affected part of the thyroid and the involved nodal groups. Fewer than half of the patients treated are permanently cured, but the tumor grows slowly and many patients live for 5 or more years after treatment. Sometimes the metastases penetrate the capsules of the nodes and invade the surrounding tissues, making it necessary to do a formal, block-dissection type of lymphadenectomy. The 5-year survival rate in 21 patients having medullary carcinoma was 54 percent (11 patients); but when followed longer, still more ultimately died of the disease or are living with incurable recurrences. Of those who died of medullary carcinoma, four lived for from 7 to 27 years after operation.

Lymphomas

Lymphomas of the thyroid respond well to radiation therapy. In recent years, because struma lymphomatosa responds well to thyroid feeding and because many lymphosarcomas arise in glands that show changes of struma lymphomatosa, we have treated all patients with lymphomas of the thyroids by a combination of radiation and suppressive doses of desiccated thyroid (3 gr daily). Whether or not the desiccated thyroid contributes to the improved results, about half of the patients treated in this way have remained well.[9] Operation is not necessary, be-

Table 24-1. Comparison of histories and physical findings in various types of thyroid tumors

	Atypical adenoma (15 patients)	Type of follicular carcinoma	
		Encapsulated (38 patients)	Invasive (15 patients)
Duration, preoperative (median)	1.5 yr	3 yr	3 yr
Sex, male	44%	32%	20%
Age, average	45 yr	47 yr	59 yr
Size of neoplasm (large)	22%	68%	57%
Follow-up data			
Postoperative metastasis	0%	11%	73%
To nodes	0%	3%	13%
Systemic	0%	8%	60%
Follow-up, 5 to 25 yr			
Living free of cancer	67%	70%	0%
Dead of cancer	0%	16%	86%
Living with recurrence	0%	3%	0%
Dead of other causes	5%	8%	7%
Untraced after 4 yr	28%	3%	7%

cause the lymphomas are so radiosensitive that persistence or local recurrence has been no problem.

HIGHLY MALIGNANT TUMORS
Anaplastic carcinoma

Anaplastic carcinomas of the thyroid are among the most malignant of all tumors. Their course, from onset to death, is usually less than 1 year and often as short as 4 months. Anaplastic carcinomas invade locally and metastasize to regional nodes and to lungs. Most of them are inoperable when first diagnosed. If attempts are made to remove them, fungating recurrences into the wound are common. Needle biopsy to establish the diagnosis, followed by radiation therapy is the most effective way of controlling the local lesion until the patient dies of metastases.

Only one of 24 patients with anaplastic carcinomas has remained well after operation. The tumor was considered inoperable, but part of it was removed and the rest treated by what is now thought to have been inadequate roentgenotherapy. For unexplained reasons the patient has remained well for more than 10 years.

SUMMARY

Those who know the natural histories of the various types of cancer of the thyroid recognize that their variability makes it impossible to define any single method of treatment applicable to all types. If biological predeterminism exists, it is most apparent in these types of cancer. The highly malignant tumors are rarely cured no matter how early or extensive the operations, and the ones of low malignancy may be cured by simple operations even after long delay.

This does not condone either delay or inadequate surgery, but it does mean that in case of doubt there is time for a few months' trial of medical treatment of benign-appearing nodules. Classic radical operations rarely are required in the treatment of tumors of low malignancy, and rarely are of value in malignancies of the highest grade.

REFERENCES

1. Crile, G., Jr., Hazard, J. B., and Dinsmore, R. S.: Carcinoma of thyroid gland with special reference to clinicopathologic classification. J. Clin. Endocrinol. **8**:762-765, 1948.
2. Crile, G., Jr.: Survival of patients with papillary carcinoma of the thyroid after conservative operations. Amer. J. Surg. **108**:862-866, 1964.
3. Hazard, J. B.: Small papillary carcinoma of the thyroid; a study with special reference to so-called nonencapsulated sclerosing tumor. Lab. Invest. **9**:86-87, 1960.
4. Hazard, J. B., Crile, G., Jr. and Dempsey, W. S.: Nonencapsulated sclerosing tumors of thyroid. J. Clin. Endocrinol. **9**:1216-1231, 1949.
5. Mortenson, J. D., Bennett, W. A., and Woolner, L. B.: Incidence of carcinoma in thyroid glands removed at 1000 consecutive routine necropsies. Surg. Forum (1954), **5**:659-663, 1955.
6. Hazard, J. B., and Kenyon, R.: Encapsulated angioinvasive carcinoma (angioinvasive adenoma) of thyroid gland. Amer. J. Clin. Path. **24**:755-766, 1954.
7. Hazard, J. B., and Kenyon, R.: Atypical adenoma of thyroid, A.M.A. Arch. Path. **58**:554-563, 1954.
8. Hazard, J. B., Hawk, W. A., and Crile, G., Jr.: Medullary (solid) carcinoma of thyroid—a clinicopathologic entity. J. Clin. Endocrinol. **19**:152-161, 1959.
9. Crile, G., Jr.: Lymphosarcoma and reticulum cell sarcoma of the thyroid. Surg. Gynec. Obstet. **116**:449-450, 1963.

Chapter 25

Panel discussion

Moderator: John C. Gaisford, M.D.

Dr. Georgiade, Professor of Plastic and Maxillofacial Oral Surgery, Duke University;
Dr. Richards, Chief of Radiology, Greater Baltimore Medical Center; Dr. Chambers,
Assistant Professor of Plastic Surgery, The Johns Hopkins University; and Dr. Ogura,
Professor of Otolaryngology, Washington University

Dr. Gaisford: We all run into the problem case. I don't care how long you work in this area or how astute and erudite you might be, some of these problems are going to remain problems for you, and there are going to be areas of differences. Many of these problems may be and possibly will be treated by more than one approach; many times there is no one perfect approach.

Surgeons dealing with cancer of the head and neck acquire a good idea of what might be accomplished by radiotherapy. The radiotherapist must have a good idea of what might be accomplished by surgery. It is absolutely impossible to run a tumor service unless there is proper rapport between the two services; it is a lot like trying to do surgery in an operating room where the surgeon doesn't speak to the anesthesiologist. The patient with a tumor cannot always be cured by surgery, and he cannot always be cured by radiation. Many times, both the radiotherapist and the surgeon must enter into the final treatment.

HEMANGIOMA

Dr. Gaisford: Hemangioma—simple, straightforward hemangioma—is a very common problem. This tumor is probably the most common one in childhood. Dr. Georgiade, how would you treat the child shown in Fig. 25-1, *A?*

Dr. Georgiade: The hemangioma is changing. I would not do anything to this child.

Dr. Gaisford: How long do you think it might be before it goes away, assuming you believe it will go away?

Dr. Georgiade: My experience is that this type of lesion will not actually go away; it will regress, but there will remain an area of scar that will have to be dealt with at a later date. My only question is whether the surgery should be done at this time. Surgically, it is better to wait; if the hemangioma regresses, the reconstruction would be a lot easier in an older child than it would be in this infant.

Dr. Gaisford: Dr. Richards, is there any reason for using radiation for this particular tumor?

Dr. Richards: You know that 85% of these tumors will regress, many of them completely by the time the child is 2 years of age. The major question of radiotherapists about capillary hemangiomas in children concerns the existence of two definite indications for treatment: are the hemangiomas subject to constant trauma, and do they therefore bleed constantly; or are they subject to constant infection? Since it is located in this particular area of the child's body, I would doubt very much that this hemangioma is subject to a great deal of trauma. I can't be sure of how much it involves the sclera or conjunctiva, so I

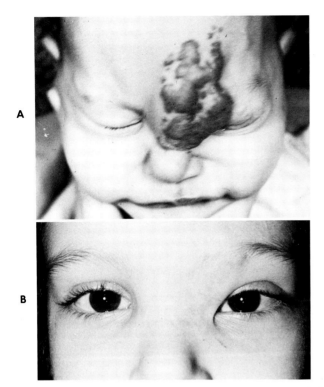

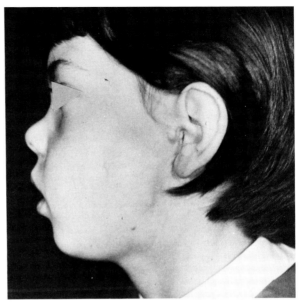

Fig. 25-2. Facial nerve paralysis after infection at age 3 months.

Fig. 25-1. A, Hemangioma of the face. **B,** Hemangioma of the face after spontaneous regression with some scarring.

would be inclined not to treat this particular one. These hemangiomas can be safely treated on the basis of good indication, and all you do is nudge them with a very small dose of superficial irradiation. We tend to use a beta plaque in the form of a strontium beta applicator to nudge them with about 100 to 150 beta rads.

Dr. Gaisford: Fig. 25-1, *B,* shows the child about 18 months later, and you are both absolutely correct. There still is a physical deformity, and there was no problem. These can be, as you know, absolutely horrendous problems at the time.

PAROTID ABSCESS

Dr. Gaisford: Fig. 25-2 shows a child who had a parotid abscess resulting in facial paralysis at the age of 11 months. Dr. Chambers, would you consider a nerve graft for this particular child?

Dr. Chambers: I would tend to go ahead and do a nerve graft and suspension as soon as possible.

Dr. Gaisford: I agree. I think a nerve graft would be the treatment of choice if one has a quiescent lesion and an appropriate time has elapsed.

LIP CANCER

Dr. Gaisford: Fig. 25-3 shows a squamous cell cancer of the lip; another small cancer is here, and leukoplakia of the entire vermilion is present. It is a very common problem and a local one. Dr. Ogura, do you expect trouble from something like this?

Dr. Ogura: Did you say that the malignancy of the lesion in the center was proved by biopsy?

Dr. Gaisford: It was treated, and when biopsied, it was diagnosed as squamous cell cancer. There are two separate lesions, and they are tiny, very superficial.

Dr. Ogura: Very superficial?

Dr. Gaisford: Yes.

Dr. Ogura: It looks as though there is leukoplakia throughout the entire rest of the lip; is that right?

Dr. Gaisford: That's right.

Dr. Ogura: You can excise the lesions and advance mucosa from the mouth; just strip all of it if the tumor is superficial.

Dr. Gaisford: This particular patient did have metastases from these tiny squamous cells to both sides of the neck and had a bilateral radical neck dissection. Then he had one metastatic lesion in the lung.

Dr. Ogura: Was that after you did this?

Dr. Gaisford: Yes, some months later. Would you

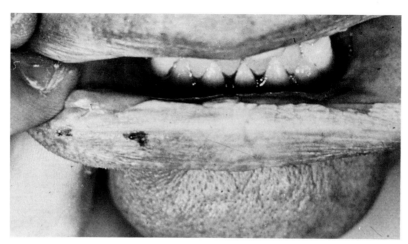

Fig. 25-3. Cancer and leukoplakia of the lower lip.

continue to treat this patient? We have followed him this far; we have done bilateral neck dissections, and he has a lesion in the lung. Dr. Richards, do you think it would be worthwhile to consider a pneumonectomy, or would you consider radiation?

Dr. Richards: Dr. Chambers and I are frequently faced with this problem. If the patient has a solitary pulmonary nodule and it has been proved by multiple tomography of the entire lung and by lung scanning that this is indeed a solitary nodule, we would suggest a lobectomy or even a pneumonectomy if necessary. On the other hand, if the patient refuses such treatment, we would have no qualms about using direct, small-field irradiation to that portion of the lung and carrying it to a tumoricidal dose of 6,000 rads; we would probably supplement this treatment with hydroxyurea.

Dr. Gaisford: This paient succumbed to his pulmonary disease; he was not treated because he refused further treatment.

Dr. Ogura: What did you do the first time?

Dr. Gaisford: Just what you suggested. He had a resection of just what you see there, and intraoral mucosa was advanced.

Dr. Ogura: How soon after that did the lesion metastasize?

Dr. Gaisford: Several months.

Dr. Ogura: You were surprised, too.

Dr. Gaisford: Very much so. Is there anyone here who would do a so-called prophylactic neck dissection for a lip cancer?

Dr. Georgiade: No.

Dr. Ogura: I would take exception there. With a large lesion infiltrating into the orbicularis muscle, I would do a bilateral suprahyoid diagnostic node removal, and depending on the findings, I would do a neck dissection. I have never heard of a small superficial lesion like that metastasizing.

OSTEOGENIC SARCOMA

Dr. Gaisford: Fig. 25-4 shows a young boy with a tumor of the left mandible; it was resected with no wide excision. An osteogenic sarcoma involved almost the entire left mandible.

Dr. Ogura: This resection was done without a biopsy?

Dr. Gaisford: Without a biopsy.

Dr. Georgiade: The treatment of choice in osteogenic sarcoma of the mandible is surgery and radiation therapy in combination. Even at that, the survival rate is only about 25%.

Dr. Gaisford: This case is presented to make the differentiation between the survival rate of osteogenic sarcoma of the mandible and osteogenic sarcoma of other bones of the body. What is your opinion about this?

Dr. Richards: Sitting next to me is one of the world authorities on the treatment of osteogenic sarcomas of the mandible. I would like to have Dr. Chambers say how he feels osteogenic sarcomas of the mandible should be treated and comment on the survival rate of his group.

Dr. Chambers: The radium element should be implanted directly into the tumor; the dose should be necrotizing, the resection is done on the day

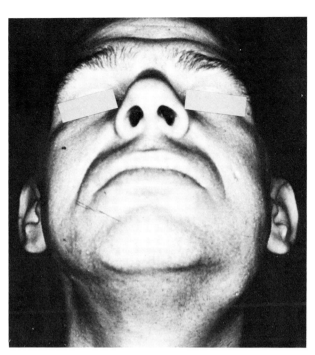

Fig. 25-4. Osteogenic sarcoma of the left mandible.

the needles come out. Our survival rate is 75% for 5 years and 72% for 1C years.

Dr. Gaisford: Do you think there is a marked difference between the survival rates of patients with osteogenic sarcoma of the mandible and patients with osteogenic sarcoma of other bones?

Dr. Chambers: They really are not the same type of tumor, and the orthopedic surgeons are loath to work with osteogenic sarcoma. On one or two occasions under pressure, they have given a necrotizing dose of irradiation and done an amputation; but as a rule, they won't.

Dr. Richards: Len Johnson, the AFIP pathologist who probably is more knowledgeable about osteogenic sarcoma than anybody anywhere, feels that all osteogenic sarcomas in every part of the body should receive a necrotizing dose of preoperative irradiation. You don't give them anything for nausea, and you don't give them anything for skin reaction; you just burn the hell out of the tumor. He feels that you change some immunologic factors.

Dr. Gaisford: Do you treat the mandible as one bone or two, Dr. Chambers? Do you treat the entire mandible with radiation and surgery, or do you just treat part of the mandible?

Dr. Chambers: I think you ought to go to the other side of the embryonic plate; in other words, the

other side of the symphysis. For instance, if you had a lesion in the horizontal ramus at about the first molar area, I would go beyond the symphysis anteriorly and disarticulate posteriorly. You preserve what you can safely. I think you can fairly accurately give yourself a wide margin.

Dr. Richards: Dr. Chambers drills holes right into the mandibular body and ramus, and we put the needles right into the bony tumor after extracting the teeth. The needles are sutured into the mandible. If the tumor extends into the floor of the mouth, a second plane of needles is put into this tumor of the floor of the mouth; occasionally, a third plane is placed on the lateral aspect of the buccal mucosa.

Dr. Gaisford: But this tumor was completely contained and hadn't broken through. It was really very localized and presented no difficulty in removal. Is there any change in your attitude regarding preoperative irradiation for this particular variety rather than one that has extended outside the bone?

Dr. Chambers: We treat all osteogenic sarcomas of the mandible the same regardless of what they look like. How did he do?

Dr. Gaisford: He did fine, with no radiation and no preoperative biopsy. It has been approximately 24 years since he was treated.

TRAUMA AND CANCER

Dr. Gaisford: Fig. 25-5 shows a farmer who was kicked in the head by a cow about 3 weeks before he developed a fungating tumor. How do you feel about trauma as a possible cause of cancer? Have you ever seen it? Do you believe it is possible? Here is an actual case. It is only 3 weeks, and he already has a metastasis in his parotid gland. We don't know the accuracy of the history, but we have had patients who gave an accurate history of rapidly growing tumors after relatively slight injuries. What do you think?

Dr. Richards: We can document cases of trauma that have developed a metastatic "take" at the site of the trauma. In this institution [Greater Baltimore Medical Center] Dr. Wood demonstrated how circulating cancer cells take in traumatized tissue. We see this very definitely in radiated areas; metastases will often develop in tissue traumatized by radiation. I think there is some evidence to relate trauma and metastatic take but not trauma and primary tumors.

Dr. Gaisford: Dr. Ogura, do you feel that manipu-

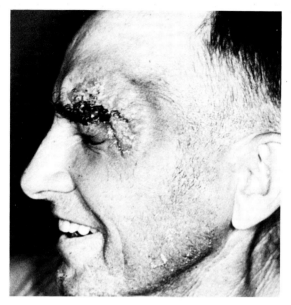

Fig. 25-5. Cancer of the forehead and metastases of the parotid gland area and neck after trauma to the head.

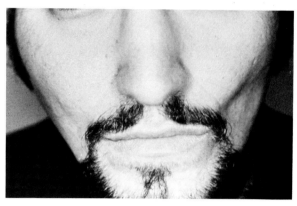

Fig. 25-6. Flattened left side of the face caused by irradiation for malignant granular cell myoblastoma of the tongue.

lation of a metastatic cancerous node is a hazardous thing? Do you think that it is a dangerous technique to push on the node, possibly pushing on it too hard, when you are examining the patient?

Dr. Ogura: I don't really know that we have any good evidence that this causes spread. I would think that it is not a good practice.

GRANULAR CELL MYOBLASTOMA

Dr. Gaisford: Fig. 25-6 shows a young man who had a malignant granular cell myoblastoma at the age of 12; at that point he had no metastatic cancerous nodes.

Dr. Chambers: Did you say malignant or granular cell myoblastoma?

Dr. Gaisford: Malignant granular cell.

Dr. Chambers: You are separating a benign granular cell and malignant one?

Dr. Gaisford: Right. Would you treat him surgically? Would you treat him by radiation?

Dr. Chambers: I would openly excise it and then irradiate it.

Dr. Richards: Local excision is the treatment of choice for this particular age group. Whether or not it is radiated afterward depends on your feeling about the spread of these things; our experience is that these lesions have a high incidence of local recurrence and can spread lymphatically,

so we have tended to irradiate them postsurgically.

Dr. Gaisford: This patient was treated by radiation initially, and no surgery was performed on the tongue. The lesion metastasized to the opposite side of the neck several years later, and the patient had a neck dissection. Now, 10 years after the operation, the patient is free of disease. This is the only lesion of this type that we have ever seen on the tongue. The left side of his face is flat as a result of the radiation.

PALLIATIVE TREATMENT

Dr. Gaisford: Fig. 25-7 shows the mother of one of our nursing supervisors at the age of about 75. At the age of 65 she had a lesion of the maxilla and was turned down for surgery because of her age. At this point the woman was not in bad shape as far as her general condition was concerned. The stench was horrible. She held her dentures in to eat, but she ate. Her daughter at this point was living with her. Dr. Georgiade, how do you feel about doing anything for these people?

Dr. Georgiade: I would ask Dr. Richards if he thinks irradiation therapy may be of value. It would clean up some of these lesions quite satisfactorily, but I would ask his opinion before making a judgment as to what I would do.

Dr. Gaisford: We have no one in our area who treats or uses Dr. Moh's chemosurgery technique. We have seen it demonstrated a number of times. I think it would be something worth considering. The one point I would like to make here

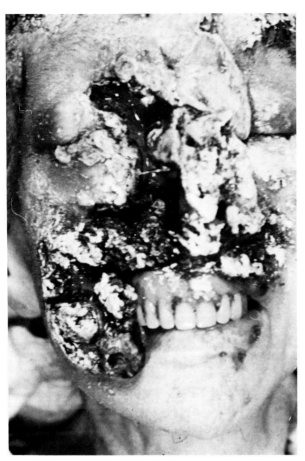

Fig. 25-7. Extensive cancer of the face.

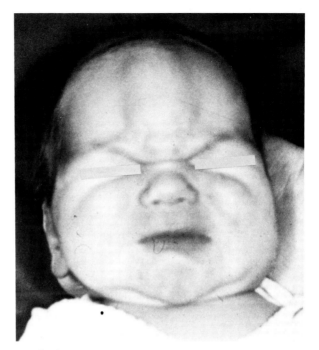

Fig. 25-8. Newborn baby with liposarcoma of the fore-head.

concerns the treatment for cancer of the head and neck in people who are in the older age group. Sixty-five is a relatively young age, and 75 is not particularly old when it comes to some head and neck problems. Many physicians are reluctant to do very much for people in the older age group; but when you see that some of these lesions can go on for many years and result in a disaster like this, there is some reason for going ahead with surgery before the disease gets to this particular state.

Dr. Richards: We would treat the lesions with very low dose, long, fractionated treatment. The radiotherapeutic point of view is to avoid being too heroic, too vigorous, too radical. The French managed these things for many generations by treating them as infrequently as once or twice a week and going very, very slowly. It is amazing how quickly they will clear up; possibly, definitive grafting can be accomplished later.

Dr. Gaisford: I'm glad to hear you say that, Dr. Richards. Some radiotherapists and surgeons only go for complete cures and won't treat people if it is going to be on a short-term basis. I think that we still have to treat them for their symptoms and hope to keep them as comfortable as we can for as long as we can.

LIPOSARCOMA

Dr. Gaisford: Fig. 25-8 shows a baby about 10 hours old who had a sausage-shaped mass in the forehead; it turned out to be a liposarcoma. I thought it was a meningocele and suggested to the pediatrician that a neurosurgeon be asked to see the child. The pediatrician didn't pay any attention to the mass, and eventually I saw the baby again when he was about 1 year old, after a general surgeon had biopsied the mass and diagnosed it as a liposarcoma. There was no skull defect, just a soft tissue tumor. This tumor was widely excised locally. The child is alive and well approximately 10 years after local excision.

FIBROSARCOMA

Dr. Gaisford: Fig. 25-9 shows another newborn. This one had a fibrosarcoma of the right cheek.

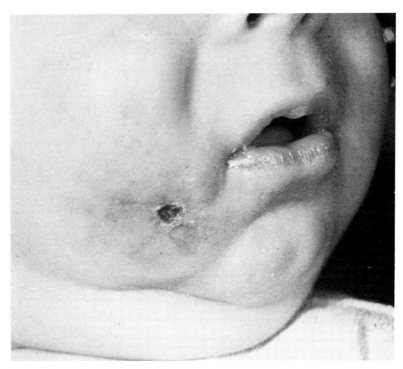

Fig. 25-9. Newborn baby with fibrosarcoma of the right cheek.

Dr. Chambers, how much surgery would you do for this one, assuming you would treat it surgically?

Dr. Chambers: I would give it about a 2-cm. margin.

Dr. Gaisford: Dr. Richards, what about using radiation for one of these? Would you consider it at all?

Dr. Richards: The only time we would consider irradiation for children would be after multiple recurrences.

Dr. Gaisford: This fibrosarcoma was treated as Dr. Chambers suggested, with relatively wide local excision; there was no recurrence. These are the only two cases we have seen like this in newborns.

MELANOMA

Dr. Gaisford: Fig. 25-10, *A,* shows a melanoma of the scalp in a red-headed girl. It was widely excised, and in 25-10, *B,* we see almost immediate recurrences along the periphery. What we are really concerned with here, however, is a nodular deep melanoma. This melanoma was superficial but did recur. It recurred three times, as a matter of fact.

Dr. Georgiade: I would do another local excision,

but I would also do a neck dissection and consider this patient for one of the immunosuppressive drugs, either BCG or some type of treatment that has become prominent in recent years in dealing with these melanomas. Once you start having recurrences they become more and more malignant and cause increasing difficulty. After I operate on patients who have melanomas, I turn them over to an immunologist.

Dr. Gaisford: Histologically, this was a so-called superficial melanoma; it was not in the dermis. I recognize that not all pathologists look at and report these melanomas in the same way, and this is why I feel that the one who is treating them should be perfectly adequately prepared to examine the slides himself so that he knows what he is treating. Have you seen these melanomas metastasize?

Dr. Georgiade: When they recur, they are no longer superficial. Once they recur, your treatment must be more radical, regardless of the initial diagnosis.

MENINGOCELE

Dr. Gaisford: Fig. 25-11 shows a little girl about 8 years old who had an asymptomatic lump in the midline of the neck. I excised this lump without

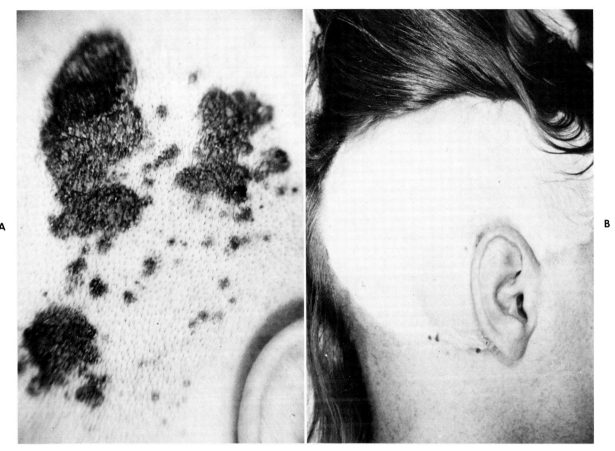

Fig. 25-10. A, Superficial spreading melanoma of the right side of the scalp. **B,** Recurrent melanoma of the right side of the scalp.

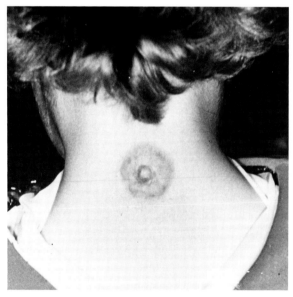

Fig. 25-11. Meningocele of the middle of the posterior wall of the neck.

a biopsy; it was a meningocele. Dr. Ogura, do you always biopsy every lump you see before you remove it? Do you ever remove any on the basis of your clinical diagnosis alone? How do you feel about that?

Dr. Ogura: Your telling me what this lump is makes the problem easier; hindsight is always better. Now that I know what it is, I would have had a neurosurgeon see the patient, too.

Dr. Gaisford: That is exactly what I should have done, because we have learned that something in the midline, particularly a lump or bump in the glabellar area, can be a developmental problem and is very apt to be connected with cord or brain.

CYSTIC HYGROMA

Dr. Gaisford: Fig. 25-12 shows a cystic hygroma that is getting this little boy into trouble. His mediastinum and chest are filled with this tumor. We consulted with thoracic surgeons who felt

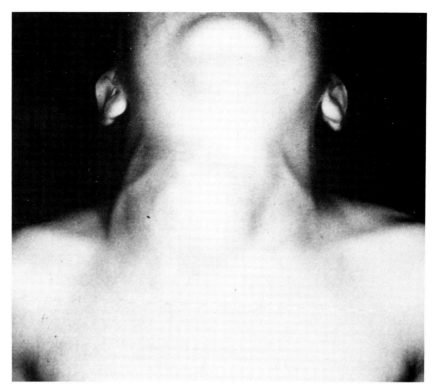

Fig. 25-12. Cystic hygroma of the neck.

that technically they could do nothing for this child and suggested radiation. Dr. Richards, how do you feel about radiation for cystic hygroma?

Dr. Richards: We have a tendency to do diagnostic procedures, namely lymphangiograms, to try to ascertain the feeding channels leading into the thoracic duct. Cystic hygroma most certainly is a surgical problem; if it can be removed surgically, then one should exercise as much vigor as one can and remove it surgically. If it recurs, it should be removed surgically a second time. In a situation such as in this particular patient, where there was no alternative, one would undertake irradiation on the basis that maybe 45% to 50% of them will show some degree of response. Sometimes the response is enough that the surgeon can remove the residual.

Dr. Gaisford: Would you like to say a word about the possibility of cancer of the thyroid being related to radiation?

Dr. Richards: The experience that was written up by the Roswell Park people did show a significant incidence of carcinoma of the thyroid in those children who had received some irradiation. The Roswell Park study showed it to be definitely dose related. The higher the dose of irradiation to the thyroid, the higher the incidence of carcinoma of the thyroid. Still, it is a small percentage, less than about 3% or 4%; it does not contraindicate this type of procedure, which was lifesaving for this child.

NEUROBLASTOMA

Dr. Gaisford: Fig. 25-13 shows a neuroblastoma of the mandible. It was radioresistant; the patient had had a full course of radiation with no effect. Would you resect it? What do you think your chances of cure are?

Dr. Chambers: These lesions can be extremely sensitive to various chemotherapeutic agents. We did a series of work on neuroblastomas in nursery children. Dr. Ward and I, back in the 1940's, used phenylphosphoramide. I still see some of those patients now, and they are well up in their 20's and have had children. Since this lesion is the only evidence that this particular little girl has of a neuroblastoma and because it's had a lot of irradiation, I would be tempted to go ahead

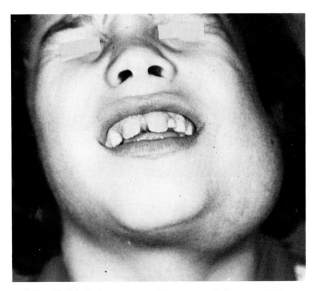

Fig. 25-13. Primary neuroblastoma of the mandible.

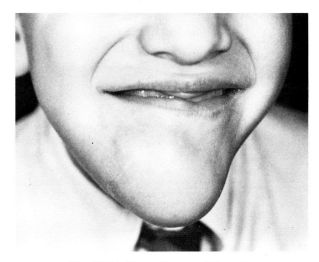

Fig. 25-14. Neurofibroma of the chin.

and resect it and then administer whatever drug the chemotherapist thought was the most appropriate.

Dr. Richards: I would agree with Dr. Chambers. If this thing did not respond to radiation, it is not going to respond to the chemotherapeutic drugs, either. The radiomimetic drugs all pretty much mimic what radiation does for most tumors, especially the neuroblastoma, which is a sensitive tumor.

Dr. Gaisford: This patient's tumor was resected, a delayed neck and chest flap was grafted to the area, and then a bone graft was done. The patient has done well over quite a number of years. The pedicle flap is the only evidence that the patient previously had a tumor.

NEUROFIBROMA

Dr. Gaisford: Fig. 25-14 shows the problem of massive neurofibroma—everybody sees some of these sometime in his career. Dr. Chambers, what are the problems that we get into in the surgical management of this particular problem?

Dr. Chambers: The most horrendous complexity is that you don't know where to stop and where to start. I have had them go all the way around the head and neck. You end up taking out what you can for the patient's comfort and appearance. The worst complication, of course, is malignant degeneration.

Dr. Gaisford: This tumor remained harmless as far

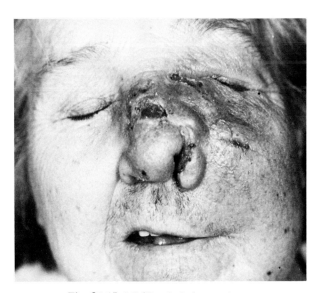

Fig. 25-15. Midline lethal granuloma.

as that was concerned. The vascularity of a tumor like this is severe, and we have had technical problems with some of the veins in these tumors. It is difficult to make people who have these tumors look right.

LETHAL MIDLINE GRANULOMA

Dr. Gaisford: Midline lethal granuloma. Dr. Richards, do you have anything to offer the patient shown in Fig. 25-15?

Dr. Richards: The former Chief of Radiotherapy at this institution, Dr. Robert Dixon, compiled a series of about 15 to 20 midline granulomas and Wegener's granulomas of the head and neck and published them in the *Journal of the Faculty of Radiologists in England*. His experience was that this is an inflammatory type of lesion rather than a malignant lesion. It was his experience and his recommendation that we stop treating these lesions as malignancies and treat them as inflammatory conditions. He recommends that we treat them not with a vigorous, radical dose of radiation, but with a so-called anti-inflammatory dose of radiation ranging between 1,800 and 3,500 rads.

Dr. Chambers: The main thing is to keep the surgeon's hands off. After you do a wide resection, it is just a matter of weeks or months.

Dr. Gaisford: The patient promptly succumbed. As a matter of fact, we haven't had very many patients with this lesion, but we haven't seen any survive.

Chapter 26

Role of immediate reconstruction in treatment of head and neck cancer

Milton T. Edgerton, M.D.

The increasing use of reconstructive surgery by the faculty members of this symposium represents a great change from the attitudes of cancer surgeons 2 decades ago. Charles Harrold has significantly referred to "many late-staged reconstructions that are often planned and rarely completed." Dwight Hanna has cited figures to suggest that recently there may be an increasing tendency to treat the primary sites of oral cavity cancer by radiotherapy techniques despite repeated and reliable studies from numerous clinics that show the importance of surgical excision in the achievement of maximum cure rates. We must ask, "Have we as surgeons failed to reduce surgical morbidity and deformity (that accompanies curative resection of cancer about the head and neck) to a sufficient degree that will make surgery an acceptable first choice of treatment in the eyes of both doctors and patients?"

Over the past 2 decades there has been an improved definition of the role of immediate reconstructive techniques after surgical resection of cancer of the head and neck. Despite frequent predictions that better understanding of cancer biology would soon eliminate surgery as one of the main treatments of malignancy, wide surgical resection continues to be our best single weapon in the cure of maxillofacial cancer. It may be many years before doctors can replace the surgical excision of cancer with metabolic or biochemical control methods.

Physicians have always appreciated that deformity and loss of function about the face and jaws are awesome prices to pay for even lifesaving control of cancer. The will to live, however, is of such strength in the average human that this price will be accepted by most persons, especially if it will increase their chances of ridding themselves of this dreaded disease.

In certain types of head and neck cancer, radical surgery may improve the patient's chances of cure only by a modest amount (5% to 10%) in comparison with treatment by radiotherapy. At other times apparently *both* surgery and radiotherapy are required to produce the maximum chance for survival. Then the tissue receives a double insult that increases deformity and discomfort and complicates reconstruction. Hopefully, the concerned cancer surgeon will not flinch from electing *any* treatment or combination of treatments that will seemingly provide more chance for cure or a better quality of life. Knowledge of and experience with all of the immediate reconstructive techniques commonly used in plastic surgery give the surgeon additional courage in counseling his patient. All of us must estimate realistically the deformity and handicap that the patient may experience to obtain the best chance for cure. We must convey those estimates accurately to the patient and let him become a partner in the decision-making process. He must *not* be allowed to believe that radiotherapy will give him "an equal chance for cure" (or vice versa) if this is not the case!

Surgeons are fully aware of the morbidity and limitations of radiotherapy, but they must also remain sensitive to the problems of body imagery associated with the surgical loss of a lip, tongue, or

Text continued on p. 174.

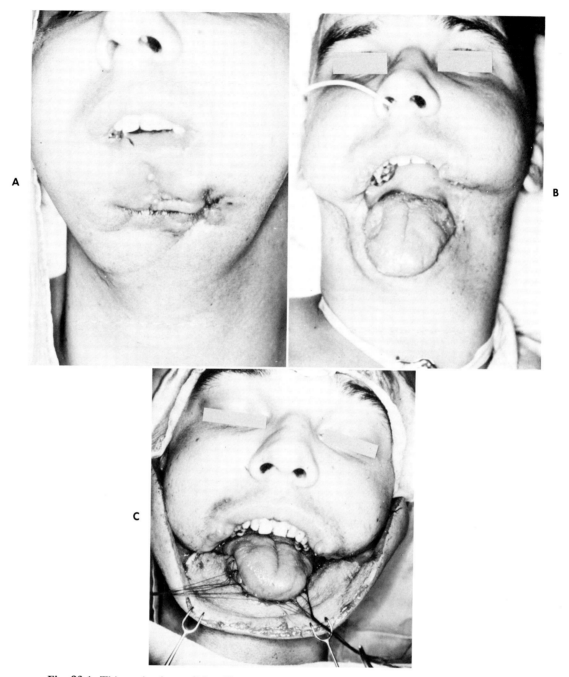

Fig. 26-1. This patient's condition illustrates the value of immediate reconstructon because of the high likelihood that no further treatment would be successful in the event of further recurrence. The immediate reconstruction reduced total economic cost and allowed pattern biopsy on two separate occasions when the flap was inset into the floor of the mouth and lip regions. **A,** Recurrent osteogenic sarcoma of the mandible in a 28-year-old man after surgery and 6,500 rads of cobalt therapy. **B,** Wide resection of the lower third of the face with an immediate skin graft to line the bipedicled forehead flap. **C,** Transfer of the lined visor flap to reconstruct the floor of the mouth, the chin, and the lip 10 days after delay of the flap and excision of the tumor. **D,** (Front and lateral views.) Pedicles of the forehead flap have been divided and turned forward to provide additional bulk of tissue for the chin and lip. A split-thickness graft from the upper part of the chest has been applied to the forehead to provide a good color match. **E,** (Front lateral views.) Result of immediate reconstruction after excision of the tumor. Patient immediately returned to work, but developed metastasis in the lungs 3 years later and died without recurrence of local disease.

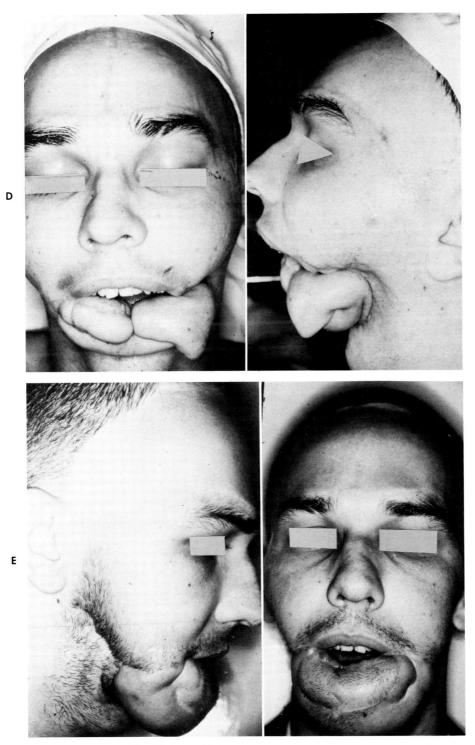

Fig. 26-1, cont'd. For legend see opposite page.

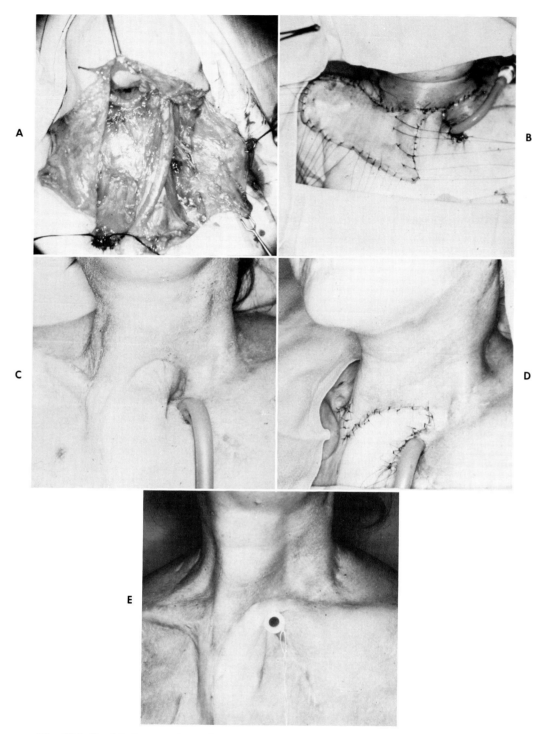

Fig. 26-2. In this instance immediate reconstruction resulted in a reduction of the total number of operatons required for repair, was extremely helpful in convincing the patient of the doctor's optimism about the possibilities of cure, and was carried out immediately so as to avoid having the patient endure a dangerous period of salivary fistula and later further surgical dissection of the neck. **A,** Defect produced by total laryngopharyngectomy with a radical neck dissection for a patient with carcinoma of the cervical esophagus and postcricoid larynx with metastases to the left side of the neck. **B,** Immediate reconstruction of the esophagus with a deltopectoral flap and split-thickness skin graft applied to the chest and right shoulder provided the easiest and safest method of reconstruction. **C,** Closure of the esophageal fistula 4 weeks later. Skin graft is now healed below the right side of the clavicle. **D,** With the patient under local anesthesia, the esophageal wall has been closed and the pedicle of the flap fitted about the permanent tracheal stoma. **E,** Small teflon button may be used in the tracheal stoma to reduce contraction and provide patient security.

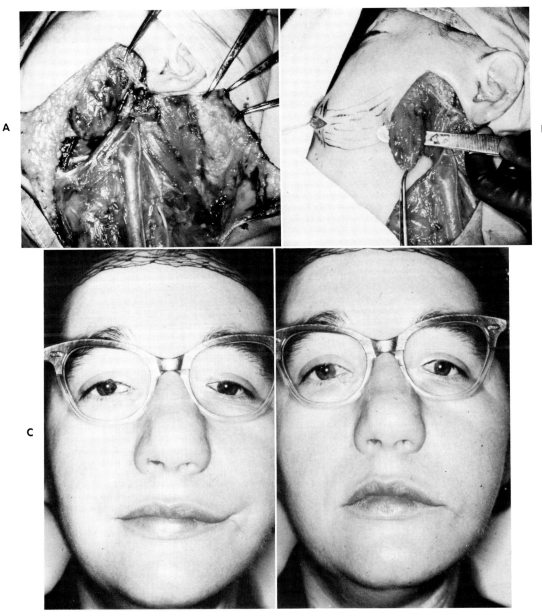

Fig. 26-3. This patient's immediate reconstruction allowed her to regain much of the function lost by sacrifice of the facial nerve and reduced her period of deformity. It also made possible the maintenance of contour of certain facial features not achievable by late repair of this type of defect. **A,** Radical neck dissection and parotidectomy, sacrificing the facial nerve and overlying skin for a patient with epidermoid carcinoma of the left parotid gland and metastases in the left side of the neck. **B,** Immediate reconstruction of the surgically produced facial paralysis achieved by using the active masseter muscle present in the base of the wound. The muscle is attached appropriately to the newly paralyzed muscles of the left corner of the mouth. **C,** Postoperative result 8 weeks later. View on left shows position of the lips when the patient tightens the masseter muscle transfer. View on right shows the face in repose.

nose or with facial palsy, drooling, or a permanent tracheostomy. How may immediate reconstructive surgery best reduce the burdens of surgical or radiation therapy? When should we withhold these techniques for weeks or months? Which techniques are not likely to interfere with later postoperative care or with treatment of a subsequent recurrence of the cancer? What reconstructive measures are of such value that they should be used immediately, even if palliation is all that may be expected?

To develop a sensible approach to these problems, surgeons must carefully examine both the advantages and disadvantages of doing an immediate reconstruction at the time of resection of the primary cancer. It is obvious that almost every patient will prefer immediate repair unless it will in some way worsen his prognosis.

Cancers of the head and neck create the maximum indications for immediate reconstruction because of: (1) the exposed location of the surgical defect; (2) the multiple functional disturbances in speech, swallowing, breathing, chewing, and facial expression that are commonly produced; (3) the critical "loss of identity" disturbances associated with facial deformities; and (4) the feasibility of using primary undelayed flaps and grafts in that part of the body that has anatomically the greatest amount of vigorous peripheral circulation. The head and neck have thus become the logical regions for testing basic concepts about the role of plastic surgery in the treatment of cancer.

For a time, surgeons voiced the fear that early reconstruction might, in some way, obscure the early detection of any recurrent tumor and make the subsequent treatment of such a patient difficult. Experience has taught us that a patient with oropharyngeal or paranasal sinus cancer almost never has two realistic chances to be cured by surgery. Once a truly radical resection has been carried out on a major cancer of the oral cavity, salivary glands, or upper

respiratory tract, few surgical cures are obtained (approximately 3%) by a second operation for local recurrence. This poor prognosis holds true whether or not the patient received any formal reconstruction with the primary operation. Furthermore, there is little evidence that the presence of a flap or graft in the defect has adversely affected either the detection or the treatment (usually palliative) of such a recurrence.

The primary advantages and disadvantages of doing immediate reconstruction are listed below. In actual practice the disadvantages of immediate reconstruction have seldom matched the numerous advantages of such an approach.

Advantages
1. Reduces total amount and number of operations
2. Reduces length of time patients endure deformity and morbidity (short life expectancy)
3. Protects and preserves vital structures exposed by tumor removal
4. Is most convincing possible evidence to patients of surgeon's expectations of cure
5. In event of failure to cure, gives longest and best palliation
6. Reduces total economic cost (lessens hospital, physicians' and nurses' fees; enables earlier return to job)
7. Keeps patient physically and functionally acceptable to family, friends, and self
8. Allows pattern biopsy at each reconstructive step; may reveal any occult tumor recurrence earlier than by routine follow-up
9. Maintains some features and functions not possible to regain by late reconstruction

Disadvantages
1. May cover recurrence of tumor
2. May make a repeated reconstruction necessary later
3. May preempt best repair method prior to cure
4. May make initial operation too long
5. May open up new tissue planes with seeding
6. Limited number of trained plastic surgeons available

Skin grafts and even many soft and pliable flaps have been found to *reveal* (by virtue of absence of

Fig. 26-4. In this instance immediate reconstruction was carried out with confidence, partly because of the low likelihood of recurrent tumor and also to protect the cornea and conjunctiva from injury associated with delayed reconstruction. **A,** Patient with basal cell carcinoma involving all layers of the central part of the lower lid. **B,** Four fifths of the lower lid, including the skin, tarsus, and conjunctiva, has been totally excised. The upper lid has been split between the skin and the outer surface of the tarsal plate. This flap of cartilage and conjunctiva is sutured to the remaining bulbar conjunctiva behind the lower lid. **C,** The skin of the upper lid is dressed superiorly, and a full-thickness graft from the upper part of the neck is fitted over the tarsal conjunctival flap. **D,** Five weeks later the eyelids are divided, leaving the skin graft, upper tarsus, and conjunctiva in the lower lid region. **E,** The lower lid in opened and closed positions has excellent function after reconstruction.

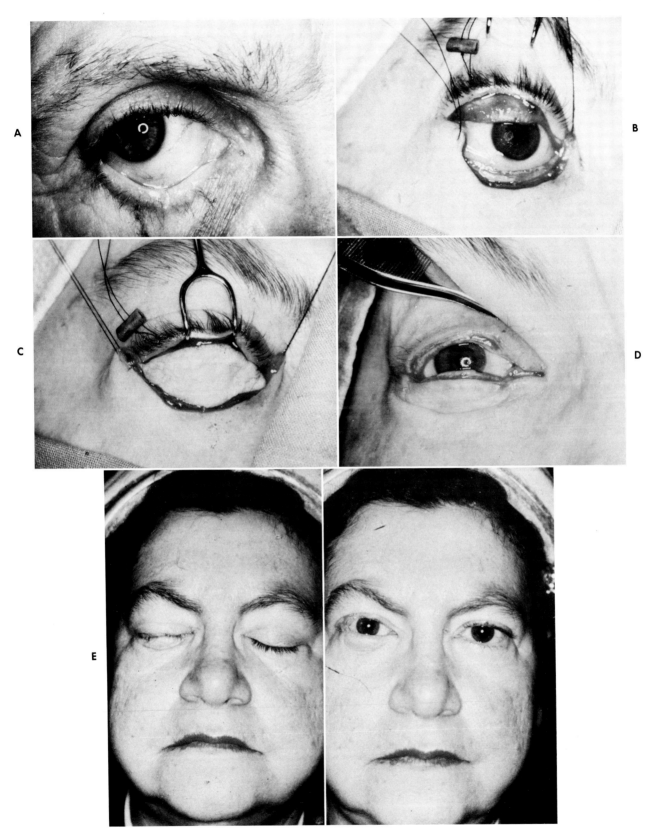

Fig. 26-4. For legend see opposite page.

fibrosis and induration) underlying tumor recurrences more often than they delay detection.

A second or even third reconstruction of the part may be required in some patients with uncontrolled primary tumors; but often this need occurs years later, and the patient is kept in "socioeconomic circulation" during the interval. I have noted that when a second accelerated or immediate reconstruction is clinically indicated after a recurrent tumor has destroyed an earlier repair, the patient consistently wants us to undertake it.

Delayed reconstruction not only forces the surgeon to redissect the original area, but this dissection has been made much more dangerous by the delay. The anatomy has been distorted. Contracture of unsupported soft tissues has increased the difficulty encountered in returning all remaining parts to their normal positions. Scar contractions have distorted the positions of the larynx and trachea, and anesthesia is thus more dangerous. Frequently nutrition and morale suffer by any delay in repair, and the patient's wound-healing problems and nursing needs will be magnified.

Surgeons have always been fearful that additional dissection (required with immediate reconstructions) would open up new tissue planes and allow seeding of the cancer in other areas. The experimental studies of Harry Greene and the work of Robert Smith and his associates at the National Institute of Health on wound washings for tumor cells would indicate that this must indeed be a rare clinical occurrence. Over the past 20 years I have used extensive primary reconstructions. Although I have certainly seen my share of local tumor recurrences, I have yet to see (or hear reported) a *single* local recurrence in the bed of a primary forehead flap, beneath the pedicle of a deltopectoral flap, in the closed donor wound of a nasolabial fold flap, or on the healed split-thickness skin graft donor site. (An exception is malignant melanoma where such seed implantability is known to occur.)

Certainly the vast majority of local recurrences from epidermoid cancer of the head and neck are caused by a residual unresected tumor within the wound and *not* by uprooted, accidentally dropped nests of tumor cells that fall from the knife or scissors and get washed by irrigation into remote corners of the wound where they survive and grow again. Such seedlings are fragile and are usually damaged by drying or by the osmotic injuries of irrigation; statistically, they seldom succeed in establishing a new beachhead of cancer.

Perhaps our greatest limitation in the effective use of immediate reconstruction in head and neck cancer is the need for more surgeons trained in tissue transfer techniques. The safe movement of long and slender flaps of tissue in elderly, often malnourished individuals requires gentleness, skill, and a constant sense of awareness of the fragility of these tissues and their vital vascular architecture. These skills can be learned, but their use requires repeated emphasis on the basics of surgery. Too often surgeons have simply read of a new plastic surgery technique and attempted to apply it in the care of one of their patients. If the flap is handled roughly, allowed to dry during a long operation, has its pedicle kinked for 20 to 30 minutes during another phase of the surgery, is passed through a too-narrow tunnel to reach its new site, or is stretched only a few micrograms too much in being sutured into place, disaster will follow. Often such an experience will lead that surgeon to condemn the operation rather than his own inept execution. Attention to detail is the sine qua non of good reconstruction. Fortunately, general surgeons and otolaryngologists are taking greater interest and are getting more training in plastic surgery techniques, and we are now seeing more routine success in the use of these methods.

Figs. 26-1 to 26-4 illustrate several practical reasons for choosing immediate reconstructive techniques. At times, several compelling reasons for early repair may be indicated in a single patient. Each must be judged individually.

SUMMARY

In developing a repair plan for any given patient with head and neck cancer, the surgeon must review many considerations. The biology of the particular tumor, the stage of the disease, the general condition of the patient, the complexity of the required plan of reconstruction, and the ability of that individual patient to tolerate given degrees of deformity and malfunction are all part of the critical evaluation that will help the surgeon determine how much—or how little—immediate repair will give the patient the easiest postoperative course, the maximum chance for cure, the optimum preservation of function and self-image, and the greatest hope.

Although more immediate reconstructions are used each year, there is still a tendency to underestimate the value of this approach. Clearly, more training programs are needed to increase experience and confidence in the use of accelerated flap techniques, muscle transfers, and implant surgery. If surgeons do not employ fastidious plastic surgery techniques and pay close attention to minute details, many techniques of immediate reconstruction will fail, and many surgeons will be discouraged from attempting these methods again. *One should first learn to do any given operation successfully before passing judgment on its potential value!*

In the treatment of a disease as poorly understood as cancer, it is always difficult to be certain that the curative effort (whether by surgery or irradiation) will improve the patient's overall welfare, but the correction of any deformity or dysfunction that results from the curative effort will predictably benefit the quality of life. We must continue to find reasonable ways of better, faster, and safer reconstruction for the patient with cancer.

REFERENCES

1. Bakamjian, V. Y.: A two stage method for pharyngoesophageal reconstruction with a primary pectoral skin flap, Plast. Reconstr. Surg. **36:**173, 1965.
2. Bowers, D. G.: Double cross lip flaps for lower lip reconstruction, Plast. Reconstr. Surg. **47:**209, 1971.
3. Edgerton, M. T.: Surgical methods of reducing deformity and loss of function in patients with head and neck cancer; quality of survival of the cancer patient, Hartford, Conn., 1969, American Cancer Society, Inc.
4. Edgerton, M. T.: Rehabilitation of the oral cavity by plastic surgery after cancer resections; proceedings of the Seventh National Cancer Conference, September, 1972, Philadelphia, 1973, J. B. Lippincott Co.
5. Edgerton, M. T., Cohen, I. K., and Holmes, E. C.: Parotid duct transplantation for correction of drooling in patients with cancer of the head and neck, Surg. Gynecol. Obstet. **133:**663-665, October, 1971.
6. Hancock, D. M.: The repair of facial defects resulting from surgery for locally advanced buccal carcinoma, Plast. Reconstr. Surg. **20:**117, 1957.
7. McGregor, I. A., and Reed, W. H.: Simultaneous temporal and deltopectoral flaps for full thickness defects of the cheek, Plast. Reconstr. Surg. **45:**326, 1970.
8. Paletta, F. X.: Early and late repair of facial defects following treatment of malignancy, Plast. Reconstr. Surg. **13:**95, 1953.
9. Smith, F.: Flaps utilized in facial and cervical reconstruction, Plast. Reconstr. Surg. **7:**415-445, 1951.
10. Von Deilen, A. W.: Methods of immediate repair after major resections of the face and jaws, Plast. and Reconstr. Surg. **11:**152, 1952.

Chapter 27

Techniques and tissues for treatment of head and neck cancer

Charles E. Horton, M.D.
K. Guler Gursu, M.D.
Jerome E. Adamson, M.D.
Richard A. Mladick, M.D.
James H. Carraway, M.D.

Techniques and tissues utilized in surgery for head and neck cancer have been well established in the past. The proper application of the surgeon's basic knowledge is more essential in surgery of this area than in surgery of other anatomical areas that may be hidden from view and have less important functional requirements. The surgeon must be aware of the disadvantages as well as the advantages of all techniques available, and he should carefully choose procedures that give improved functional and esthetic results to the already compromised patient. The main motive of surgery for head and neck cancer must be to cure the patient; however, consideration must also be given to restoration of function, the patients' cosmetic appearance, and his social rehabilitation.

In the treatment of cancer of the skin of the head and neck, several new modalities have recently been shown to have therapeutic benefit. Since skin lesions may be either superficial or deep, and because most superficial lesions are normally easily cured by any modality that removes the superficial skin, many papers have recently been written extolling unusual and new treatments. For superficial basal cell lesions, excision remains the historic standard treatment of choice, although dermatologists have long favored curettage or cautery, or both. Radiation, topical or systemic chemotherapy, cryotherapy, and the use of the laser beam have all been suggested for use in the treatment of skin cancers; however, no treatment to date has exceeded the cure rate of adequate excisional surgery.

Regardless of the initial treatment used, recurrences are reported. These recurrences may be caused by a physician's unfamiliarity with a technique; certainly, some surgeons excise more radically than others, and some radiologists treat with heavier dosages than others. We must admit that individual variances exist in the adaptation of techniques to certain problems and that one physician may be much more adept at surgery than at curettage, and vice versa.

The surgeon's ego should not preclude a careful assessment of personal standards of care; and if unfamiliarity or lack of dexterity deters proper treatment, the honest physician must seek consultation from teams with more proficient therapists and refer all complicated cases to cancer treatment centers.

It is our feeling that *once a skin tumor recurs, no treatment should be used other than surgery if a cure is desired.* Once the tissue planes have been violated by scar tissue, other treatments become unreliable. On the other hand, if palliation is desired, radiation, chemotherapy, the laser beam, or other modalities of treatment may be desirable.

The selection of the technique for repair after treatment of head and neck cancer depends greatly on the initial therapy. For example, radiation causes intense fibrosis accompanied by a diminution in the local blood supply to adjacent tissues, and reconstruction from a distant tissue is usually required.

Many materials can be used in the repair of defects after cancer therapy. Among these are split-thickness grafts, full-thickness grafts, dermal grafts, mucous membrane grafts, local flaps, distant flaps, composite grafts (cartilage and bone), and tissue substitutes, such as Silastic and nonautogenous grafts, as well as metallic prostheses.

The advantages of a split-thickness skin graft are well known: (1) it is easily available; (2) it provides a good color match if taken from adjacent donor sites; (3) it grows easily, even in the mouth; (4) the donor site heals spontaneously; (5) a large amount is available; (6) visible facial muscular motion is transmitted through the graft; (7) it does not camouflage a recurrence; and (8) it does not need to be applied immediately after primary surgery. The disadvantages of a Split-thickness skin graft are: (1) the surface contour is not reconstructed; (2) it contracts and may distort; (3) it may have a different color and texture; (4) the graft sensation is imperfect; and (5) there is no hair growth.

A full-thickness skin graft has many advantages: (1) it is easily available; (2) it provides a better-color match than split-thickness skin grafts; (3) there is muscular motion transmitted through the graft; (4) it will grow in the mouth; and (5) it will not contract. They also have certain disadvantages: (1) the surface contour is not reconstructed; (2) the graft may have a different texture and color; (3) sensation return is imperfect; (4) the donor site must be closed; (5) they are more difficult to grow than other grafts; (6) the donor areas are limited; (7) hair growth is imperfect; and (8) the chance of the graft taking is less.

Dermal grafts are occasionally used in head and neck reconstruction. (1) They are readily available; (2) donor sites can usually be closed; (3) they provide bulk; and (4) they provide a protective covering for the arteries. Their disadvantages are that (1) the bulk may not remain (because of resorption); (2) there are donor site scars; and (3) the recipient area must be ideal and have a good blood supply.

Mucous membrane grafts are also utilized in head and neck reconstruction. They (1) grow easily, (2) do not contract, and (3) can be used to reconstruct normal tissues in the mouth. Their disadvantages are that (1) the donor sites are limited; (2) taking tissue from the donor sites is painful; and (3) the grafts are of little use outside of the mouth and lid area.

When free grafts cannot be used in head and neck reconstruction, flaps should be considered. Local flaps have the following advantages: (1) they have an abundant blood supply; (2) they provide a good color and texture match; (3) surface contours are reestablished; (4) protective sensation is regained; (5) they will grow in less than ideal conditions; (6) donor sites are easily closed; (7) the repair is completed in one operation; and (8) they grow well in the mouth. They have the following disadvantages: (1) they may mask recurrences; (2) the donor area defect may distort; (3) the flap may "pincushion"; (4) the flap will not transmit facial motion; (5) the flap may need delay; (6) flap hair may grow in the mouth; and (7) they have restricted length and availability.

When local flaps cannot be used because the adjacent tissue has been damaged or because there is not sufficient tissue within the immediate area, a distant flap can be utilized. These flaps have the following advantages: (1) they provide abundant tissue; (2) they can be used in less than ideal recipient areas; (3) they can be lined to provide two surfaces; (4) they provide an adequate covering for other tissue transplants (bone, cartilage, and so on); and (5) they do not contract. Their disadvantages are: (1) they occasionally require delay; (2) they require careful technique; (3) donor areas are limited and scarred; (4) donor areas must be closed; (5) contour and color match is often imperfect; (6) sensation return is imperfect; and (7) hair growth is imperfect.

Composite grafts are occasionally useful in head and neck tissue reconstruction. They have the following advantages: (1) the contour is reestablished; (2) hair growth may be reestablished; (3) color and texture are normal; (4) the repair is completed in one operation; and (5) tissue support is provided. The disadvantages of composite grafts are: (1) donor sites are limited; (2) graft size is limited; (3) they are difficult to grow; and (4) the donor site may be distorted.

Basic principles of surgical technique are important. Tissues should be handled carefully and not crushed and traumatized by heavy clamps. Excess tension should be avoided in closure. Suture materials should be as small as skin tension will allow, to diminish foreign body reaction in the healing wound.

The use of Z-plasties, W-plasties, V-Y advancements, rotation flaps, advancement flaps, tongue flaps, and muscle, skin, and bone flaps have all been reported for selected problems; however, their specific indications are too individualized for detailed discussion. The tibial bolt or Kirschner pin used to hold the hemimandible in place temporarily has been of great assistance in preventing postoperative deformity after resection of the mandibular bone. Wiring of the teeth to prevent displacement malocclusion of the mandibular segment has been widely utilized. Less postoperative scar tissue pull has been noted when flaps are utilized to reconstruct oral defects, and severe deformities such as those that were encountered in the past are not now occurring. Contoured Silastic implants for repair of the forehead, cheek, and mandible are useful.

Facial prostheses play an essential part in the total rehabilitation of the patient with head and neck cancer. Prostheses to replace the palate, the ear, and the nose are particularly useful.

When hairless skin has been used in the reconstruction of a man's face, tatooing to simulate a light beard may give a better appearance to the face.

Fascial slings and muscular transfers around the face may occasionally be necessary and useful to support facial tissues.

Recently, microvascular free flap transfers have been popularized, particularly in Japan, China, Australia, and the United States. These techniques have much to offer and will be used extensively in the future, as soon as more surgeons become familiar with the microvascular technique. Free intestinal segments have been used to restore esophageal continuity, and free omental transfer to the head and neck area on a microvascular pedicle have been utilized so that a split-thickness graft can be placed on top of the vascularized omentum to provide epithelial coverage.

In treatment of head and neck cancer, the idea of allowing a patient to die with dignity cannot be overemphasized. The patient with uncontrolled head and neck cancer whose deformity and interruption of functional activities are obvious to even the casual visitor becomes a dilemma to the conscientious surgeon and to the patient's family. The patient with head and neck cancer who must struggle to eat or breathe, is in constant pain, and yet has no impairment of other vital body functions remains one of modern medicine's unsolved problems. The patient who wishes to die and cannot compromises the conscientious physician who recognizes the inevitable outcome and the interim problem of persistent pain, discomfort, and humiliation to the patient. Energetic systemic chemotherapy has occasionally been a blessing even in its failures, for occasionally in the absence of a favorable response, the suffering patient may have a hastened death that is not unappreciated if cure cannot be effected.

The conscientious physician must evaluate each patient with head and neck cancer according to the family background, the physical condition of the patient, and other circumstances that would be affected by the type of cancer therapy chosen. The patient with an invalid dependent at home should not be subjected to an unnecessarily prolonged hospitalization, just as the patient with a severe cardiac condition should not be subjected to a hazardous prolonged surgery. There is no standard way to care for the many problems associated with the destructive process of removing cancer tissue from the body. Concerned surgeons should be aware of all new therapeutic modalities and should be able to consider the individual patient in choosing the appropriate technique and tissue to restore function, hasten rehabilitation, and return the patient as intact as possible to society.

Chapter 28

Reconstruction after excision of skin cancer

Shattuck W. Hartwell, Jr., M.D.

In closing cutaneous defects about the face after removal of malignant disease, the reconstructive surgeon is challenged to provide the best possible postoperative appearance. The face is as much exposed as any other part of a human being, and as a person one is recognized more by his facial features than by any other trait. This chapter introduces the reader to many methods, both simple and complex, of repairing cutaneous defects. The experienced reconstructive surgeon may see more readily the "best way" to repair them. However, the beginner can also find the "best way" and execute his reconstructive plan to achieve the best possible result if he is well informed, well trained, and brings good sense and some imagination to his task.

The expectation of both patient and surgeon must be reasonable. It is unfortunate but unavoidable that the best possible reconstruction sometimes falls short of restoring normal appearance. The physician should prepare his patient for this possibility by giving him a sensible explanation of what the problem and the reconstruction entail. No such explanation is possible unless the surgeon has a clear idea of how to plan wound closure and understands the options available. Simple closure by approximation, free grafts, and flaps are basic methods that virtually flash through the mind of the surgeon when he ponders over how to close or how to reconstruct. He must sort out the choices available and consider types and subtypes of basic methods that might apply. If two or three choices are suitable, he must ask himself why might one be better. If his first plan should fail, he must consider what his second plan would be. This chapter will be successful to the extent that the reader is reminded to

be orderly, self-critical, and realistic in planning skin coverage about the face.[1] The many drawings of several kinds of flaps are meant to be useful only to the extent that they stimulate the imagination and provide the reader with ideas. I have successfully used every kind of flap described, some of them rarely and some often. In this work necessity is indeed the mother of invention. To contrive a clever flap is exhilarating, even though one may suspect that this clever flap has also been made by other surgeons in other times and other places. We grow in the craft of surgery from our own experience and from the experience of others, here and there recalling difficulties and modifying ideas.

The scope of this chapter does not include methods for the total reconstruction of the nose, ears, and eyelids. These techniques are elaborate and difficult, even for the few plastic surgeons and reconstructive ophthalmologists who undertake this work with special interest. Rather, this presentation of general principles of closure of cutaneous defects about the face should prove helpful to the cancer surgeon. The references are modern, and the flaps illustrated are keyed to the references for convenience, but it must be remembered that many of these flaps are much older than the references and that recent publications point out significant applications or modifications of some useful designs of a venerable age. The reader is therefore encouraged to use the references but should avoid naming the flaps according to the surgeons.

SIMPLE CLOSURE

Wherever possible, simple closure of facial defects is desirable. Laxity of facial skin in elderly pa-

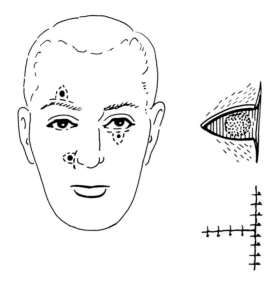

Fig. 28-1. ⊤ closure for defects at a margin.[10] Undercutting permits advancement and edge-to-edge approximation. Note the excision is an incomplete ellipse.

tients makes possible the approximation of wound edges without deformity. Youthful skin is not so accommodating; but then, malignant disease is not so common in younger persons. Simple closure can be done in the young, but it may not be so readily done. In any event, after resection of malignancy, the surgeon will recognize the situations where simple wound closure would be satisfactory (Fig. 28-1) and when such edge-to-edge closure would create a deformity, unacceptable asymmetry, or impaired function; then a skin graft or a flap must be used to repair a defect.

FREE SKIN GRAFTS
Definitive reconstruction

Donor sites for free grafts are of two sorts, regional and distant. Regional grafts are advantageous because of the color match they provide; grafts from the postauricular area, the upper eyelids, and the neck should be thick split-thickness or full-thickness skin grafts. The color of facial skin is similar, and these grafts can give excellent cosmetic results. An important precaution is to avoid trimming these grafts too much. Thin grafts, even though from these areas, will not provide a good color and texture match to blend with facial skin.

Distant free grafts from the abdomen, buttock, or thigh have the disadvantage of not matching facial skin. Their advantage in definitive resurfacing of the head and neck lies in the abundant supply of

this skin. Although these free grafts may be all that is desired in the reconstruction of cutaneous defects, a disadvantage of split-thickness grafts is that they may shrink or wrinkle unpredictably. These changes in the graft may be deforming to adjacent tissue, causing eyelid ectropion or labial asymmetry in addition to the unesthetic appearance of the graft. What was hoped to be definitive reconstruction must then be redone.

Staged reconstruction

Skin grafts may serve to obtain a "clean closed wound" in the course of staged reconstruction. Whereas the surgeon will often choose to follow a plan of reconstruction that is as complete as possible in one procedure by using either a free graft or a flap where the wound edges cannot be approximated without deformity, there are times when a free graft will be used to obtain closure that is temporary. For example, when the limits of reasonable resection have been reached and increased morbidity may result from an operation prolonged by reconstruction, a free skin graft will provide closure. Also, there are times when complete confidence in an adequate resection is lacking. Although some surgeons will elect to reconstruct with flaps immediately (hoping that the best has been achieved), others will prefer to use a skin graft. Skin grafts have a transparent quality that allows persistent or recurrent malignancy to be noticed or felt within an interval of time (a few weeks to a few months) prior to definitive reconstruction.

FLAPS

For purposes of this chapter (dealing with cutaneous defects) there are only three types of flaps, but among them are some important subtypes. The three types are local (direct) flaps, bridged (indirect) flaps, and distant (carried) flaps.

Local (direct) flaps

Local flaps all have one common feature: they are designed from tip to base within immediately adjacent tissue; when shifted in such a way as to cover defects, they are forced to lie completely in the plane of normal contour. There are five subtypes of local flaps.

Advancement flaps. Laxity of adjacent skin is more important than its plasticity in this kind of flap. All flaps take advantage of the property of skin that gives it some stretching and adaptability, but the advancement flap simply requires an excess or

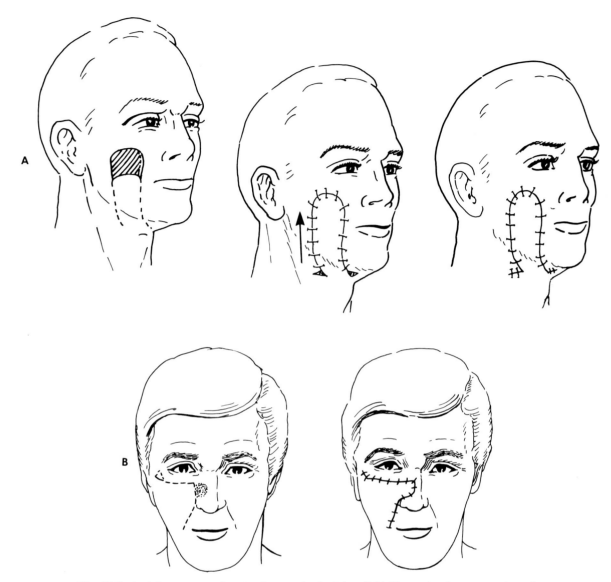

Fig. 28-2. A, Advancement flap to close a cheek defect.[11,14] Note triangles removed at the base of the donor site to facilitate an even closure. **B,** Advancement flap to restore defects in the midpart of the cheek and the side of the nose. Facial laxity is important for utilization of this flap.

abundance of skin. It therefore has limited usefulness and will generally require triangular excisions of the margins of the donor site (Fig. 28-2). Advancement flaps are commonly used to close defects in the cheek centrally or toward the nose. Skin grafts are never required to close donor sites.

Rotation flaps. Although these flaps may be partially advanced into defects, by far the more important maneuver is *turning* these flaps to achieve closure. Whereas the advancement flap is simply undercut and pulled into a defect to close it, adjacent skin in the rotational flap is turned to some degree into the wound. This rotation may be slight or obvious (Figs. 28-3 to 28-5), and donor areas may be closed edge to edge or by skin grafts. The design of rotational flaps requires a practiced eye, an understanding of stresses created in the closure of the donor site, and a realization that the area of the flap must be much larger than the area of the defect.

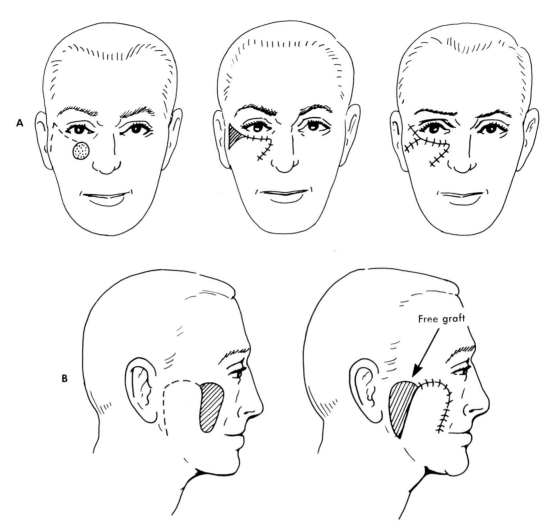

Fig. 28-3. A, Flap with both rotational and advancement characteristics.[11] The donor site may be grafted or closed primarily. **B,** Flap to cover a cheek defect.[11] Skin grafts are usually used to close donor sites.

Transposition flaps. The best example of a transposition flap is the Z-plasty, which is familiar to every plastic surgeon. The Z-plasty requires that flaps be elevated and transposed, ideally at an angle of 60 degrees. Similarly, all transposition flaps are elevated and switched in their direction at a significant angle from the donor site (Figs. 28-6 to 28-8, 28-10, and 28-11), often permitting edge-to-edge closure of the donor site. What are termed rotation flaps may be seen as being similar to transposition flaps; transposition flaps are turned, of course, but the donor site is usually farther away from the defect than it is in rotation flaps and is usually closed edge to edge (Fig. 28-7). It is always necessary that a surgical defect extend to the pedicle to permit

reconstruction with a local flap; that is, if the wound to be covered is not continuous with the skin defect created by the elevation of a flap, then conditions for a local flap do not exist. Occasionally extending the defect beyond that area needed for adequate excision of a lesion provides a shape allowing special techniques for closure that are effective and esthetic (Figs. 28-7 and 28-8).

Island and kite flaps. Island and kite flaps descriptively name important skin flaps (Fig. 28-9) that are nourished on a vascular stalk of subcutaneous tissue beneath the flap. The "island" of skin is free to move only so far as the tether of its pedicle permits. Fig. 28-9 illustrates the practical use to which these flaps are put. Surgical defects in the

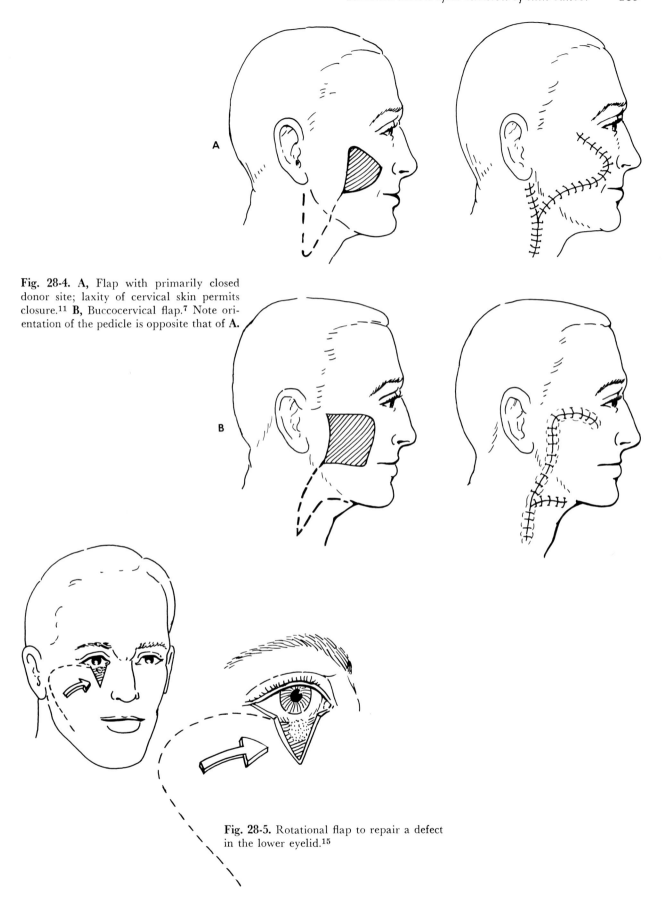

Fig. 28-4. A, Flap with primarily closed donor site; laxity of cervical skin permits closure.[11] **B,** Buccocervical flap.[7] Note orientation of the pedicle is opposite that of **A.**

Fig. 28-5. Rotational flap to repair a defect in the lower eyelid.[15]

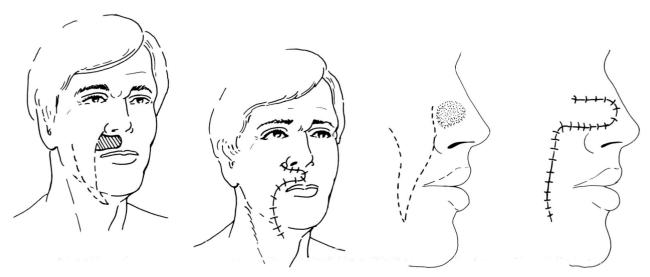

Fig. 28-6. Transposition flap to close an upper labial defect.[17]

Fig. 28-7. Transposition flap from the nasolabial crease to resurface nasal defects. Nasolabial fold is a donor site easily closed; esthetic results are good.

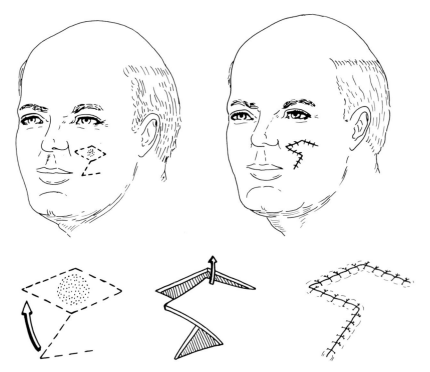

Fig. 28-8. L shaped flap to repair a lozenge-shaped defect.[4,5] A lozenge-shaped defect is created to permit an L shaped flap to close the defect. All sides of defect and flap are equal in length.

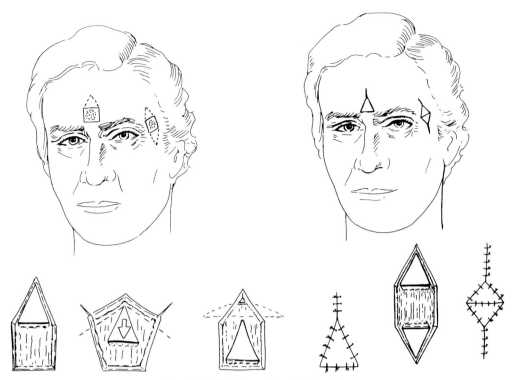

Fig. 28-9. Single and double kite flap.[6]

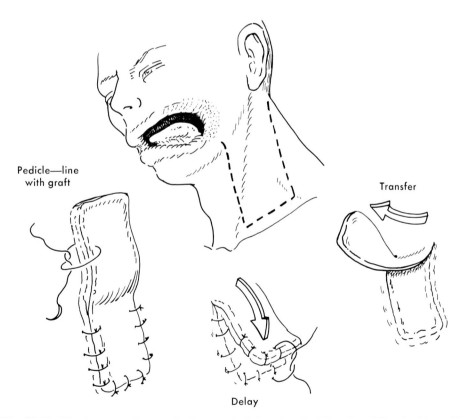

Pedicle—line with graft

Transfer

Delay

Fig. 28-10. Cheek restoration employing cervical flap that is delayed and lined with a skin graft.[9,16]

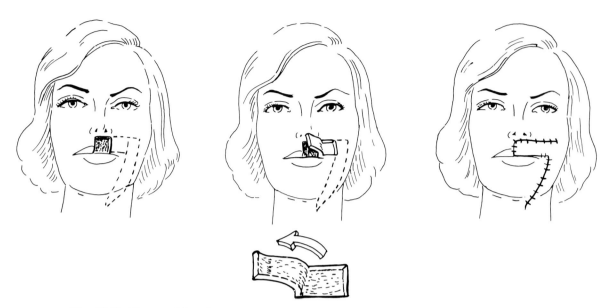

Fig. 28-11. Transposition flap to repair an upper labial defect.[18] Note lining of the flap is obtained from adjacent skin and tumbles backward into wound. Bearing whiskers, such flaps are not advantageous.

forehead and temples that would otherwise require a skin graft or a deforming edge-to-edge closure are suitably closed with a kite flap.

Lined flaps. Most local flaps do not require an inner as well as an outer epithelial surface; but when they do, plans must be made to line them. Certain eyelid defects and full-thickness lip and cheek defects will need an inner or deeper epithelium as well as an outer epithelium. Free skin grafts (Fig. 28-10) can line a flap prior to its final elevation and transfer, or two local flaps may serve to line one another (Fig. 28-11).

Bridged (indirect) flaps

The identifying feature of bridged flaps is the remoteness of the pedicle from the surgical defect. These flaps, somewhere between their base and tip, span normal tissue or spaces. The donor site and the recipient site are entirely separate wounds, as can be seen in Figs. 28-12 to 28-17. These donor sites often require a split skin graft. Wherever possible, the central span of a bridged flap is closed; simple tubing of the flap is often the easiest method of achieving such closure. The distal end of the flap may be lined or unlined, depending on the nature of the defect to be closed or reconstructed. After the flap is securely established in its new location, the bridge to the base is detached and discarded or returned and set back in the donor site.

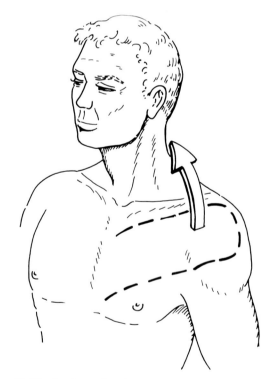

Fig. 28-12. Outline of a large deltopectoral flap that is useful in resurfacing the neck and face.[2,13]

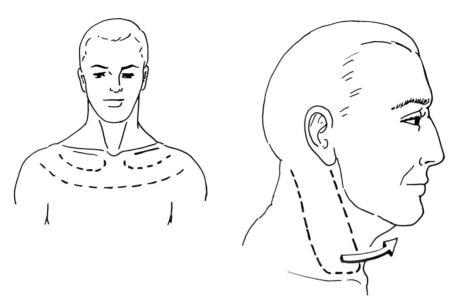

Fig. 28-13. Pectoral and cervical flaps to provide large amounts of tissue for cervical closure.[19]

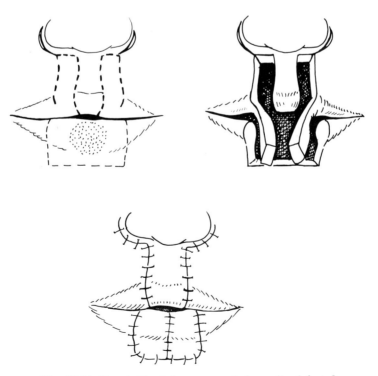

Fig. 28-14. Two bridged flaps to repair lower lip defects.[3]

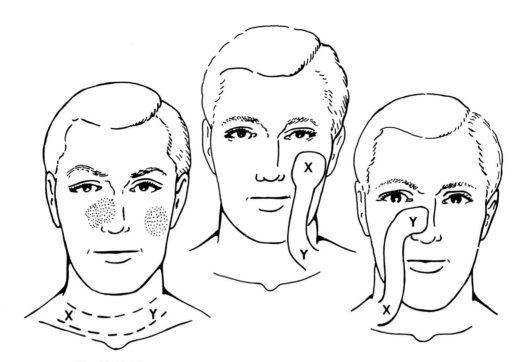

Fig. 28-15. Tubed cervical flaps providing tissue to repair facial defects.[12]

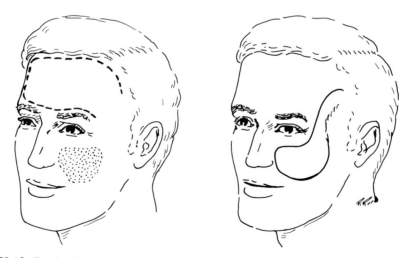

Fig. 28-16. Forehead flap to cover a large facial defect.[10a] A totally resurfaced forehead provides esthetic symmetry even though the full extent of a forehead flap may not be required. Forehead flaps extending part way across the breadth of the brow may suffice.

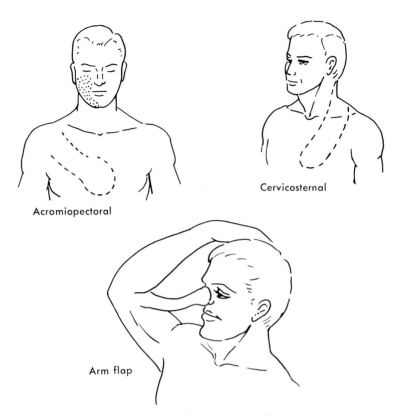

Acromiopectoral

Cervicosternal

Arm flap

Fig. 28-17. Bridged flaps.[8]

Distant (carried) flaps

Kazanjian has written,

A tubed flap from a distant area is to be considered as a last resort. It is indicated when a pedicled flap from the face and neck is not available. There are many such conditions; for instance, the skin of the neck may be scarred and the viability of a flap may be questioned. Secondly, when deforming tissues are scattered over various parts of the face . . . tube flaps may have to be transferred from one area to the other; third, when it becomes necessary to supply an interlining of the mouth and nose; and fourth, when a large amount of skin has been lost, shifting a local flap may leave a secondary defect which is hard to close. The disadvantage of tube flaps are: color, thickness and texture which may not harmonize with the skin of the face, and risk of multiple operations and long hospitalizations. However, in spite of these handicaps, tubed flaps have been useful procedures when indicated. . . .[11]

There are instances where abdominal skin must be brought to the head and neck on a vehicle such as the forearm or arm, but such instances usually relate to secondary reconstruction in the burn patient or to other posttraumatic defects requiring large reconstructions. Such flaps deserve mention only for the sake of completeness. They are not illustrated in this chapter. To manage closure of defects after operations to remove cancer, the local and bridged flaps will serve in practically all instances where simple closure or free skin grafts are not ideal.

REFERENCES

1. Adams, W. M.: The use of neighboring tissues in the correction of an extensive facial deformity, Plast. Reconstr. Surg. **2:**105, 1946.
2. Bakamjian, V. Y.: A two stage method for pharyngo-esophageal reconstruction with a primary pectoral skin flap, Plast. Reconstr. Surg. **36:**173, 1965.
3. Bowers, D. G.: Double cross lip flaps for lower lip reconstruction, Plast. Reconstr. Surg. **47:**209, 1971.
4. Dufourmental, C.: La fermeture des pertes de substance cutanée limitées, Ann Chir. Plast. (Paris) **7:**60, 1962.
5. Dufourmentel, C.: Traitement chirurgical des naevi pigmentaires bénins, Ann Chir. Plast. (Paris) **7:**105, 1962.
6. Dufourmentel, C., and Talatt, S. M.: The kite flap. In Hueston, J. T., editor: Fifth International Congress of Plastic and Reconstructive Surgery, Melbourne, 1971, Butterworth & Co. p. 1223.

7. Esser, J. F. S.: Cheek rotation, Rev. Chir. Plast. 3:298, 1934.

8. Furnas, D. W., and Conway, H.: Correction of major facial defects by pedicle flaps, Plast. Reconstr. Surg. 31:407, 1963.

9. Hancock, D. M.: The repair of facial defects resulting from surgery for locally advanced buccal carcinoma, Plast. Reconstr. Surg. 20:117, 1957.

10. Hirshowitz, B., and Mahler, D.: T-plasty technique for excisions in the face, Plast. Reconstr. Surg. 37:453, 1966

10a. Hoopes, J. E., and Edgerton, M. T.: Immediate forehead flap repair and resection for oropharyngeal cancer, Am. J. Surg. 112:527, 1966.

11. Kazanjian, V. H.: The use of skin flaps in the repair of facial deformities, Plast. Reconstr. Surg. 5:337, 1949.

12. Macomber, W. B., and Wang, M. H.: Tubed neck flaps in facial reconstruction, Plast. Reconstr. Surg. 45:346, 1970.

13. McGregor, I. A., ad Reed, W. H.: Simultaneous temporal and deltopectoral flaps for full thickness defects of the cheek, Plast. Reconstr. Surg. 45:326, 1970.

14. Mouly, R.: Le lambeau en "U" jugal pour la réparation des pertes de substance mentonniéres, Ann. Chir. Plast. (Paris) 8:209, 1963.

15. Mustardé, J. C.: The use of flaps in the orbital region, Plast. Reconstr. Surg. 45:146, 1970.

16. Owens, N.: A compound neck pedicle designed for the repair of massive facial defects. Plat. Reconstr. Surg. 15:367, 1955.

17. Paletta, F. X.: Early and late repair of facial defects following treatment of malignancy, Plast. Reconstr. Surg. 13:95, 1953.

18. Smith, F.: Flaps utilized in facial and cervical reconstruction, Plast. Reconstr. Surg. 7:415, 1951.

19. Von Deilen, A. W.: Methods of immediate repair after major resections of the face and jaws, Plast. Reconstr. Surg. 11:152, 1952.

Chapter 29

The forehead flap in intraoral reconstruction

John E. Hoopes, M.D.

No longer can the cancer surgeon look to survival data alone as a measure of his success. Alteration of either function or appearance to the point of precluding an individual's right to pursue a meaningful existence is in violation of current concepts. Quality of survival is at least as important as length of survival. The surgeon with a complete reconstructive armamentarium at his disposal may direct his total effort toward cure without fear of producing an "oral cripple."

Increased emphasis on *primary* reconstruction has provided the impetus for increased utilization of the "temporal flap."[2-8,11,12,14] The anatomy of the forehead vasculature has been described.[4] Routine ligation of the external carotid artery in the course of radical neck dissection is not necessary and should be avoided to preserve the option for forehead flap reconstruction. The superficial temporal artery may be spared in virtually all instances. A hemi-forehead flap may be based entirely anterior to the hairline on the zygomatico-orbital branch of the superficial temporal artery. A total forehead flap need not be delayed, provided that the pedicle includes both the superficial temporal and posterior auricular arteries. Necrosis of the flap will result from elevation of an undelayed total forehead flap in the absence of an intact superficial temporal artery.

Distinct advantages are offered by immediate forehead flap reconstruction: (1) patients whose disease has a poor prognosis are subjected to minimal hospitalization and operative procedures; (2) salivary fistulas are avoided; (3) intraoral anatomical relationships are preserved; and (4) postoperative administration of radiation therapy is facilitated.

SURGICAL TECHNIQUE

The forehead flap has been maligned on the basis that it is not acceptable esthetically. This criticism may be overcome simply by a proper design of the flap.

Hemi-forehead flap

The pedicle lies on a transverse line at the level of the external canthus and extends either to the temporal hairline or to the anterior margin of the auricle. Placement of the pedicle entirely anterior to the hairline allows a one-staged procedure by means of deepithelialization of that portion of the pedicle not contributing to replacement of oral mucosa. The flap extends precisely from the superior margin of the eyebrow to the hairline and terminates in the midline of the forehead.

Total forehead flap

The forehead must be visualized as a *single* esthetic unit. The pedicle of the flap lies on a transverse line at the level of the lateral canthus and extends from the eyebrow to a point 2 cm. posterior to the ear. The transverse dimension of the flap must extend precisely from the superior margin of the eyebrow to the hairline. The distal extremity of the flap must follow the temporal hairline and terminate on a transverse line at the level of the contralateral external canthus.

Elevation of either the hemi-forehead flap or the total forehead flap usually is accomplished at the level of the pericranium; this plane of dissection allows rapid elevation of the flap with minimal blood loss. Several authors, however, advocate elevation of the flap at a level superficial to the frontalis muscle.[10] Utilizing the principle that the quality of color match is related to the proximity of recipient and donor site, the surgeon obtains the skin graft to be applied to the forehead from the supraclavicular area.

Several techniques have been described for introduction of the forehead flap into the oral cavity.[1,4,7,9,12] I prefer using either a cheek tunnel lateral to the zygomatic arch or the avascular plane medial to the zygomatic arch. Utilization of the avascular plane medial to the zygomatic arch requires detachment of the temporalis insertion; occasionally, resection of the zygomatic arch is required to ensure lack of compression of the pedicle. The reliability of the forehead flap is impressive; marginal necrosis of the most distal extremity of the flap occurs infrequently, and major loss of flap tissue is a rarity.

Mandibular resection is never performed solely for the purpose of facilitating either exposure or wound closure. The indications for mandibular resection are based entirely on considerations regarding adequate tumor margin; progressively increasing attention is being directed to "marginal mandibular resections," particularly in the management of tumors involving the retromolar triangle.

When utilizing the total forehead flap, the surgeon should direct his attention to possible usages for the pedicle at the time of the second-stage procedure for retrieval of the pedicle. Ordinarily, the pedicle of the total forehead flap is retrieved and discarded. In extended resections, however, the pedicle may be utilized for closure of antral fistulas or for reconstruction of the soft palate.[3] Division of the pedicle is performed 3 weeks after the primary procedure. The pedicle is transected intraorally, and only the hair-bearing portion of the flap is returned to the temporal region.

The distal extremity of a total forehead flap will reach the sternoclavicular joint and provide adequate coverage for an exposed carotid artery. Smalley has described the resurfacing of an exposed carotid artery with a total forehead flap,[15] and I have utilized this technique.

Mandibular reconstruction

The necessity for mandibular stabilization after mandibular resection is reduced by an adequate replacement of intraoral lining. Routinely, dental impressions are obtained preoperatively, and guide-plane appliances are utilized during the immediate postoperative period. The concept that primary re-

construction of the mandible seems both unwise and generally unnecessary appears to be correct.[13] Reconstruction of the mandible, if indicated, is performed at some convenient interval after resection. Many patients will not require reconstruction of the mandible.

SUMMARY

Primary reconstruction provides optimal management for patients with intraoral cancer.

The forehead flap provides immediately available, highly dependable tissue for primary reconstruction. The palliative value of forehead flap reconstruction has been emphasized by Toomey.[16]

REFERENCES

1. Davis, G. N., and Hoopes, J. E.: New route for passage of forehead flap to inside of mouth, Plast. Reconstr. Surg. **47**:390, 1971.
2. DesPrez, J. D., and Kiehn, C. L.: Methods of reconstruction following resection of anterior oral cavity and mandible for malignancy, Plast. Reconstr. Surg. **24**:238, 1959.
3. Hoopes, J. E.: Uses for the forehead flap. In Conley, J., and Dickinson, J. T., editors: Plastic and reconstructive surgery of the face and neck, vol. 2, New York, 1972, Grune & Stratton, Inc. p. 144.
4. Hoopes, J. E., and Edgerton, M. T.: Immediate forehead flap repair in resection for oral pharyngeal cancer, Am. J. Surg. **112**:527, 1966.
5. McGregor, I. A.: The temporal flap in intraoral cancer; its use in repairing the post-excisional defect, Br. J. Plast. Surg. **16**:318, 1963.
6. McGregor, I. A.: The temporal flap in facial cancer. In: Transactions of the Third International Congress of Plastic Surgery, International Congress Series No. 66, Amsterdam, 1964, Excerpta Medica Foundation, p. 1096.
7. McGregor, I. A.: The temporal flap in intraoral reconstruction. In Gaisford, J. C., editor: Symposium on Cancer of the head and neck, St. Louis, 1969, The C. V. Mosby Co.
8. McGregor, I. A., and Reid, W. H.: The use of the temporal flap in the primary repair of full-thickness defects of the cheek, Plast. Reconstr. Surg. **38**:1, 1966.
9. McGregor, I. A., and Reid, W. H.: Simultaneous temporal and delto-pectoral flaps for full-thickness defects of the cheek, Plast. Reconstr. Surg. **45**:326, 1970.
10. McNeill, K. A.: Forehead flap oroplasty. In Conley, J., and Dickinson, J. T., editors: Plastic and reconstructive surgery for the face and neck, vol. 2, New York, 1972, Grune & Stratton, Inc, p. 221.
11. Millard, D. R.: Forehead flap in immediate repair of head, face, and jaw, Am. J. Surg. **108**:508, 1964.
12. Millard, D. R.: Immediate reconstruction of the lower jaw, Plast. Reconstr. Surg. **35**:60, 1965.
13. Millard, D. R., Garst, W. P., Campbell, R. C., and

Stokley, S. T. H.: Composite lower jaw reconstruction, Plast. Reconstr. Surg. **46:**22, 1970.

14. Mladick, R. A., Royer, J. R., Thorne, F. L., Pickrell, K. L., and Georgiade, N. C.: Immediate reconstruction of the pharynx after combined therapy for advanced tonsillar carcinoma, Am. J. Surg. **116:**691, 1968.

15. Smalley, J. J., and Cunningham, M. P.: Forehead flap rotation to protect the carotid artery, Plast. Reconstr. Surg. **49:**96, 1972.

16. Toomey, J. M.: Forehead flap reconstruction of the floor of the mouth, Ann. Otol. Rhinol. Laryngol. **77:**94, 1968.

Chapter 30

Reconstructive management of the mandible in the treatment of head and neck cancer

Magdi S. Kodsi, M.D.
Norris K. Culf, M.D.
Stuart J. Hulnick, M.D.
Lester M. Cramer, D.M.D., M.D.

The need for immediate restoration of function after head and neck cancer resections has long been recognized; this need has been neglected, however, because of the possibility that immediate restoration will prevent early detection of tumor recurrence. However, it is well accepted that the best chance for cure in resections of cancer of the head and neck is with the initial attack; the watchful waiting approach taken toward patients operated on for cure unjustifiably denies them the opportunity of resuming normal daily activities and regaining their normal place in society.[20,21,26]

The management of the mandibular framework in head and neck cancer surgery has to be tailored to the procedure of extirpation. Present data support preservation of the mandible in a higher percentage of patients having resection for intraoral carcinoma than formerly.[4,50] Sacrifice of the mandible for the sole objective of providing soft tissue mobilization and ease of closure should be seriously questioned. The indications for mandibular resection are based solely on the extent of disease.

Determination of the extent and mode of the repair made after extirpation is based on: (1) size of the resultant defect, (2) extent of distortion of residual tissues, (3) ensuing dysfunction, and (4) disfigurement.

The primary objective in mandibular management after a resection is the reestablishment of the correct spacial relationship of the remaining tissues so that the configuration of the dental arch, the buccal mucous membrane, and the mobility of the tongue are minimally compromised. The need for additional soft tissue coverage of any residual skeletal framework or for bone grafting is dictated by these factors and has to be planned for before embarking on the resection.

Frequently, soft tissue replacement alone obviates the need for additional bone replacement,[22,52] particularly in margin resections of the anterior mandibular arch and in wedge resections of the lateral mandible. The flap that provides both adequate soft tissue lining and bulk helps maintain the proper relationship of the residual framework.

MANAGEMENT OF THE MANDIBULAR FRAGMENTS AFTER OSTEOTOMY FOR EXPOSURE

When a tumor resection requires a mandibular osteotomy, an offset or step is placed in the osteotomy line to obtain a mortise at the line of reapproximation. This fracture line is managed by direct intraosseous fixation supplemented by intermaxillary fixation.

196

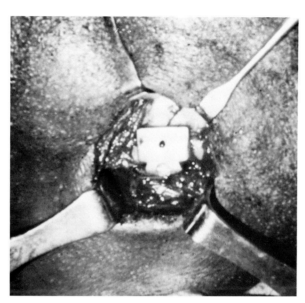

Fig. 30-1. Pericortical compression clamp, a means of intraosseous fixation.

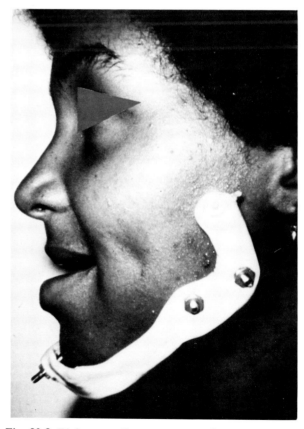

Fig. 30-2. Biphase appliance, a means of external fixation of the mandible.

Means of intraosseous fixation
  Direct wiring[19,68]
  Kirschner wire[12,19]
  Compression plates
      Pericortical clamps[8] (Fig. 30-1)
      Axial screw plates[45]
  Mandibular plates[19,44]
  Mesh cribs
      Metal cribs[8,36,37]
      Biodegradeable cribs[24]

Means of intermaxillary fixation
  Interdental wiring[19,68]
  Arch bars[19]
      Circummandibular wiring to nasal spine, pyriform aperture,[19] or transalveolar fixation

Means of external fixation
  Morris biphase appliance[64] (Fig. 30-2)
  Roger-Anderson[19,31]
  Stader splint[20,30]

MANAGEMENT OF THE MANDIBULAR FRAGMENTS AFTER BONE RESECTION

When extirpation of the intraoral tumor requires mandibular resection, the approach to the mandibular stumps will depend on the size and location of the osseous gap.

Limited mandibular resections

If the resultant bony defect is small and located posterior to the mental foramen, a soft tissue flap of moderate bulk will often be sufficient.[22,28,52]

Deviation of the residual mandible after composite jaw resections, generally attributed to loss of mandibular support, is very frequently prevented by the provision of proper soft tissue replacement[28,52] and the achievement of primary wound healing without tension. Soft tissue replacement alone can restore the proper anatomical spacial relationship to the mandibular fragments by preventing contraction and distortion of the adjacent tissues. This improves swallowing and speech abilities after the resection and provides a satisfactory cosmetic result. Patients who have had a partial hemimandibulectomy and adequate soft tissue replacement frequently turn down the opportunity for secondary bone grafting.[52] However, in mandibular resections not requiring extensive soft tissue sacrifice, such as ameloblastomas, fibrous dysplasia, tumors of dental origin, or myxomas, further refinement in cosmetic and functional result is frequently sought.

Control of mandibular drift. In limited mandibular resections after the necessary soft tissue coverage has been provided, prevention of soft tissue contraction and secondary mandibular drift is required temporarily and is achieved by maintaining the mandibular fragments in their proper spacial anatomical relationship.[30] The status of dentition in the residual mandibular fragment and the maxillary arch provides the index for the type of immobilization required (Fig. 30-3).

Adjuvant control of mandibular drift can be achieved by the use of Kirschner wires (Fig. 30-4), threaded bolts, bolts and wires, intraoral splints (Fig. 30-3, *B*), and external appliances.

Simple Kirschner wires in an intraosseous gap tend to telescope with time (Fig. 30-5) and may get dislodged. Erosion through the skin can occur secondary to wound contracture. Dislodgement incidence varies, but the need for wire removal is usually late and occurs after it has fulfilled its function. Bending the ends of the Kirschner wire at a double right angle will prevent telescoping.[9,31]

Transfixation of a Silastic rod or block[53,54] by the Kirschner wire is another means of maintaining the intraosseous gap (Figs. 30-6 and 30-7).

The use of the threaded tibial bolt[35] with nuts and washers, supplemented by a wire loop, secures immobilization of the bolt and the bone fragments.[61]

The intraoral splints that can provide a satisfactory means of control of the mandibular drift are of several varieties. The most popular one consists of an inclined guide plane on the buccal surface of the maxillary arch on the side opposite the mandibular resection (Fig. 30-3, *B*). An outrigger or a flange secured to the buccal aspect of the remaining mandible is guided to prevent mandibular devia-

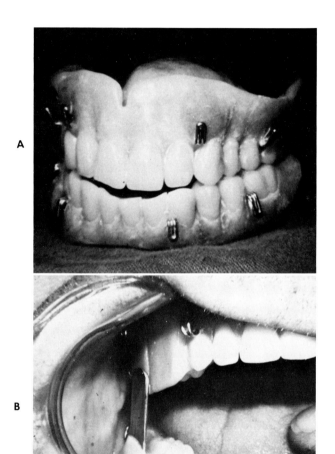

A

B

Fig. 30-3. A, Original dentures modified with hooks for intermaxillary fixation provide a good mode of stabilization in the edentulous patient. **B,** Intraoral splint, a mandibular vertical bar gliding on a maxillary guide plane, maintains the chin in the midline in an open or closed position.

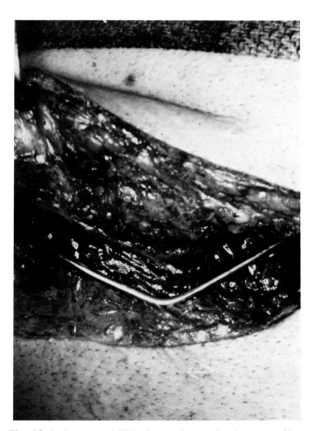

Fig. 30-4. Contoured Kirschner wire maintains centralization of the mandible.

tion.[28,31] These appliances are only needed for a period of up to 3 months. They are maintained in position by various means, ranging from clasps and gate splints to circummandibular, transalveolar, or drop-wire fixation.[28] Of the external appliances, the Morris biphase appliance is the most utilitarian. It has been used to maintain a bony gap up to a year without complications[29] except for the presence of crusting and oozing where the external threaded screws emerge through the skin.

More extensive mandibular resections and those involving anterior arch

When the tumor resection includes the anterior mandibular arch, greater disability secondary to a lack of pharyngeal support and tongue control seriously aggravates the swallowing difficulty. Salivary incontinence, speech defects, and severe facial disfigurements are also troublesome. The basic principles of reconstruction are (1) adequate intraoral lining, (2) adequate external skin surfacing, and (3) skeletal support.

Immediate control of the proximal mandibular fragments is essential to prevent the remaining mandible from being drawn upward and inward by the attached muscles and their subsequent fibrosis in this abnormal position. Here, soft tissue replacement alone will not prevent development of a significant deformity unless adequate substitution of the skele-

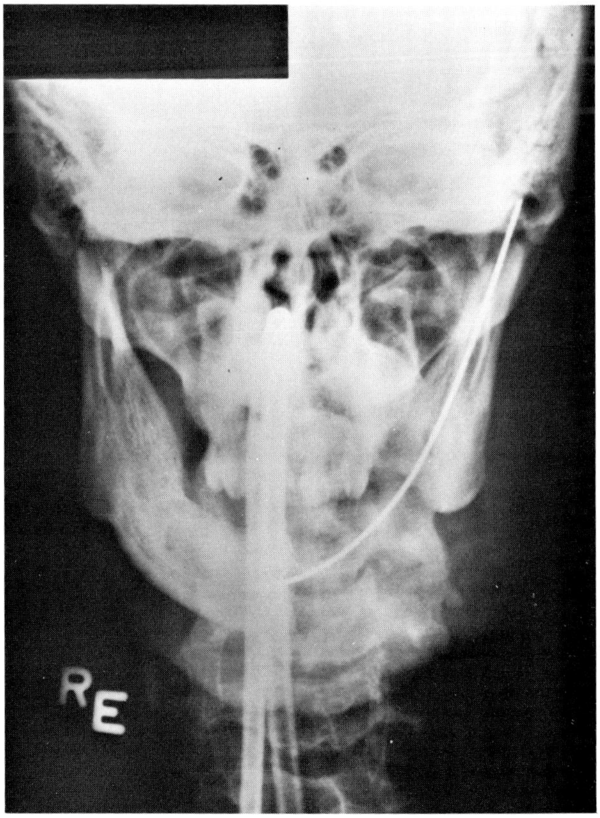

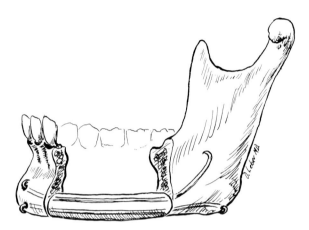

Fig. 30-6. Kirschner wires through Silastic block maintain the mandibular gap. (From McQuarrie, D. G.: Arch. Surg. **102**:448, May 1971. Copyright 1971, American Medical Association.)

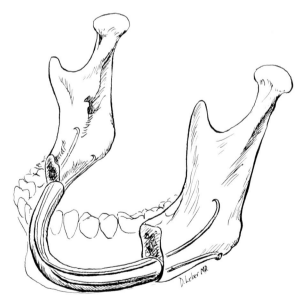

Fig. 30-7. Mandibular arch maintained by Kirschner wires and Silastic block. (From McQuarrie, D. G.: Arch. Surg. **102**:448, May 1971. Copyright 1971, American Medical Association.)

Fig. 30-5. Contoured Kirschner wire to assist mandibular centralization. Note telescoping through proximal fragment.

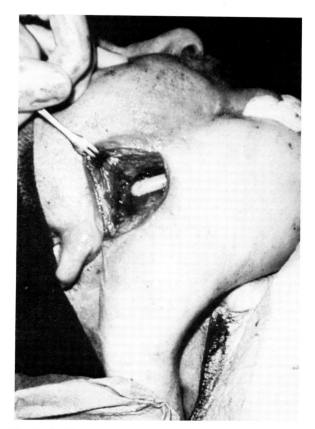

Fig. 30-8. Silastic rod, a temporary device extending from one ascending ramus to the other, exposed during a staged reconstruction.

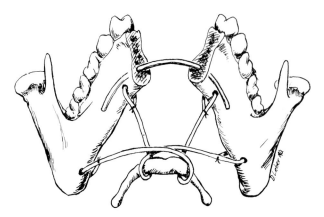

Fig. 30-9. Fascia lata strips used as a double sling around the hyoid bone assist in the restitution of the pharyngeal funnel. (From Desprez, J. D., and Kiehn, C. L.: Plast. Reconstr. Surg. **24**:244. © 1959, The Williams & Wilkins Co., Baltimore.)

arch.[26] This process will allow the maintenance of a pharyngeal funnel (Fig. 30-9).

The presence of erupted posterior molars can be taken advantage of by applying stainless steel caps to the teeth on each mandibular fragment and connecting the caps with a contoured intraoral, extramucosal bar to bridge the symphyseal gap and immobilize the proximal stumps in their proper position.[39]

RECONSTRUCTION OF THE MISSING SKELETAL FRAGMENT

World War I stimulated major efforts to restore mandibular continuity.[1,38] In World War II the use of the iliac crest as the source of bone grafts to treat mandibular defects was well established. Further experience in the ensuing years reinforced the value of autogenous bone grafts. Current available means of reconstruction of the missing skeletal fragment of the mandible are bone grafts, composite grafts and pedicled flaps, island flaps, and prostheses.

Bone grafts

Bone grafts are the most popular of these measures, and although they include autogenous homogenous, and heterogenous varieties, the autogenous bone graft is most generally preferred. Successful grafting with the other types has been very disappointing.

Homogenous bone grafts. Homogenous bone grafts are unpredictable, particularly in bridging gaps that do not have osteogenic potential. New approaches to

tal support has been achieved. The initial control of the proximal mandibular fragments is most frequently achieved by contoured Kirschner wires or tibial bolts inserted in the cut ends of the mandibular stumps.[35,61] Transfixation of a Silastic bar or rod by a Kirschner wire[53,54] provides a softer framework, additional bulk, and more ease for the draping of the soft tissue (Figs. 30-7 and 30-8). In addition, it will provide a tunnel facilitating the creation of a pocket for later bone grafting.

The application of a Steinman pin transversely between the mandibular stumps has been described by McGregor.[52]

Many authors[13,27,71] consider additional support in the form of suspension of the larynx and tongue upward and forward after resection of the symphysis important. This suspension can be achieved by encircling the hyoid bone with either stainless steel wire or fascia lata and suspending it to the center of the bar or bone graft replacing the mandibular

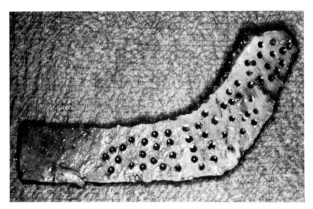

Fig. 30-10. Whole carved full-thickness segment of the ilium partially decorticated by drill holes.

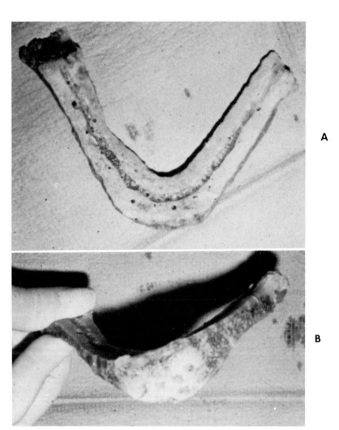

Fig. 30-11. Whole carved symphysis and body with partial decorticaton, harvested from the ilium.

homografts are being investigated. Richter and Boyne[67] have reported on a clinically successful mandibular homograft combined with autogenous marrow. More recently, freeze-dried homogenous anterior mandibles in which holes had been drilled and filled with autogenous cancellous bone and marrow from the iliac crest have been reported by DeFries, Marble, and Snell[25] to produce good cosmetic results and radiographic replacement of the homograft by new bone. This approach deserves further attention.

Heterogenous bone grafts. Hetergenous bone grafts are not in general use, because of their uncontrolled antigenicity and resorption. They act as a space-occupying barrier to osteogenesis.[7]

Autogenous bone grafts. The ideal bone graft should provide an element of stability and yet lead to rapid union by early ossification; these two objectives are best achieved by the use of corticocancellous grafts. Cortical bone by itself provides good stabilization, but its ossification is slow because the hard cortex acts only as a scaffold for new bone replacement by creeping substitution.[23,65]

Cancellous bone has a simple network of spongy trabeculae, which support a large, active cellular mass that provides greater osteogenic potential.[43,65]

Osteocytes exposed to plasmatic circulation survive and form osteoid, which leads to rapid ossification and early union. The deeper cells, deprived of direct contact with the vascular bed, die and later disappear. Thus it is recommended that cancellous chips be provided at the line of mortise as well as along the length of the defect to be bridged.

Good blood supply of the recipient bed plus adequate soft tissue coverage and its close apposition to

the bone graft are essential for a successful take. Boyne[6] has reported a higher osteogenic potential with the use of marrow and autogenous cancellous bone combined.

Autogenous bone grafts can be utilized as whole carved segments, bone blocks, bone chips, and composite grafts or components of composite pedicle flaps.

Whole carved segments. Whole carved segments are usually obtained from the ilium, and preferences for utilization vary from a full-thickness carved reproduction of the resected mandibular segment[47,48] (Figs. 30-10 and 30-11), to a single cortical surface and its underlying cancellous bone,[10,68] to cancellous bone excluding the cortical component,[28] to the whole iliac crest with a three-sided cortical covering.[30] The area of the anterior superior iliac spine lends itself to the reproduction of the chin prominence.

Bone blocks. Cancellous bone blocks can be wired together and made to conform to the skeletal gap to which they are wired[10] (Fig. 30-12). They can also be threaded on a Kirschner wire, and the intervening spaces are packed with bone chips[26,55] (Fig. 30-13).

Bone chips. Implantation of cancellous bone chips in a soft tissue pocket of mucosa and muscle is reported to produce a fibro-osseous union adequate for mandibular stability.[2,3] Cancellous bone chips and bone marrow applied in a contoured chrome cobalt (Vitallium) mesh crib, lined by a nylon-backed cellulose filter, have been shown to ossify and unite with the mandibular fragments[49] (Fig. 30-14).

More recently, polylactic acid, a biodegradable material used experimentally on mandibular fractures,[24] is being investigated at the U.S. Army biologic research laboratory for use as a biodegradable crib to contain cancellous bone chips in the grafting of mandibular gaps.[33] The use of compound silicone implants with wire reinforcements and cancellous bone chips in the treatment of congenital, traumatic, and esthetic problems has been described by Swanson and colleagues.[73]

Autogenous mandibular grafts. The autoclaved resected mandible and its use as a buried devitalized splint, as attempted by Martin[51] and described by Harding,[36] has not gained popularity, because of its behavior as a foreign body[31,51] and its replacement by fibrous tissue. In 1967 Gaisford[30] reported the use

in selected cases of the resected mandible after it has been separated from the mucoperiosteum where a 1-cm. margin of normal tissue intervenes between the tumor and bone. It would appear that in the majority of instances the possibility of compromising the en bloc principle in harvesting the bone may be violated.

Composite grafts and flaps

Snyder and co-workers[69] have successfully used the sternoclavicular joint to replace the temporomandibular joint. Ivy[38] has reviewed the use of osteocutaneous flaps for mandibular restoration. Snyder

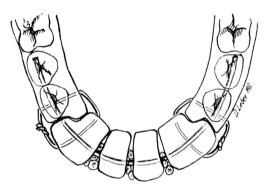

Fig. 30-13. Bone blocks threaded over a Kirschner wire; the intervening spaces are packed with bone chips. (From Desprez, J. D., and Kiehn, C. L.: Plast. Reconstr. Surg. 24:244. © 1959, The Williams & Wilkins Co., Baltimore.)

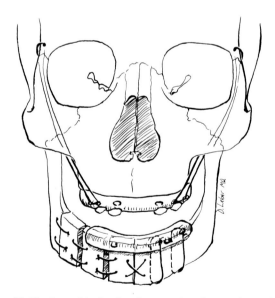

Fig. 30-12. Bone blocks fitted to each other and to the mandibular stumps by wire loops conforming to fill the skeletal gap. (From Bromberg, D. E., and others: Plast. Reconstr. Surg. 32:596. © 1963, The Williams & Wilkins Co., Baltimore.)

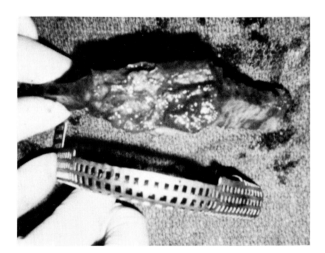

Fig. 30-14. Whole carved iliac bone graft to substitute symphysis and body; vitalium mesh tray shown was used only as a model for carving the bone. When the contour of the ilium is insufficient for one-segment replacement, the vitalium tray may be packed with cancellous chips.

and co-workers[69] have reported on eight clavicular osteocutaneous flaps, and Conley and colleagues[16,17] have reported on a variety of osteocutaneous flaps used in 50 patients.

Vascular island flaps

In 1969 Strauch, Bloomberg, and Lewin[72] presented the island artery composite rib graft in dogs. McKee[52a] reported on free rib grafting with vascular anastomosis to the neck vessels in 1971. Ketchum and co-workers[39a] gave the first case report of mandibular reconstruction using a composite island rib flap in 1973. These modalities are ingenious ones to have in the armamentarium.

Prostheses

Although reports have been made of the retention of various metal and synthetic appliances used as mandibular replacements, further follow-ups indicate a high incidence of their displacement or erosion through the soft tissue bed. Their use as a temporary device, however, can be valuable in helping to maintain proper spacial anatomical relationships. These appliances also allow for delayed bone grafting with a high rate of success.

BONE GRAFTING

The enthusiasm of primary bone grafting has waxed and waned. In combined resections primary bone grafting is not advisable[14] because of a 30% incidence of graft losses.[15,60] The exposure afforded at the time of tumor resection is unsurpassed, and it is indeed very tempting to proceed with primary bone grafting. However, the following classical requisites for successful bone grafting must be met:

1. The patient's general condition should be good, and his nitrogen content must be positively balanced.
2. Vascularity of the soft tissue receiving the bone graft must be adequate, the intraoral and extraoral seals must be watertight. Heavily irradiated tissues are not adequate,[14,32] and bone grafts have resorbed more frequently when inserted in flaps that were disconnected from their pedicles.
3. Intraoral and extraoral soft tissue coverage without tension must be adequate.
4. The recipient fragments of the host must be well vascularized, and there must be enough bleeding surface to provide a large enough area of contact with the graft.[27]
5. Fixation of the graft to the recipient fragments

with immediate postoperative immobilization must be adequate.[10,28,30]
6. Dead space must be eliminated, and hematoma about the graft must be prevented.
7. Antibiotic coverage must be adequate.[14,38]

Selection of donor site

Although the tibia, fibula, clavicle, and autogenous mandible have been used,[38,62] the ilium and the rib continue to remain the most popular donor sites for bone grafting. Provision of adequate cancellous bone offers the host a large number of viable cellular bone elements[65] and diminishes the amount of ossification by creeping substitution. A rapid union and the formation of a solid-lined framework capable of taking the stresses of the region are thus enhanced.

Ilium. The abundance of cancellous bone in the ilium accounts for its popularity as a donor site for bone grafts.[26,30,47,57] Surgeons generally prefer to retain the iliac crest when feasible, particularly if a full-thickness bone graft is to be harvested.[48,57] This procedure will prevent an ugly deformity, allow for a ledge support for the belt, prevent a landslide hernia, and prevent injury to the epiphyseal plate in the younger patient.[20,57] The inner cortical plate is satisfactory for small and medium-sized corticocancellous segments as well as for the harvest of bone chips. Sparing the outer cortical plate reduces morbidity and postoperative pain by preventing transection of the tensor fascia lata and dissection of the gluteal musculature.[40] The outer cortical plate offers an easier exposure and allows larger segments to be harvested.

Surgical approach to the ilium. The patient is positioned so that the pelvis and shoulder are rotated away from the edge of the table at a 40-degree angle. This postion is best accomplished by the use of rolled towels. The knee is maintained in extension. Routine preparation and draping are carried out. The incision is made parallel to the iliac crest and below it, starting posterior to the anterior superior iliac spine while the skin is retracted medially. This procedure will prevent injury to the lateral cutaneous nerve of the thigh and place the scar well below the belt line.[18,20] The incision is then carried down to the fascia lata.

If the inner cortical plate has been selected, the dissection is continued to expose the insertion of the abdominal muscles to the crest. Sharp dissection is then used to reflect the abdominal muscles off the iliac crest down to the periosteal attachment of the

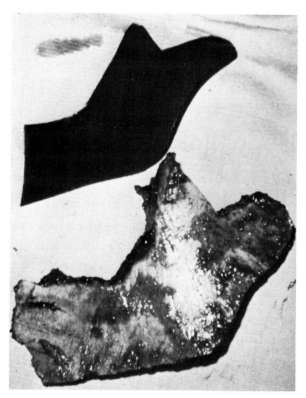

Fig. 30-15. Template and segment of the iliac bone as harvested from the donor site. Only minor adjustments will be required prior to fixation.

inner table of the ilium, which is then stripped away from the bone, with the iliac muscle. While the iliac muscle is retracted medially, an outline of the desired graft is made on the inner cortex with an osteotome or, more easily, with an air drill. The desired corticocancellous segment is then pried off. Additional bone chips can then be harvested. Special care has to be taken to prevent retro-peritoneal and intraperitoneal injuries and an expanding retroperitoneal hematoma.

If the outer cortical plate has been selected, a bold incision is made through the fascia lata and the underlying gluteal muscles down to the cortical bone 2 cm. below the curve of the crest. A subperiosteal dissection exposes the extent of bone required. It is generally desirable to have a pattern of the required graft available to position over the donor bone to determine the proper thickness and contour. Additional length has to be allowed for a satisfactory mortise to be made at the time of fixation of the graft to the host. A condyle, sigmoid notch, and even a coronoid, as described by Manchester,[47,48]

can be carved in continuity where required (Fig. 30-15). When the symphysis of the mandible is to be replaced, the area of the anterior superior iliac spine provides a very satisfactory substitute. The pattern has to be applied in such a fashion as to avoid the thin area of the iliac fossa. Millard and colleagues[57] have described bending the iliac bone graft for mandibular arch repairs by removing three wedges of the inner cortical and cancellous bone so that the graft may be bent to the proper contour. Additional bone chips should be secured to be applied at the line of the mortise as well as in the regions where the osteotomy of the graft has been needed to achieve the acquired contour. After the bone graft has been procured and the necessary hemostasis has been secured, a drain is inserted and the wound is closed in layers; special care is taken to properly approximate the tensor fascia lata to prevent the development of an abnormal gait caused by interference with the locking mechanism of the knee in extension. This approximation can be achieved by abducting the patient's hip by the addition of a rolled towel between the knees. A pressure dressing is applied at the termination of the procedure.

Rib. The rib has enjoyed a great popularity in mandibular grafting[9,56,58-60,62] because of its shape, contour, and malleability. However, its osteogenic potential and its resistance to heavy oral contamination is inferior to that of the iliac bone graft[28] probably because of the smaller amount of cancellous bone provided and the potentially poor vascularization when the graft is utilized with an intact cortex. The outer lateral curve of the rib matches the anterior curve of the horizontal portion of the mandible (Figs. 30-16 and 30-17). Whole-rib decortication compromises the strength of the graft to withstand stress. Whole ribs contoured to bridge the osseous gap have been used as rib grafts; fixation is accomplished by intramedullary Kirschner wire and wire loops at the junction. Rib and costal cartilage have also been used as rib grafts; the latter is shaped to fit into the glenoid of the temporomandibular joint.[11,28] Decortication of a single surface of the rib promotes early vascular penetration and osteogenesis. Bromberg and colleagues[9] have reported on the use of split ribs, popularized by Longacre for cranial defects.[42,43]

Surgical approach to the rib. Exposure is obtained through a standard thoracotomy approach overlying the seventh, eighth, or ninth rib. When a condylar head is needed, the cartilaginous portion of the rib is included in the extra periosteal rib resection and

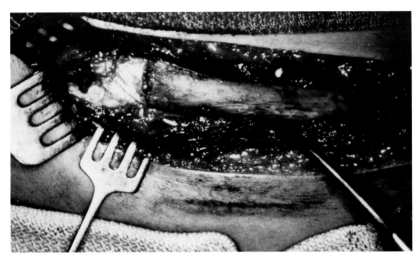

Fig. 30-16. Surgical exposure of the seventh rib and cartilage. The lateral curve of the rib matches that of the mandible. The cartilage can be carved into a condyle.

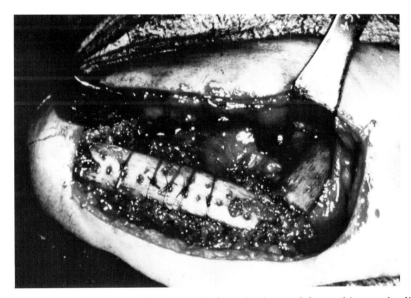

Fig. 30-17. Rib graft in its bed. Note partial decortication and bone chips at the line of mortise. Catgut ties reinforce deeper soft tissue approximation to the inner surface of the graft.

the outer surface of the periosteum is maintained with the graft. This procedure adds to the support of the external cortical layer at the time that the graft is contoured. When the rib is to be used as a whole graft, a Kirschner wire is drilled through it, and wedges of cortical cancellous bone are excised from the inner concave surface of the rib.[56,58-60] This procedure will allow the graft to match the contour of the symphysis.

Another method of approaching the rib consists of the insertion of a Kirschner wire in the rib graft and decortication of the anterior convex surface with a vertical osteotomy not extending into the posterior cortex to obtain the desired contour. The resultant open wedges are filled with cancellous iliac bone chips, which provide viable bone at the farthest point from the line of junction to the host. Additional bone chips at the mortise line will help

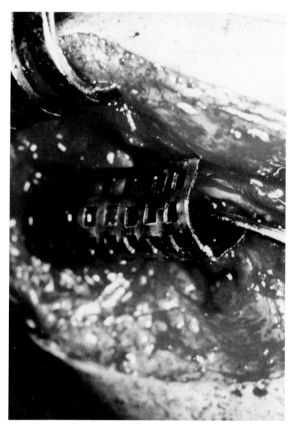

Fig. 30-18. Vitalium crib, a means of reinforcement of the lines of mortise, is fixed by screws to the mandibular stump and the graft.

promote union. Difficulty may be encountered in the proper insertion of the Kirschner wire when the rib graft is long and its natural curve is accentuated.

Bromberg and colleagues[9] have advocated fixating the host fragments with a Kirschner wire and the use of the two halves of the split rib bone grafts alongside the Kirschner wire; the cancellous portion of each is in direct contact with the soft tissue. These are then fixated to the host fragments.

Fixation of the bone graft to the mandibular stumps

The extraoral approach is usually preferred, particularly in delayed bone grafting; it prevents intraoral contamination and subsequent bone graft infection and loss. Skin and subcutaneous tissue offer better coverage and closure than the tenuous oral mucosa. Successful grafting can be achieved by the intraoral approach, but this method carries a higher incidence of complications.

In secondary bone grafting, soft tissue shrinkage has taken place; the bone graft must therefore be less bulky than the originally resected mandibular segment.

The graft bed must be adequately vascularized and free of infection. Scar tissue when present must be excised without penetration into the mouth. The ends of the stump must be denuded of the fibrous

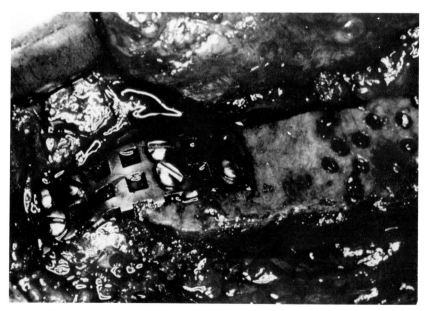

Fig. 30-19. Perforated Vitalium sheet immobilizes graft with screws.

tissue and freshened by partial decortication affording a contact surface of at least 2 to 3 cm. for the graft. A mortise has to be provided at the line of junction between the recipient fragments and the host, and is most easily achieved by surface-to-surface apposition of the cancellous bone (onlay of the graft on the host).[27,28,71] It can also be obtained by providing a slot in each mandibular stump into which the graft is fitted,[58,59] by providing the slot in the graft itself,[57] or by stepping. The preference in technique will depend on the configuration of the opposing bone ends.

Intraosseous fixation of the graft to the mandibular stump is achieved by transfixing the Kirschner wire (when used through the graft) by engaging the protruding ends of the wire into the mandibular stumps. Fixation is also achieved by the use of transosseous wire loops,[30] an additional small Kirschner wire, mesh cribs and screws,[8,36,37,62] or metal plates[14] (Figs. 30-18 and 30-19).

The addition of cancellous bone chips at the junctional area as well as along the course of the graft, particularly at the farthest point from the line of junction, promotes early vascular penetration and osteogenesis.

Drainage has been recommended,[48] particularly after primary bone grafting.[26] There is always a certain amount of resorption in the graft.

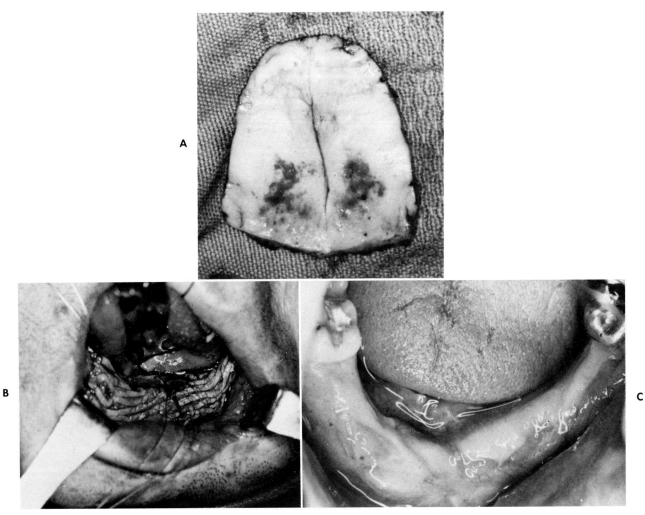

Fig. 30-20. A, Harvested palatal mucoperiosteum prior to meshing. **B,** Meshed palatal mucoperiosteal graft in recipient bed. **C,** Mandibular ridge after grafting. (From Morgan, R. L. and others: Plast. Reconstr. Surg. **51:**359. © 1973, The Williams & Wilkins Co., Baltimore.)

Postoperative immobilization

Adjuvant methods of immobilizing the grafted mandible are necessary until union between the graft and the host bone stumps occurs, usually in 8 to 12 weeks.[11] Persistence of the graft is dependent on adequate vascularization and the provision of undisturbed bony contact. The ultimate strength of the bone graft is dependent on the stress to which it is subjected.

When teeth are present in the mandibular stump and the maxillary arch, previously placed arch bars are put into intermaxillary fixation. When there are no teeth, acrylic splints are secured to the stable arch structure and put into intermaxillary fixation.[10]

In extensive grafts or where access to the oral cavity is needed postoperatively, the use of external fixation by the Morris biphase appliance has been very satisfactory.[5,29,66] Gaisford has reported the use of the Stader and Roger-Anderson splints.[30] The Morris biphase appliance is less bulky and obviates most of the problems encountered with the latter two splints.

Satisfactory contour and function are restored after the successful take of the mandibular bone graft.

RESTORATION OF AN ADEQUATE ALVEOLAR RIDGE AND SULCUS

Interference with the use of a satisfactory stable denture because of an inadequate sulcus or alveolar ridge is not infrequent. Gaisford[30] recommended cutting the overlying soft tissues, pushing them downward, and covering the bare bone with heavy aluminum foil, which is secured to the bone with wires. Normal-appearing mucosa creeps under the foil and over the bone graft, providing a satisfactory alveolar ridge.

MacIntosh and Obwegeser[46] have recommended vestibuloplasty by the use of skin grafts. Hall and O'Steen[34] have used free grafts of palatal mucosa (Fig. 30-20, *A*). To obtain better draping and more coverage, Morgan and colleagues[63] have illustrated the use of meshed free grafts of hard palate mucoperiosteum in seven patients, six of whom had received extensive bone grafts for submental losses of mandibular substance (Fig. 30-20, *B* and *C*). Extensive mobilization of the gingival edges is required on both sides of the mandible. The edges are maintained in their position by sutures fastened to the floor of the mouth and tied over the skin of the upper neck. Immobilization of the graft on the mandibular ridge is achieved by the use of a soft dental compound, which is kept on for 14 days. Although this method

seems very successful, it cannot be recommended in patients who have had leukoplakia of the palate.

SUMMARY

The major importance of the residual mandible in the management of patients with head and neck cancer has not been fully appreciated. Proper control of this bone and adequate replacement of the intraoral lining are our objectives at the time of the resection of the primary tumor; they may obviate the need for replacing the missing mandibular segment. If the bone must be replaced, this replacement is best accomplished by a secondary procedure using a carefully carved corticocancellous iliac bone graft supplemented by bone chips.

REFERENCES

1. Alonso, M. R., and Bailey, B. J.: Reconstruction of the mandible, Otolaryngol. Clin. North Am. **5:**501, 1972.
2. Anlyan, A. J.: Immediate reconstruction of mandibular defects with autogenous bone chip grafts, Am. J. Surg. **110:**564, 1965.
3. Anlyan, A. J., and Mannis, J. R.: Re-evaluation of bone chip grafts for mandibular defects, Am. Surg. **116:**606, 1968.
4. Ariel, I. M.: The treatment of tumors of the tongue. In Pack, G. T., and Ariel, I. M., editors: Treatment of cancer and allied diseases, vol. 3, ed. 2, New York, 1959, Paul Hoeber, Inc., p. 121.
5. Baumgarten, R. S., and Desprez, J. D.: The Morris bi-phasic external splint for mandible fixation, Plast. Reconstr. Surg. **50:**66, 1972.
6. Boyne, P. J.: Autogenous cancellous bone and marrow transplant, Clin. Orthop. **73:**119, 1970.
7. Boyne, P. J.: Transplantation, implantation and grafts, Dent. Clin. North Am. **15:**433, 1971.
8. Boyne, P. J., and Morgan, F.: Evaluation of a compression intraosseous fixation device in mandibular fractures, Oral Surg. **33:**695, 1972.
9. Bromberg, B. E., Song, I. C., and Craig, G. T.: Split rib mandibular reconstruction, Plast. Reconstr. **50:**357, 1972.
10. Bromberg, B. E., Walden, R. H., and Rubin, L. R.: Mandibular bone grafts; a Technique in fixation, Plast. Reconstr. Surg. **32:**589, 1963.
11. Brown, J. B., and Fryer, M. P.: Bone grafts for large gaps in the mandible, Am. J. Surg. **85:**401, 1953.
12. Brown, J. B., Fryer, M. P., and McDowell, F.: Internal wire pin immobilization of jaw fractures, Plast. Reconstr. Surg. **4:**30, 1949.
13. Byars, L. T., and McDowell, F.: Preservation of jaw function following surgery and trauma, Surg. Gynecol. Obstet. **84:**870, 1947.
14. Conley, J.: A technique of immediate bone grafting in the treatment of benign and malignant tumors of the mandible and the review of seventeen consecutive cases, Cancer **6:**568, 1953.
15. Conley, J.: The crippled oral cavity, Plast. Reconstr. Surg. **30:**469, 1962.

16. Conley, J.: Use of composite flaps containing bone for major repairs in the head and neck, Plast. Reconstr. Surg. **49:**522, 1972.

17. Conley, J., Cinelli, P. B., Johnson, P. M., and Koss, M.: Investigation in bone changes in composite flaps after transfer to the head and neck region, Plast. Reconstr. Surg. **51:**658, 1973.

18. Converse, J. M.: Reconstructive plastic surgery, vol. 1, Philadelphia, 1964, W. B. Saunders Co., p. 153.

19. Converse, J. M.: Reconstructive plastic surgery, vol. 2, Philadelphia, 1964, W. B. Saunders Co., pp. 450-496.

20. Converse, J. M., and Crockford, B. A.: The ilium as a source of bonegrafts in children, Plast. Reconstr. Surg. **50:**270, 1972.

21. Conway, H., and Murray, J. E.: Indications for reconstruction at the time of surgical excision of cancer of the oral cavity, Cancer **6:**46, 1953.

22. Cramer, L. M., and Culf, N. K.: Use of pedicle flap tissues in conjunction with a neck dissection. In Gaisford, J., editor: Symposium on cancer of the head and neck, St. Lous, 1969, The C. V. Mosby Co., p. 61.

23. Crenshaw, A. H.: Campbell's operative orthopedics, ed. 4, St. Louis, 1963, The C. V. Mosby Co., p. 57.

24. Cutright, D. E., Humsuck, E. E., and Beasley, J. D.: Fracture reduction using biodegradable material, polylactic acid, J. Oral Surg. **29:**393, 1971.

25. DeFries, H. O., Marble, H. B., and Shell, K. W.: Reconstruction of the mandible, Arch. Otolaryngol. **93:**426, 1971.

26. Desprez, J. D., and Kiehn, C. L.: Methods of reconstruction following resection of anterior oral cavity and mandible for malignancy, Plast. Reconstr. Surg. **24:**238, 1959.

27. Edgerton, M. T.: The mouth, tongue, jaws and salivary glands. In Sabiston, D. C., editor: Davis-Christopher textbook of surgery, Philadelphia, 1972, W. B. Saunders Co., p. 1265.

28. Edgerton, M. T., and Desprez, J. B.: Reconstruction of the oral cavity in the treatment of cancer: Plast. Reconstr. Surg. **19:**89, 1957.

29. Flemming, I. D., and Morris J. H.: Use of acrylic external splint after mandibular resection, Am. J. Surg. **118:**708, 1969.

30. Gaisford, J. C.: Reconstruction of head and neck deformities, Surg. Clin. North Am. **47:**295, 1967.

31. Gaisford, J. C., Hanna, D. C., and Gutman, D.: Management of the mandibular fragments following resection, Plast. Reconstr. Surg. **28:**192, 1961.

32. Gaisford, J. C., and Rueckert, F.: Osteoradionecrosis of the mandible, Plast. Reconstr. Surg. **18:**436, 1956.

33. Getter, R. L.: Fifth Annual Biomaterial Symposium, Clemson, S. C., April, 1973.

34. Hall, H. D., and O'Steen, A. N.: Free crafts of palatal mucosa in mandibular vestibuloplasty, J. Oral Surg. **28:**565, 1970.

35. Hamilton, J. M., and Hardy, S. B.: The use of the Webb bolt as a space maintaining appliance in defects of the mandible, Plast. Reconstr. Surg. **22:**296, 1958.

36. Harding, R. L.: Replantation of the mandible in cancer surgery, Plast. Reconstr. Surg. **19:**373, 1957; Plast. Reconstr. Surg. **48:**586, 1971.

37. Hinds, E. C., Spira, M., Sills, A. H., and Galbreath, J. C.: Use of tantalum trays in mandibular surgery, Plast. Reconstr. Surg. **32:**439, 1963.

38. Ivy, R. H.: Collective review; bone grafting for restoration of defects of the mandible, Plast. Reconstr. Surg. **7:**333, 1951.

39. Ivy, R. H.: Iliac bone graft to bridge a mandibular defect; 49 year clinical and radiological follow-up, Plast. Reconstr. Surg. **50:**483, 1972.

39a. Ketchum, L. D., Masters, F. W., Robinson, D. W.: Mandibular reconstruction using a composite island rib flap, Plast. Reconstr. Surg. **53:**471, 1974.

40. Leake, D. L., and Rappaport, M.: Mandibular reconstruction; bone induction in aloplastic tray, Surgery **72:**332, 1972.

41. Levy, R. N., and Siffert, R. S.: Inner table Iliac bone grafts, Surg. Gynecol. Obstet. **128:**605, 1969.

42. Longacre, J. J.: Surgical correction of extensive defects of scalp and cranium with autogenous tissues; transactions First International Congress, Plastic Surgery, Baltimore, Md., 1957; p. 346. The Williams & Wilkins Co.

43. Longacre, J. J., and DeStefano, G. A.: Further observations of the behavior of autogenous split rib grafts in reconstruction of extensive defects of the cranium and face, Plast. Reconstr. Surg. **20:**281, 1957.

44. Loré, J. M.: An atlas of head and neck surgery, Philadelphia, 1962, W. B. Saunders Co., p. 153.

45. Luhr, H. G.: In Conley, J. and Dickinson, J. T. editors: Plastic and reconstructive surgery of the face and neck; proceedings of the First International Symposium, Vol. 2, New York, 1972, Grune & Stratton, Inc., p. 47.

46. MacIntosh, R. B., and Obwegeser, H. L.: Preprosthetic surgery; a scheme for its effective employment, J. Oral Surg. **25:**397, 1967.

47. Manchester, W. M.: Immediate reconstruction of the mandible and temporomandibular joint, Br. J. Plast. Surg. **18:**291, 1965.

48. Manchester, W. M.: Some technical improvement in the reconstructions of the mandible and temporomandibular joint, Plast. Reconstr. Surg. **50:**249, 1972.

49. Marble, H. B., Boyne, P. J., and others: Grafts of cancellous bone and marrow for restoration of avulsion defects of the mandible; report of two cases, J. Oral Surg. **28:**138, 1970.

50. Marchetta, F. C., Sako, K., and Murphy, J. B.: The periosteum of the mandible and intraoral carcinoma, Am. J. Surg. **122:**711, 1971.

51. Martin, H.: Surgery of head and neck tumors, New York, 1957, P. B. Hoeber Inc., p. 59.

52. McGregor, I. A.: The temporal flap in intraoral reconstruction. In: Gaisford, J. C., editor: Symposium on cancer of the head and neck, St. Louis, 1969, The C. V. Mosby Co., p. 72-88.

52a. McKee, D.: Microvascular rib transposition for reconstruction of the mandible. Presented at the annual meeting of the American Society of Plastic and Reconstructive Surgeons, Montreal, Canada, 1971.

53. McQuarrie, D. G.: Reconstruction of the mandible with a simple prosthesis at the time of radical surgery

for oral carcinoma; report of thirteen cases, Lancet 88:282, 1968

54. McQuarrie, D. G.: Immediate functional restoration of the mandible after surgical treatment of advanced oral cancer; a simple prosthesis, Arch. Surg. **102**:447, 1971.

55. Millard, D. R.: Immediate reconstruction of the lower jaw, Plast. Reconstr. Surg. **35**:60, 1965.

56. Millard, D. R., Campbell, R. C., Stokely, P., and Garst, W.: Interim report on immediate mandibular repair, Am. J. Surg. **118**:729, 1969.

57. Millard, D. R., Deane, M., and Garst, W. T.: Bending an iliac bone graft for anterior mandibular arch repair, Plast. Reconstr. Surg. **48**:600, 1971.

58. Millard, D. R., Maisels, D. O., and Batstone, J. H. F.: Immediate repair of radical resection of the anterior arch of the lower jaw, Plast. Reconstr. Surg. **39**:153, 1967.

59. Millard, D. R., and others: Immediate reconstruction of the resected mandibular arch, Am. J. of Surg. **114**:605, 1967.

60. Millard, D. R., and others: Composite lower jaw reconstruction, Plast. Reconstr. Surg. **46**:22, 1970.

61. Mladick, R. A., and others: A simple technique for securing a K-wire to the mandible, Plast. Reconstr. Surg. **49**:228, 1972.

62. Mohnac, A. M.: Gross loss of mandibular hard structure, J. Oral Surg. **27**:508, 1969.

63. Morgan, L. R., Gallegos, L. T., and Frileck, S. P.: Mandibular vestibuloplasty with a free graft of the mucoperioteal layer from the hard palate, Plast. Reconstr. Surg. **51**:359, 1973.

64. Morris, J. H.: Biphase connector, external skeletal splint for reduction and fixation of mandibular fractures, Oral Surg. **11**:1382, 1949.

65. Mowlem, R.: Bone grafting, Br. J. Plast. Surg. **16**:293, 1963.

66. Parsons, R. W., and others: Surgical rehabilitation after extensive losses in the lower face from war injuries, Plast. Reconstr. Surg. **49**:533, 1972.

67. Richter, H. E., and Boyne, P. J.: New concepts in facial bone healing and grafting procedures, J. Oral Surg. **27**:557, 1969.

68. Rowe, N. L., and Killey, H. C.: Fractures of the facial skeleton, ed. 2, Baltimore, Md., 1968, The Williams & Wilkins Co.

69. Snyder, C. C., Bateman, J. M., and others: Mandibulofacial restoration with live osteocutaneous flaps, Plast. Reconstr. Surg. **45**:14, 1970.

70. Snyder, C. C., Levine, G. E., and Dingman, D. L.: Trial of a sternoclavicular whole joint graft as a substitute for the temporomandibular joint, Plast. Reconstr. Surg. **48**:447, 1971.

71. Straith, C. L.: A morticed mandibular bone graft following giant cell tumor removal, Plast. Reconstr. Surg. **4**:282, 1949.

72. Strauch, B., Bloomberg, A., and Lewin, M.: Artery island, composite rib grafts for mandibular replacement, Surg. Forum **20**:516, 1969.

73. Swanson, L. T., Habel, M. B., and others: compound silicone-bone implants for mandibular reconstruction, Plast. Reconstr. Surg. **51**:402, 1973.

Chapter 31

Role of surgical measures in voice restoration after laryngectomy

Donald P. Shedd, M.D.

The inclusion of a chapter on speech rehabilitation in a book on head and neck surgery is indicative of the present level of interest in surgical measures in this field. This wave of interest followed the work of Asai[1] of Japan, whose report described a three-staged method of creating a pharyngotracheal fistula.

The reasons for a resurgence of interest in surgical measures for speech rehabilitation are:

1. A significant number of laryngectomees, possibly 50%, do not achieve good esophageal speech.
2. The electrolarynx is not acceptable to many patients as a substitute voice.
3. An increasing number of patients are now undergoing an extended pharyngolaryngectomy, and these patients only rarely have enough muscle function to develop esophageal speech.
4. Some investigators working with the new air tunnel methods are strongly impressed with the fact that most patients so treated can obtain a strong, dependable voice within a few weeks of operation.

HISTORICAL SUMMARY

Surgical approaches to speech rehabilitation are not new. In the earliest laryngectomies a fistula was deliberately left in the patient to be used for speech purposes. The idea of putting reed sound through the fistula was reported in the United States as early as 1886 by Roswell Park of Buffalo, N.Y.[6] The idea of transferring air alone from the trachea to the esophagus was utilized early by a patient who made the fistula himself, using an ice pick. Over a considerable period of years, fistula methods were not used, largely because primary closure of the pharynx had become the standard practice. The prevailing method of speech rehabilitation was esophageal speech, and later the electrolarynx was added.

In 1958 Briani[2] of Italy described a simple method using an appliance to transfer air from the trachea to the pharynx, and later various other workers attempted to use this method by creating surgical tunnels in stages. The work of Asai was impressive in this area and was corroborated by Miller[4] in the United States. It was apparent to those working in this field that there were problems involved in the construction of dependable air tunnels and that the three stages were a disadvantage.

Taub[8] reintroduced the idea of using a reed, but then shifted over to an air tunnel method. The reed concept was developed further by the group at the Roswell Park Memorial Institute (RPMI),[7] where there were a number of pharyngolaryngectomy patients who needed such a method if they were to talk at all.

McGrail and Oldfield,[3] Montgomery,[5] and Taub described useful variations of air tunnel methods. Each of these variations was an attempt to eliminate some of the problems and disadvantages associated with previous air tunnel methods. Montgomery described a two-staged procedure that he used on suitable patients. He created a small pharyngocutaneous fistula at the time of the laryngectomy, and a few weeks after this procedure he made a surgical tunnel connecting the cutaneous outlet to the tracheostomy.

Taub utilized a lateral esophageal fistula and also developed a differential valve that eliminated the need for the patient to use his finger for occlusion of the tracheal outflow in speech. McGrail and Oldfield utilized a deltopectoral flap to make a tracheopharyngeal air tunnel at the time of laryngectomy.

RECENT STUDIES AT THE RPMI
Investigators

The work described was done by a group consisting of: (1) surgeons—D. Shedd, K. Sako, and V. Bakamjian of the RPMI; (2) maxillofacial prosthodontists—N. Schaaf and W. Carl of the RPMI; and (3) Speech pathologist—M. Mann of the Department of Speech Communications, State University of New York at Buffalo, and B. Weinberg, Director, Speech Research Laboratory, University of Indiana.

Reed-fistula methods

The original report from the RPMI described a reed-fistula method used on seven patients. In this method a fistula is made at the time of the pharyngolaryngectomy as part of the deltopectoral flap

reconstruction. This fistula is subsequently used as a route for the introduction of sound that is produced in an external appliance containing a reed. The reed is actuated by expired air from the trachea. In one patient who was carefully tested, the quality of speech was very good, ranking slightly above a comparison sample of excellent esophageal speech. Since the first report, four additional patients have been studied, and the place of the method has been further defined. The patients in the original report were all men, but one of the later patients was a woman. We were concerned about whether a satisfactory female pitch could be obtained and found that modifying the reed made this pitch possible.

There are problems and pitfalls involved with procedures of this complexity, the most important of which is the management of the fistula. Making a good fistula in which the appliance can control salivary leakage is not easy, but it is now possible to do so. Careful selection of patients is important, because managing the fistula and the appliance require motivation and skill; a few of the older patients have not possessed the degree of skill necessary to handle the appliance. For the successful pa-

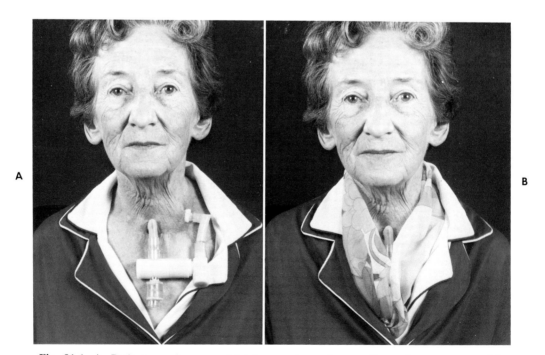

Fig. 31-1. A, Patient wearing a reed-fistula speech appliance after a laryngectomy with extensive pharyngoesophageal resection. **B,** Patient with a speech appliance partly concealed by overlying clothing.

tients the inconvenience of the fistula is a small price to pay for good vocal communication (Fig. 31-1).

Air tunnel method

For patients undergoing straight laryngectomy, a method that would be simple and dependable was sought. A system that would not involve a permanent direct tracheal esophageal fistula was desired. We decided to make a simple pharyngocutaneous fistula at the time of the laryngectomy, and we then used an external appliance to connect the fistula to the trachea. Some of our fistulas were made in the manner of Montgomery, which depends on the presence of an adequate residual esophageal mucosa at the end of the resection. Others were made from tubulated flaps of cervical skin. In patients with the best fistulas, leakage was a negligible problem; in others it was an inconvenience. Some patients wore foam plastic plugs to control the leakage.

The appliances are made by the Department of Maxillo Facial Prosthetics of Silastic (Dow Corning Co.), and are a simple **T** connection from the trachea

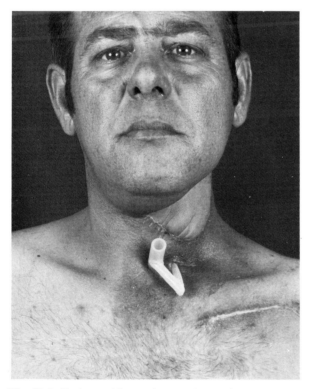

Fig. 31-2. Patient with an air tunnel speech appliance in place. Fistula is a low upward-directed tunnel close to the tracheal opening.

to the fistula. The patient breathes through one limb of the **T**, and when he wishes to talk, he occludes with his finger the tracheal outflow, diverting expired air into the pharynx, where vibrations are set up for speech purposes (Fig. 31-2). A commercially made valve is available for the patient who wishes to eliminate the use of the finger.

Eleven patients have been managed in this manner to date. It is impressive to see a competent patient begin to speak immediately when the appliance is fitted a few weeks after the laryngectomy; at this time he can speak with relative ease and with minimal instruction. We do recommend instruction, however, because communication of a much better quality will result. The voice has about the same quality as esophageal speech, but the phrasing is longer, and some can achieve good volume because of the strong air supply from the trachea.

The problems of air tunnel methods are less complicated than those of the reed-fistula method, because smaller fistulas and a simpler appliance are used. We have had the difficulty of stenosis of the tunnel occurring in one patient who had an inflammatory stricture. Patients with severe chronic bronchitis who have a heavy output of sputum have problems wearing any type of appliance that connects to the trachea.

On the whole, our impression is that the air tunnel method is useful in carefully selected patients who are intelligent and have good motivation. Such a patient can be assured of satisfactory speech a few weeks after the laryngectomy. If he should develop over the course of time good esophageal speech by the traditional method, the fistula can simply be closed.

PRESENT VIEWS ON PROCEDURES OF CHOICE

Experience with surgical methods of speech rehabilitation at the RPMI has led us to the conclusion that such approaches have a place in appropriate laryngectomees. For the patient undergoing a pharyngolaryngectomy, the reed-fistula method is a way of restoring good communication. For patients having a standard laryngectomy, the air tunnel technique will provide early restoration of vocal communication in a dependable manner. Both methods involve pitfalls and difficulties that the surgeons and the patient must acknowledge and accept as the price for speech rehabilitation.

For the patient who has undergone laryngectomy in the past and who has failed to develop adequate esophageal speech despite good teaching, one can consider rehabilitation by the air tunnel method if the patient is found to be suitable.

REFERENCES

1. Asai, R.: Laryngoplasty after total laryngectomy, Arch. Otolaryngol. **95:**114-119, 1972.
2. Briani, A. A.: Il ricupero sociale dei laryngectomizzati attraverso un metodo personale operatorio, Medicina Sociale **8:**265-269, 1958.
3. McGrail, J., and Oldfield, D.: One stage operation for vocal rehabilitation at laryngectomy, Trans. Am. Acad. Ophthalmol. Otolaryngol. **75:**510-512, 1971.
4. Miller, A.: Experience with Asai technique, J. Laryngol. Otol. **85:**567-567, 1971.
5. Montgomery, W.: Postlaryngectomy vocal rehabilitation, Arch. Otolaryngol. **95:**76-83, 1972.
6. Park, R.: A case of total extirpation of the larynx, Ann. Surg. **3:**28, 1886.
7. Shedd, D., Bakamjian, V., Sako, K., Mann, M., Barba, S., and Schaaf, N.: Reed fistula method of speech rehabilitation after laryngectomy, Am. J. Surg. **124:**510-514, 1972.
8. Taub, S., and Bergner, L.: Air bypass voice prosthesis, Am. J. Surg. **125:**748-756, 1973.

Chapter 32

Social rehabilitation of the patient with head and neck cancer

William P. Graham III, M.D.
Ronald H. Rosillo, M.D.

Cancer should be considered a chronic illness. The prognosis of maxillofacial cancer is often more favorable than the prognosis of a variety of other chronic illnesses or disabilities. Consequently, the social rehabilitation of the patient with maxillofacial cancer should not be much different from that of patients with rheumatoid arthritis or chronic heart disease.

The presence of maxillofacial cancer and its treatment often threaten almost every aspect of the patient's life, affecting his financial security, social behavior, and familiar patterns of adaptation. The loss or the threat of loss of certain senses, a source of important functions and pleasures, (taste, smell, and vision), occurs either through treatment or the cancer itself. The organs involved not only create attendant body image problems, but in addition they are publicly exposed, which produces an additional burden for the patient to bear.

The psychologic impact of head and neck cancer in a large number of patients leads to a significant decrement in work, social, and sexual activities beyond that caused by the physical disabilities resulting from the lesion and its treatment.[6]

Obviously, a low morale in patients is significantly related to poor progress in rehabilitation. Imboden and colleagues have shown that in certain illnesses the patients with slow recoveries can be dif-

ferentiated from the ones with faster recoveries early in their treatment by the state of their morale.[4]

Those patients who are likely to return to work after successful treatment of their cancer can be predicted by psychologic tests that assess their morale level and their degree of covert anxiety at the onset of therapy.[8]

The social rehabilitation of the patient with head and neck cancer begins the first moment he makes contact with his physician. The presence or absence of a hopeful attitude on the part of the physician might weigh heavily in the success or failure of the patient's eventual reintegration into the community. Attempts at rehabilitation should not begin when social problems or maladjustments appear; rather, these attempts should begin before the problems do appear. By raising issues in a considerate manner with the patient, the physician does not create additional problems; rather, he tries to prevent them.

The better the surgeon and the team know the patient, the more effective their approach will be. Knowledge of the patient's personality, patterns of adaptation, and previous and present coping behavior is essential. No less essential is the determination of the importance of the appearance and function of those organs affected by the malignancy and its treatment in maintaining the patient's self-esteem.

Good psychologic preparation prior to treatment is mandatory for allaying realistic and unrealistic fears. Encouraging the patient to verbalize feelings

Supported in part by a grant from the Irvin Zubar Memorial Cancer Fund.

215

includes asking the patient to repeat back what has been explained to him.

Almost all patients initially attempt to maintain the same pattern of adaptation and behavior that they displayed prior to the appearance of disease. Such behavior should be encouraged only to the extent that it is realistic. The patient must be encouraged to take the initiative in seeking solutions. Changes in his pattern of coping should be brought about in a progressive and gentle fashion so that the patient does not reject the changes and experience further deepening of any attendant depression.

While hospitalized, if feasible, the patient should be encouraged to go on outings with relatives or friends. Such social activities will assist him in becoming reintegrated in his community. On his return to the hospital from every outing, an opportunity to vocalize his feelings should be provided, as well as emotional support if needed.

Not only must emotional support be given to these patients, but the results and complications of their treatment must be anticipated and managed. Attention must be directed to future cosmetic and functional defects. Treating these losses requires a team approach (see list below) and individualization of the treatment based on the particular patient, the duration of the proposed rehabilitation program, economic factors, and the availability of appropriate specialists.[1]

Family physician
Surgeon
   Head and neck surgeon
   Oral surgeon
   Otolaryngologist
   Plastic and reconstructive surgeon
   Surgical oncologist
Radiotherapist
Dentist
Prosthodontist
Physical therapist
Psychiatrist
Psychologist
Speech therapist
Nurse
Dietician
Social worker
Vocational rehabilitator
Medical oncologist

Many of the problems of these patients after treatment can be likened to those of the individual with a severe craniofacial anomaly. Lessons can be taken from F. Monasterio's fine analysis of the specialist's role in treating craniofacial anomalies.[5] Monasterio has graphically illustrated the points in therapy at which a certain specialist might become involved in treating individuals with congenital maxillofacial disorders. A similar analysis could be made for treating the patient with maxillofacial cancer. This integrated therapy, given from the preoperative period to the final phase of rehabilitation, involves anticipation, execution, and follow-up. In the midst of the specialists the family physician, who may have to counsel and console the patient or his family at times of unexpected stress (even after a successful recovery), will be most important.

The physical rehabilitation of the patient may be surgical, prosthetic, or a combination of the two (Figs. 32-1 to 32-3). A better decision for management might be made by a team of specialists than by an individual specialist alone. No two patients' problems are identical, and rote treatment may yield unsatisfactory overall results.

When a protracted course of reconstructive surgery is undertaken, several considerations are paramount. The individual hospitalizations for each surgical procedure must be kept as brief as possible, and the projected number of surgical procedures must be as accurate as possible; the ability of the patient to remain a social being between procedures is imperative, and possible complications should be accurately portrayed. With each future operation, no matter how minor, the patient might reexperience the anxieties that he endured at the time of the initial operation for the removal of cancer. Similarly, when additional operative steps become necessary in the course of reconstruction, the unprepared patient may lose confidence and decide that he is no longer free of cancer.

The patient's appearance during his reconstructive phase is important, because as long as he can physically face the public, either with skillful dressings or a temporary prosthesis, he is more likely to do so. The use of a cervical pharyngostomy avoids the tell-tale "elephant trunk" appearance of a nasogastric feed tube that turns patients with head and neck cancer into recluses[2] (Fig. 32-4).

Not to be overlooked are the prospects of retraining the employable individual, but employability cannot be the only yardstick by which successful treatment is gauged. Rosillo and Graham[6] have shown that nearly half (44%) of their patients cured of maxillofacial cancer display a poor long-term adjustment in the areas of work, social, and sexual functioning. Schonfield,[7] in evaluating patients who had no recurrence of cancer 9 months after initial treatment concluded "that a patient's psychological status

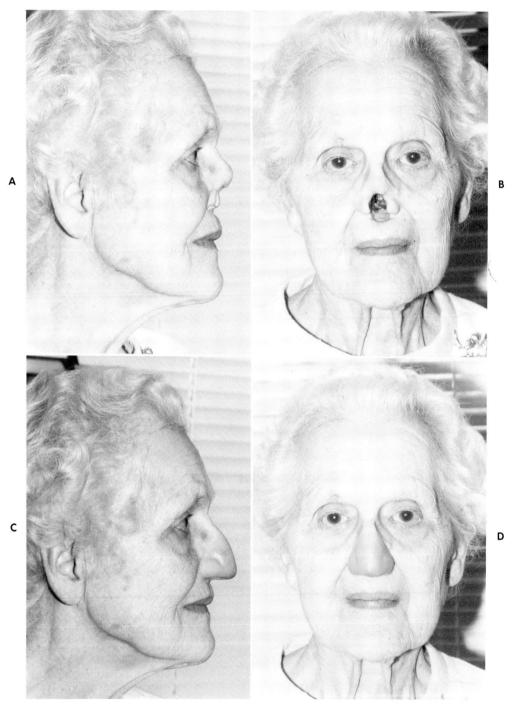

Fig. 32-1. Prosthetic replacement of the nose of an elderly lady who was treated by excision and radiation therapy for squamous cell carcinoma of the nasal septum.

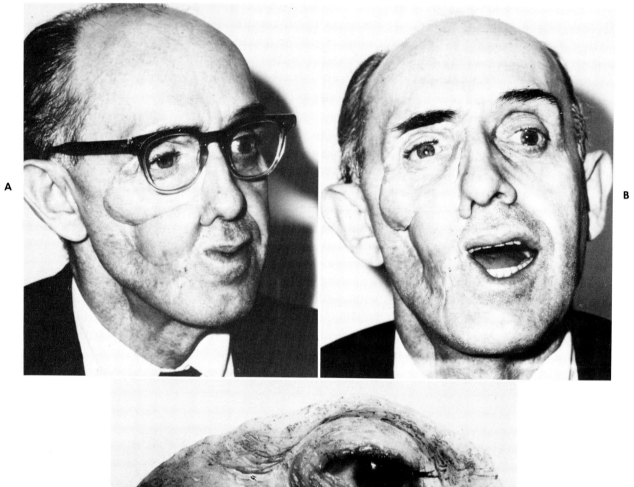

Fig. 32-2. Elderly gentleman with squamous cell carcinoma of the maxillary antrum who was treated by surgical excision, reconstruction of the cheek skin with a thoracic flap, and the fabrication of a prosthetic eye and malar prominence. (**B** From Welty, M. J., Graham, W. P. III, and Rosillo, R. H.: Nurs. Clin. North Am. **8**(1):137-151, 1973, W. B. Saunders Co., Philadelphia.)

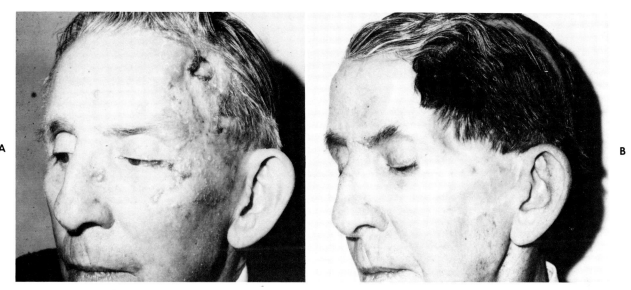

Fig. 32-3. Elderly gentleman who was treated for diffuse facial basal cell carcinoma by excision, skin grafting, and a rotated scalp flap.

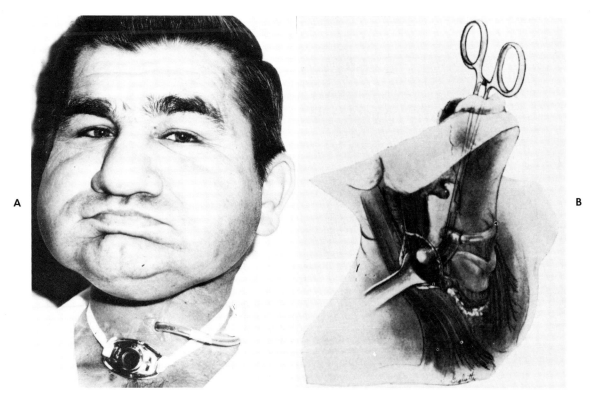

Fig. 32-4. A, Patient with a cervical pharyngostomy tube in place. The low placement of the tube makes it easily concealed by clothing. **B,** Cervical pharyngostomy technique. (**B** From Royster, H. P., and others: Am. J. Surg. **116:**611, 1968.)

at the time of diagnosis and initiation of treatment may influence his subsequent return to an earlier life style."

Last, the etiologic factors in these malignancies must be considered. Because many of the patients who acquire squamous cell carcinoma of the oral cavity are alcoholics, rehabilitation may be a doubly difficult task.[3] Continued personal abuse with alcohol and tobacco may increase the patient's future susceptibility to oral, esophageal, or lung cancer. It is frustrating to the physician and demoralizing to the patient if he survives one malignancy only to experience a second one several years later.

The use of many community resources, such as workshops, retaining, counseling, and joint meetings with patients and families, as needed along the course of the patient's rehabilitation will significantly assist in his resocialization. The ultimate goal is to help the patient maintain his morale and return to as productive and meaningful a life as possible.

REFERENCES

1. Graham, W. P., and Lapidus, S. M.: Rehabilitation of the head and neck cancer patient, J. Pa. Osteo. Med. Assoc. **15**(4):6, 1973.

2. Graham, W. P., and Royster, H. P.: Simplified cervical esophagostomy for long term extra-oral feeding, Surg. Gynecol. Obstet. **125**:127, 1967.

3. Kissin, B. Kaley, M. M., Su, W. H., and Lerner, R.: Head and neck cancer in alcoholics; the relationship to drinking, smoking and dietary patterns, J.A.M.A. **224**:1174, 1973.

4. Miller, R. N.: Psychological problems of patients with head and neck cancer. In: Rehabilitation of the cancer patient, Chicago, 1972, Year Book Medical Publishers, Inc., p. 19.

5. Monasterio, F.: A system for the training of a team for craniofacial surgery. Presented at the Fifty-second Annual Meeting of the American Association of Plastic Surgeons, New York, 1973.

6. Rosillo, R. H., and Graham, W. P.: The long term adjustment of the patient with head and neck cancer following successful treatment. I. Work, social and heterosexual activity levels, J. Surg. Oncol. **4**:439, 1972.

7. Schonfield, J.: Psychological and other factors affecting return to gainful employment after remission of cancer following radiotherapy. Presented at the Forty-seventh Annual Meeting of the American Congress of Rehabilitation Medicine, New York, 1970.

8. Schonfield, J.: Psychological factors related to delayed return to an earlier life-style in successfully treated cancer patients, J. Psychosom. Res. **16**:41-46, 1972.

Chapter 33

Maxillofacial prosthetics for the patient with head and neck cancer

Norman G. Schaaf, D.D.S.

The plastic and reconstructive surgeon should have available the services of a maxillofacial prosthodontist for complete reconstruction of the patient with head and neck cancer to be accomplished. The multidisciplinary approach, with a realization of fuller cooperation between plastic surgeons and prosthodontists, is certainly more of a reality today.

By definition, "Maxillofacial Prosthetics is the art and science of anatomic, functional and cosmetic reconstruction, by the use of non-living substitutes, of those regions in the maxillae, mandible and face that are missing or defective."[1] The maxillofacial prosthodontist is usually a dentist who has had 2 years of postgraduate training in prosthodontics, the study of prostheses to be used in the oral cavity, plus an additional hospital-oriented year of experience in the use of the prostheses for the head and neck area in general (maxillofacial prosthetics). The National Cancer Institute is now supporting the training of these specialists and that of laboratory technicians; additional help for cancer centers and hospitals is thus on its way.

At various times during his course of treatment, the patient with head and neck cancer can be benefitted by the use of prostheses.

CLASSIFICATION

The following is one method of classifying prostheses for the patient with head and neck cancer:

A. Facial prostheses
   1. Nasal
   2. Orbital
   3. Auricular
   4. Composite
B. Intraoral prostheses
   1. Obturators (postoperative)
   2. Speech aids
   3. Complete and partial dentures (modified)
   4. Feeding prostheses
C. Treatment prostheses
   1. Obturators (surgical)
   2. Stents
   3. Splints
   4. Flange prostheses
   5. Prosthetic dressings
   6. Mandibular exercisers
D. Implants
   1. Mandibular (metal)
   2. Facial (silicone rubber)

To clarify this classification, each type of prosthesis is discussed.

Facial prostheses

The most commonly used materials for facial prostheses are silicone rubber (Silastic), polyvinyl chloride, acrylic, or polyurethane. All of the materials have certain shortcomings but are successfully used. The prostheses are usually held on the face by the use of skin adhesives, but occasionally they can be retained by undercuts in the facial defect or by mechanical means (elastics around the head).

Nasal. The loss of external nasal tissue is quite common because of the necessary treatment of basal cell carcinoma in this area. The surgeon frequently

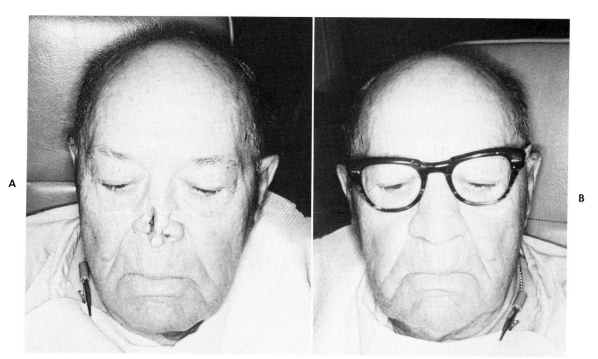

Fig. 33-1. A, Nasal defect after chemosurgery for basal cell carcinoma. **B,** Silicone rubber nose prosthesis colored by a tattooing procedure.

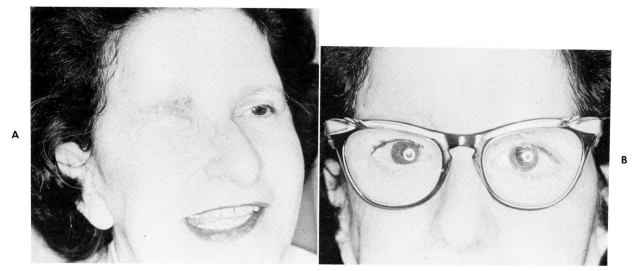

Fig. 33-2. A, Facial defect after surgical exenteration of the orbit. **B,** Silicone rubber orbital prosthesis with an acrylic ocular section.

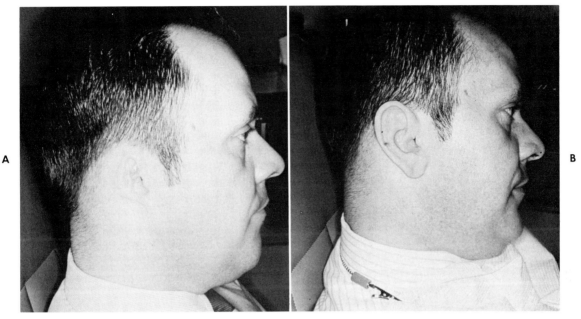

Fig. 33-3. A, Loss of all of the external ear structure after necessary cancer surgery. **B,** Silicone rubber auricular prosthesis retained by skin adhesive.

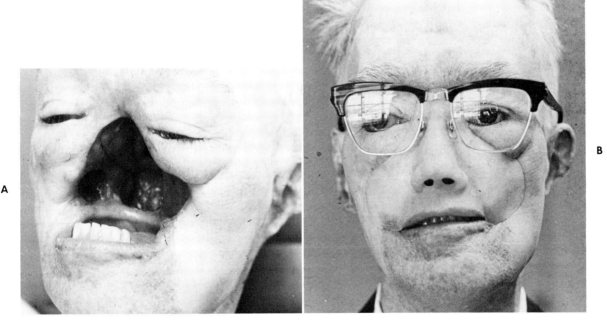

Fig. 33-4. A, Facial defect after many years of treatment for both basal cell and squamous cell carcinoma. **B,** Polyvinyl chloride facial prosthesis allows the patient to return to work.

delays reconstruction in many patients because of the possibility that the disease will continue. Because the nose is a rather discrete portion of the face, the use of a prosthesis makes the patient's appearance acceptable (Fig. 33-1).

Orbital. There is as yet no surgical reconstructive procedure to replace the total eye with its attachments. The patient in whom all of the orbital contents have been removed as a result of necessary tumor surgery is suited for a prosthesis because of the definitively outlined margins. These prostheses

are frequently successful; however, the patient must accept certain limitations. The eyeball will not move in harmony with the other eye, nor will the eyelids blink. Eyeglasses with heavy rims and possibly tinted lenses help to enhance the overall appearance (Fig. 33-2).

Auricular. When all of the external ear has been lost because of necessary cancer surgery, the area does not lend itself easily to surgical reconstruction. On the other hand, the prosthetic ear is perhaps the most readily accepted facial prosthesis that is con-

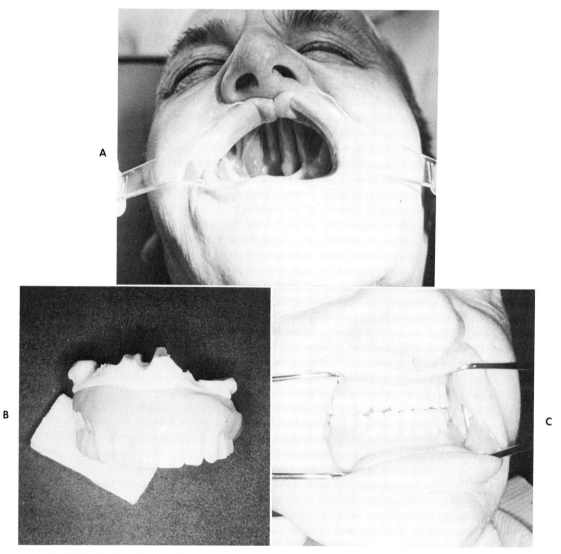

Fig. 33-5. **A,** Maxillary defect after surgical treatment for squamous cell carcinoma of the palate. **B,** Maxillary obturator with silicone rubber tissue section. **C,** Maxillary obturator separates the nasal cavity from the oral cavity for appropriate speech and mastication.

structed. It is also the facial prosthesis most often retained by adhesives, although surgically prepared skin loops can be used where possible (Fig. 33-3).

Composite. With more extensive surgery to save the cancer patient, larger facial defects are encountered. Although larger prostheses are not as esthetically acceptable, they can be used in situations where surgical reconstruction is not possible. In addition to creating esthetic problems, the larger facial defects frequently compromise vital functions such as speech and mastication, so patients usually accept the prosthesis as an integral part of their rehabilitation (Fig. 33-4).

Intraoral prostheses

Most prostheses used in the oral cavity are dependent on the teeth or a stable denture for stability. It is important for the cancer patient to retain every tooth possible so that a prosthesis can be retained. Consultation with the prosthodontist prior to the cancer surgery can be helpful in getting the patient in the best possible dental and oral condition to receive a prosthesis after surgery.

Obturators (postoperative). When the surgical defect is an extension of the oral cavity, numerous oral functions of the patient are disturbed. Speech is defective because air flows into other cavities in an uncontrolled fashion; mastication is difficult because food goes into the surgical defect; deglutition is disturbed because of the difficulty in managing the defect. A prosthesis that closes an opening is called an obturator. Palatal obturators are most commonly prepared for patients who have had a maxillectomy. The restoration of appropriate speech generally gives the patient a significant psychologic boost (Fig. 33-5).

Speech aids. With the loss of appropriate function of the velopharyngeal opening because of a pharyngectomy or soft palate surgery, the patient exhibits nasal emission of air and nasality of speech. The speech aid is an extension of an oral prosthesis (complete denture or partial denture) and functionally reacts with residual pharyngeal musculature to approach normal speech.

Complete and partial dentures (modified). Because of the many varied surgical procedures that are done in the oral cavity, it is necessary to construct unusual modifications of oral prostheses. Dentures that plump the lips after surgery and supply missing portions of the alveolar process and teeth are commonly prepared.

Food guides. Difficulties in deglutition result from surgical procedures that involve the floor of the mouth, base of the tongue, and epiglottis. Surgical or prosthetic reconstruction of the tongue have not been very successful, but it is possible to construct prostheses that will guide liquids and semiliquids into the esophagus (Fig. 33-6). In these instances the patient cannot chew, because the tongue is not available to continually replace the food onto the chewing surfaces of the teeth.

Treatment prostheses

Although the definition of maxillofacial prosthetics states that the prosthetic reconstruction re-

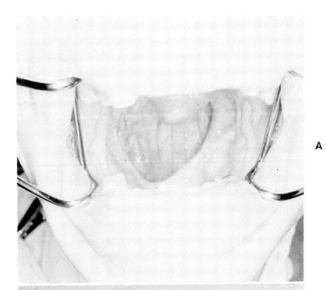

A

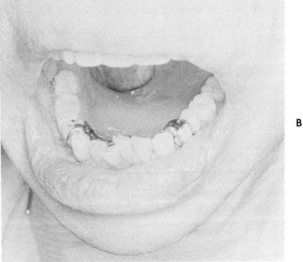

B

Fig. 33-6. A, Floor of the mouth area showing airway and foodway after complete glossectomy. **B,** Prosthesis is in place to guide food into the esophagus.

places portions of the head and neck that are missing or defective, many prostheses are prepared that are actually necessary in the active treatment of the patient. Most often these prostheses are used to fill out tissue spaces or hold two tissue fragments in relation to each other.

Obturators (surgical). Like the postoperative obturator, the surgical obturator most commonly closes an opening in the palate. However, it is put into place while the patient is in the operating room and thus also serves to hold packs in place and support the face on the side being operated on. With such a prosthesis the patient is not faced with the defect on awakening from anesthesia and frequently does not require a nasogastric tube for feeding (Fig. 33-7).

Stents. These prostheses are used to plump out or fill in tissue spaces. Frequently they are an extension of another oral prosthesis that serves to carry a split-thickness skin graft to place, such as into the floor of the mouth after a hemiglossectomy or into the maxilla after an antrectomy.

Splints. When it has been necessary to split the mandible during cancer surgery, a dental splint is useful to maintain the mandibular segments in relation to each other until union has occurred. The splint can be accurately attached to the teeth or wired to the bony segments for rigid stability.

Flange prostheses. Frequently when one side of the mandible has been resected, the remaining segment deviates toward the affected side because of

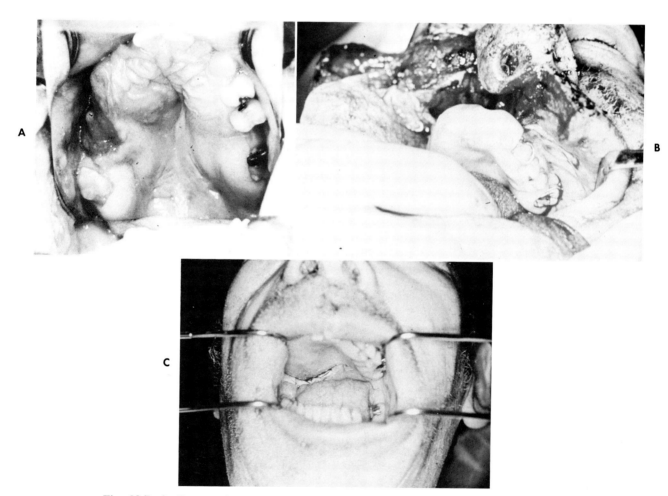

Fig. 33-7. A, Preoperative appearance of a maxillary tumor. **B,** Placement of surgical prosthesis. **C,** Immediate postoperative appearance. This prosthesis restores the palatal contours and allows appropriate function.

the muscle pull. The result is a patient who has difficulty in mastication and speech. When the patient has a sufficient number of stable teeth, it is possible to construct a prosthesis that will return the mandibular segment to an appropriate relationship with the maxilla and maintain it there while the patient chews in a nearly normal fashion (Fig. 33-8).

Prosthetic dressings. Immediately after surgery, when it is impractical to construct a definitive facial prosthesis because of rapid tissue change, a simulated dressing is a useful adjunct to the patient's treatment. It allows the patient to remove the dressing in one piece rather than using a complicated adhesive and gauze dressing. This treatment prosthesis is also useful for patients who work in a very dusty atmosphere where a delicate facial prosthesis would be impractical (Fig. 33-9).

Mandibular exercisers. To combat the trismus that occasionally occurs after radiation and surgery, a simple prosthesis that uses the principle of the screw and inclined plane can be prepared. With this prosthesis the patient can increasingly put the mandibular musculature under stress to improve his ability to depress the mandible (Fig. 33-10).

Implants

The use of prostheses or nonliving substitutes to supplement tissues in the head is well established. The availability of metals that are tolerated by the

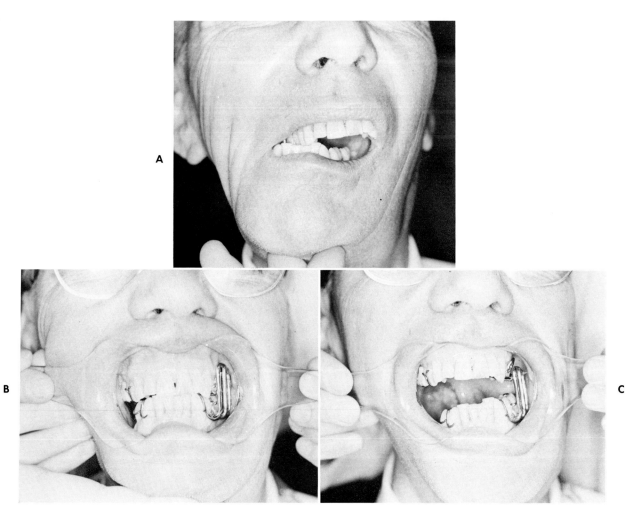

Fig. 33-8. A, Deviation of the mandibular segment after resection. **B,** Flange prosthesis places the mandibular segment into an appropriate relationship with the maxilla. **C,** Flange prosthesis also allows the patient to open and close the mouth appropriately.

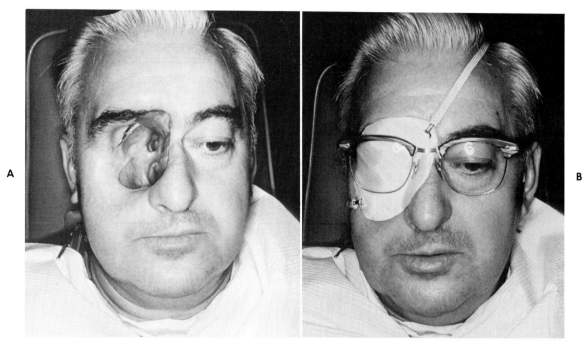

Fig. 33-9. **A,** Facial defect after surgery for cancer. **B,** Prosthetic dressing that the patient uses while working in a dusty atmosphere.

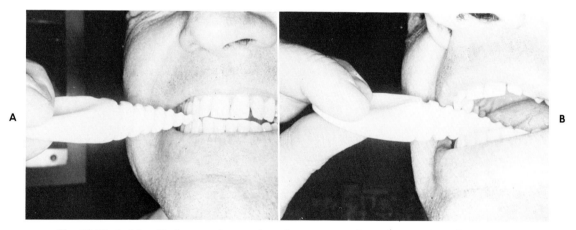

Fig. 33-10. **A,** Mandibular exerciser ready to be turned to force the opening of the mouth. **B,** Mouth forced open by the turning of the exerciser.

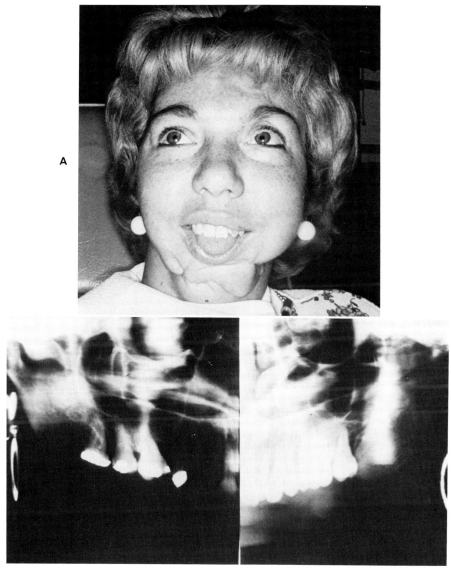

Continued.

Fig. 33-11. A, Patient who has had complete removal of the body of the mandible. **B,** Panorex radiograph showing the remaining mandibular ramus segments. **C,** Vitallium mesh tray implant to replace the body of the mandible. **D,** Patient has some mandibular contour with the implant in place.

body (Vitallium, Ticonium, titanium, and tantalum) and other materials that do not cause a foreign body reaction (medical grade silicone rubber) has allowed the plastic surgeon and maxillofacial prosthodontist to enhance the rehabilitation of the patient with head and neck cancer.

Mandibular implants (metal). Metal implants, prepared in a tray form, can be custom cast to fit a particular patient or prepared from available pre-

formed sections. Since loss of continuity of the mandible is rather debilitating for the patient, these implants offer a definite opportunity not only for reconstructing the mandible but also for recontouring the patient's face (Fig. 33-11).

Facial implants (silicone rubber). The facial defects left by loss of bony support of the face can be recontoured by the placement of custom-prepared medical grade silicone rubber. This material is

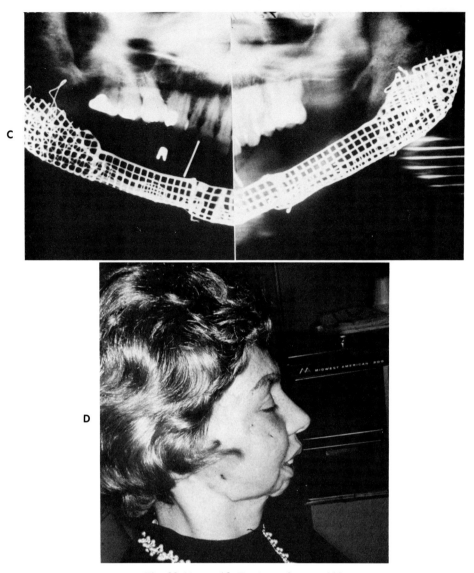

Fig. 33-11, cont'd. For legend see p. 229.

readily accepted by the body and does not resorb with time (Fig. 33-12).

INDICATIONS FOR THE USE OF A PROSTHESIS

The patient who has a very large defect, has been irradiated, and is a poor risk for surgery because of advanced age or poor health has all of the contraindications for plastic and reconstructive surgery.

The use of an interim prosthesis can readily be envisioned where a recurrence is a possibility, where radiation therapy is being considered, or where surgical reconstruction of the anatomical part is simply not possible.

Some advantages of the use of a prosthesis are that there is no physical stress on the patient, it takes less time than reconstructive surgery, and it usually looks more esthetic. No prosthesis, however, is permanent; it must be remade every year or two. Also, the patient must contend with daily removal and cleansing of the prosthesis.

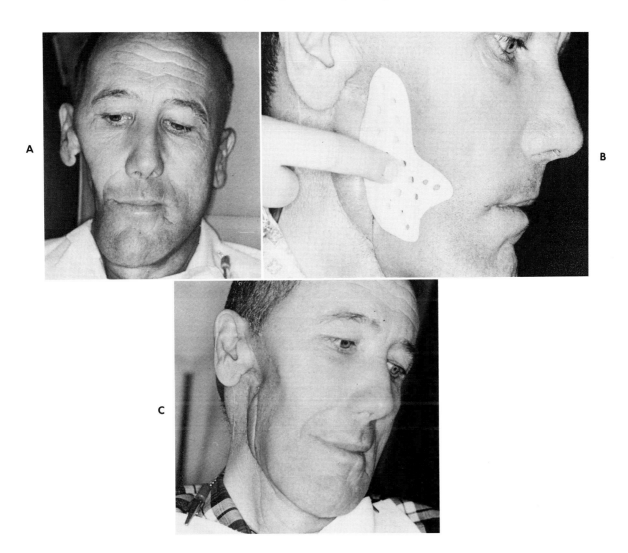

Fig. 33-12. A, Loss of facial contour after resection of the mandible. **B,** Medical grade silicone rubber implant to be placed to recontour the face. **C,** Angle of the mandible reestablished through the use of the silicone rubber implant.

CONCLUSION

At times the plastic and reconstructive surgeon is not fully aware of the many primary and supportive measures in the form of prostheses that the maxillofacial prosthodontist can perform. It is recommended that the surgeon have such a specialist on his team or consult with one prior to any head and neck cancer surgery. Not only can these measures make the patient's treatment course smoother, they can also simplify the surgeon's treatment plan and make nursing care easier.

REFERENCES

1. Bulbulian, A. H.: Maxillofacial prosthetics; evolution and practical application in patient rehabiltation, J. Prosthet. Dent. **15**(3):554-569, 1965.
2. Bulbulian, A. H.: Facial prosthetics, ed. 1, Springfield, Ill., 1973, Charles C Thomas, Publisher.
3. Chalian, V. A., Drane, J. B., and Standish, S. M.: Maxillofacial prosthetics, ed. 1, Baltimore, 1972, The Williams & Wilkins Co.
4. Schaaf, N. G.: Color characterizing silicone rubber facial prostheses, J. Prosthet. Dent. **24**(2):198-202, 1970.

Index

232